Patient Assessment and Management by the Nurse Practitioner

DEE ANN GILLIES, R.N., Ed.D.
Assistant Director of the Department of Education,
Health and Hospitals Governing Commission of Cook
County, Chicago, Illinois

IRENE B. ALYN, R.N., Ph.D.
Associate Professor of Medical Surgical Nursing,
University of Illinois College of Nursing,
Chicago, Illinois

1976

W. B. SAUNDERS COMPANY
Philadelphia, London, Toronto

W. B. Saunders Company: West Washington Square
Philadelphia, PA 19105

1 St. Anne's Road
Eastbourne, East Sussex BN21 3UN, England

833 Oxford Street
Toronto, Ontario M8Z 5T9, Canada

Library of Congress Cataloging in Publication Data

Gillies, Dee Ann.
    Patient assessment and management by the nurse practitioner.

    Includes index.
    1. Chronically ill—Care and treatment.
2. Chronic diseases—Diagnosis.   3. Nurse practitioners.   I. Alyn, Irene Barrett, joint author.
II. Title. [DNLM: 1. Patient care planning—Nursing texts. 2. Nurse practitioners. WY128 G481p]
RT120.C45G54   610.73'6   75-28793
ISBN 0-7216-4133-4

Patient Assessment and Management by the Nurse Practitioner   ISBN 0-7216-4133-4

© 1976 by W. B. Saunders Company. Copyright under the International Copyright Union. All rights reserved. This book is protected by copyright. No part of it may be reproduced, stored in a retrieval system, or transmitted in any form or by any means, electronic, mechanical, photocopying, recording, or otherwise, without written permission from the publisher. Made in the United States of America. Press of W. B. Saunders Company. Library of Congress catalog card number 75-28793

Last digit is the print number: 9   8   7   6   5   4   3   2   1

*This book is dedicated to
Rex and Fay Gillies,
without whose loving support and prayers
it would never have been written.*

Dee Ann Gillies

PREFACE

Times change, health requirements change, and health professions change.

When little was known of disease and treatment, the physician could master most health lore, diagnose illness singlehandedly, and direct both patient and nurse (to whom he had delegated responsibility for hour by hour ministrations to the patient) in what to do and how to do it.

As medical science progressed and knowledge of pathophysiology and therapeutics expanded, the physician could no longer master all medical information, so he began to specialize in restricted areas of medicine and to rely upon the nurse to collect and supply him with the vast array of patient data which was needed to diagnose illness and direct treatment. In recording and reporting this growing mass of patient information, the nurse became increasingly curious about, first, the reasons for such data collection and, then, the conclusions which could be drawn from the data. She began to ask *why* as well as *how* she was to carry out certain aspects of the patient's care. She was encouraged by the physician to ask such questions and even to use patient data that she had helped to collect in low-level problem solving on the patient's behalf; but she was not expected to decide what patient data should be collected nor to interpret patient data for the purpose of making a diagnosis.

Today, the explosion of knowledge continues and, at a time when it is impossible for any one care giver to master all medical knowledge, the patient, who now receives care from several specialists, desperately needs a single care giver to oversee his entire health program: to give health instruction; to provide primary care for each new episode of illness; to refer him to an appropriate specialist when the need arises; and to coordinate the efforts of the several specialists who contribute to his care. A generalist, rather than a specialist, is needed for his task of care coordination. Family practice physicians have filled this role satisfactorily for certain types of patients. For other types, notably chronically ill patients requiring regular and prolonged health supervision of a psychologically and socially supportive type, nurse practitioners have been as successful as or more successful than family practice physicians in providing both primary care and long term health supervision.

Thus, though this modern nurse practitioner is still, to some extent, receiving guidance from the physician (she follows a physician-constructed protocol in treating the patient), she is increasingly responsible for decision making in reference to a particular patient's needs. It is she who decides, for each patient, what data are to be collected and how they are to be interpreted. The formerly passive recipient of information is now an hypothesizer, a data gatherer and processer, and a decision maker.

Nurse practitioners are now using these skills in a variety of ambulatory settings and sometimes in acute care settings. They do screening examinations of well patients and give preventive care and advice. Nurse practitioners are particularly well suited to act as primary care givers to chronically ill patients as a result of certain skills and habits they bring from their nursing education and experience. They are accustomed to constructing long- and short-term goals to guide their patient care efforts, to writing out a care plan based upon these objectives, and to modifying that plan as the patient's condition and health requirements change. In writing care plans, nurses have learned the necessity of considering what is being done for the patient by such other care givers as physician, dietitian, social worker, and physiotherapist in order that planned nursing activities support rather than defeat the treatment efforts of others. Because most nurses have at some time in their careers been exposed to team nursing, they are accustomed to thinking of themselves as one member of a service group and have learned the necessity of prompt and accurate information exchange among group members bent on the same task. Nurses have also acquired considerable skill in interviewing, and in observation and interpretation of physical signs in the course of their nursing activities.

What is needed, then, to convert an effective and experienced nurse to a nurse practitioner who can give primary care to chronically ill patients is instruction and guided experience in obtaining a health history, in performing a physical examination, in ordering indicated diagnostic tests, in recording and reporting significant data, in making a diagnosis, and in following protocols for the treatment of patients with specific illnesses.

This book is designed to provide information on these topics, with particular relevance to the nurse who is giving primary care to chronically ill patients. It should be useful as a text and reference book both in educating nurse practitioners and in teaching interviewing and physical assessment skills to students in basic nursing programs.

DEE ANN GILLIES

IRENE B. ALYN

CONTENTS

1
TECHNIQUES OF HEALTH INTERVIEWING 1

2
THE CONTENT OF THE PATIENT'S MEDICAL HISTORY 13

3
THE PHYSICAL EXAMINATION 33
    Overview 33
    Examination of the Head and Neck 38
    Examination of the Thorax 63
    Examination of the Abdomen 86
    Examination of the Pelvis 100
    Examination of the Back 107
    Examination of the Extremities 109
    Neurological Examination 114

4
LABORATORY TESTS AND SPECIAL EXAMINATIONS 129

5
PSYCHOSOCIAL ASSESSMENT AND INTERVENTION 150

6
RECORDING DATA AND PLANNING CARE 159

7
MANAGEMENT OF THE PATIENT WITH HYPERTENSION 168

8
MANAGEMENT OF THE PATIENT WITH DIABETES MELLITUS ... 176

9
MANAGEMENT OF THE PATIENT WITH CHRONIC ARTHRITIS ... 184

10
MANAGEMENT OF THE PATIENT IN CHRONIC CONGESTIVE HEART FAILURE ... 192

11
MANAGEMENT OF THE PATIENT WITH OBESITY ... 200

12
MANAGEMENT OF THE PATIENT WITH ALCOHOLISM ... 208

NORMAL LABORATORY VALUES OF CLINICAL IMPORTANCE ... 221

INDEX ... 229

1
TECHNIQUES OF HEALTH INTERVIEWING

In order to provide quality health care for any patient, it is necessary to identify carefully his present health condition, his present life situation, his past medical history, his attitudes toward all these, and his expectations regarding the care that he seeks.

This information can be obtained from many sources: the patient himself, his family and friends, the physical examination, and laboratory and diagnostic tests. The patient however, is the best single source of information about himself. In order to tap this rich source of data, as well as to solicit the patient's active cooperation in the treatment process, the first steps in his care should be to obtain a careful and detailed medical history and to explore his present feelings about his health state. Time spent at the beginning of the nurse-patient relationship in painstaking collection of all relevant facts and sensitive exploration of the patient's feelings about his problems will eliminate many later time-consuming errors and misunderstandings.

The quality of the medical history and other information obtained depends, almost entirely, on the nurse practitioner's skills as an interviewer. There are a number of easily learned interviewing techniques that can be used to encourage patients to speak freely about their past and present health problems. However, only after much practice does the nurse acquire a sense of timing that will enable her to use each technique at exactly that moment when it will stimulate the patient to tell his story completely, accurately, and with the least possible discomfort.

The purpose of the interview is to allow a reciprocal interchange of information between the patient and the nurse practitioner. In order for this exchange to occur, the patient must first feel that his words are understood in the sense in which he conveys them, then that his concerns are being dealt with sensitively, and finally that the practitioner is capable of using the information that he gives her in his best interests.

In the health interview, as in a social conversation, the quality of the interchange depends upon the nature of the environment in which the participants find themselves. Because of this, the interview should be undertaken in pleasant, nonthreatening surroundings. A quiet private room is, of course, preferred. If the interview must be carried on in a large open area, then the patient and the nurse practitioner should be separated from others by screens or partitions, and the interview should be conducted in a tone of voice that cannot be overheard by those nearby.

The time for the interview should be carefully selected. If the information obtained in the medical history is to be used as a basis for treatment, the interview should be held shortly after the patient's arrival in the clinic or hospital unit. If, however, on arrival the patient is in pain, is extremely anxious, or is distracted by the fact that his relatives or friends must soon leave him, it would be best to postpone the interview until these concerns have been suitably dealt with.

If the nurse's facial expression, body movement, and tone of voice are those of a pleasant, unhurried, and sympathetic listener, the patient will tend toward greater self-revelation than he would if faced with an aloof, critical, or preoccupied interviewer. If a relative or close friend is with the patient when the nurse is ready to take the medical history, she may wish to invite the visitor to remain during the interview to amplify or verify certain information given by the patient. It would not be wise, however, to include more than one relative or friend in the interview situation, as greater numbers of people create confusion.

The nurse should open the interview with a courteous greeting, give her name and title, describe her role in relation to the patient, and indicate that she is going to take his health history. It will be helpful to describe the purpose for history taking with a remark such as, "Any information you can give me about your present and past health will help me to determine the exact nature of your present problem and will make it easier for me to do whatever is possible to make you more comfortable."

Since many patients will expect the physical examination to be performed by a physician, it may be helpful for the nurse to introduce herself by saying, "I am Ms. Jones, a nurse practitioner. A nurse practitioner is a nurse who has had special training and experience in taking medical histories, doing physical examinations, and in managing patients with difficulties like yours."

At the beginning of the interview, the nurse practitioner should take steps to make herself and the patient comfortable. Any discomfort or anxiety that the nurse feels will be transmitted to the patient in such manner as to block his free communication. Before beginning the interview, the nurse should recognize and attempt to reduce any anxiety which she feels concerning her interaction with the patient; should satisfy any demanding physical needs of her own, such as a need for food, for elimination, or for relief of minor pain; and should seat herself in a comfortable chair so situated that she can both see and hear the patient without strain.

Any discomfort that the patient feels may distract him so that he cannot relate a full and accurate history; consequently, it may be advisable to change the patient's position, to provide him with additional pillows, to change his dressing, to offer him a bedpan or urinal, or even to administer an analgesic before beginning the interview.

Following are several suggestions that should guide the nurse in obtaining the patient's medical history.

1. *Begin* talking about the topic that is most important to the patient.
2. *Guide* the communication to allow for expression of thought and feeling.
3. *Observe* nonverbal communications.
4. *Listen* carefully.
5. *Concentrate* on current facts and feelings.
6. *Examine* your phrasing.
7. *Speak* in terms the patient can understand.
8. *Evaluate* the patient's perception.
9. *Stay* on the same subject as the patient.
10. *Keep* your opinions to yourself.
11. *Consider* the physical and emotional distance between yourself and the patient.
12. *End* the interview with an attitude of support.

BEGIN WITH TOPIC MOST IMPORTANT TO THE PATIENT

Initiating conversation on the topic of his greatest concern subtly suggests to the patient that he is somehow in control of the interview—a conviction that will motivate him to take an active part in the conversation. The fact that the nurse, on their very first meeting, is willing to help the patient express his chief concern in some detail helps to establish a relationship of trust between the two that will facilitate the patient's later disclosure of facts and feelings about present and past illnesses. Further, by identifying the patient's chief concern during this first meeting, the nurse obtains a useful point of information to be used later in establishing priorities of care.

One way to identify the issue of chief concern to the patient is to ask, "What caused you to come here today?" The patient will usually respond to this question by expressing, in a few words, his chief complaint.

It should be noted that certain problems, such as venereal disease, frigidity, and incontinence, carry social and moral connotations that may make it difficult for the patient to express his complaint directly. A patient with such a problem may discuss another, lesser, problem at the beginning of the interview in order to test the practitioner's receptivity to his concerns and to gauge her tendency to judge patients who suffer the disorder in question.

Especially in the early part of the interview, it is desirable that the patient do most of the talking in order that the nurse does not restrict in any way the patient's expression of his most important problems. On the other hand, the patient will probably require some direction from the nurse to keep his conversation pertinent to the objectives of the interview.

GUIDE THE PATIENT'S COMMUNICATION

In guiding the patient's talk, the nurse should encourage his expression of both thought and feeling. In short, the patient should be encouraged to relate not only what has happened to him, and what was done about it, but also his reactions to these experiences.

When relating the sequence of events in his present illness, the patient should be encouraged to express what he thought about these events; that is, what explanation he gave himself as to the probable cause and effects of each symptom and sign. Such information will help the nurse determine how well informed the patient is concerning health issues in general and his problems in particular. This information will also enable her to immediately correct any gross misunderstandings or totally unrealistic expectations that might adversely affect the patient's later response to treatment.

Because many or most of the feelings provoked by illness are themselves painful and disruptive, it will be therapeutic for the patient to purge himself of these feelings by relating them to a sympathetic listener. Expressing to a concerned nurse his worries about dependence upon care givers, loss of social role and status, changes in body image, reduction in self-esteem, economic problems, and possible disability or death will reduce his anxiety level, enable him to understand better the information given him about his condition, and make it easier for him to participate actively in his treatment program.

The fact that the practitioner draws the patient out, inviting him to relate his feelings about the unpleasant things that have been happening to him, establishes a precedent for their later interactions, demonstrating that his feelings, as well as the facts of his situation, are to be reviewed in their later joint discussions.

INTERPRET NONVERBAL COMMUNICATION

Throughout the interview, the nurse should continuously compare the messages that the patient transmits in words to those conveyed through his facial expression, posture, and gestures. Because repression plays so large a part in the process of socialization, body language tends to be a more accurate expression of feeling than verbal language. Careful attention to the patient's facial expression may reveal that despite his calm recital of symptoms he is in fact shamed or disgusted by recent changes in his body's functioning. Or, despite his denials of pain, occasional grimacing or wincing may reveal that the patient does, indeed, experience discomfort. Widening of his palpebral fissure and increase in his respiratory rate may signify an increase in the patient's anxiety, thereby indicating the emotional importance of the issue under discussion. Dropping his eyes may indicate that the patient wishes to avoid discussion of the current topic, is embarrassed, perceives or expects the nurse's disapproval of his actions, or needs time to collect his thoughts before continuing. Movement away from the interviewer, by pushing backward in his chair, or turning his head to one side or the other, may demonstrate that the patient wishes to change the subject or conclude the interview, that he rejects a potentially helpful ally.

Gestures used by the patient to describe his symptoms are extremely useful diagnostic tools. Typically, patients with duodenal peptic ulcer locate the site of their pain by pointing with one finger, patients with coronary occlusion describe their chest pain by clenching and unclenching a fist, and patients with cardiac arrhythmias demonstrate their increased heart rate and skipped beats by a syncopated waggling of a finger.

LISTEN ACTIVELY, TALK SPARINGLY

Since throughout the interview it is desirable that the patient do most of the talking, the nurse practitioner should spend most of her time listening. Her listening, however, is not to be merely a passive reception of messages transmitted willy-nilly by the patient; rather her listening should be an active process through which, by prolonged eye contact and appropriate gestures and silences, she leads the patient to a free, full, purposeful narration of his story.

At the beginning of the interview, after asking the patient to describe his chief complaint ("What was it that caused you to come here today for help?") and after inviting him to describe his present illness in some detail ("Tell me about this diarrhea, from the time that it first developed until now") the nurse should remain quiet in order that the patient may describe his problem without interruption, distraction, or external suggestion. When the patient pauses from time to time in his story, the nurse may remain quiet while he collects his thoughts or, if his silence is prolonged, she may indicate her continuing attention and her acceptance of what has been said by a nod of her head or a comment such as "Yes," "I see," "Go on," or "Tell me more." While the patient will need a moment of silence every now and again to reflect on some idea or feeling, or to organize his thoughts for the next revelation, he will react to an excessively long silence with anxiety and will look to the nurse for direction in resuming the interview.

EMPHASIZE CURRENT CONCERNS

In conducting the interview, the nurse practitioner should direct the patient's conversation toward current facts and feelings, while at the same time encouraging him to relate each aspect of his present experience to past events in his life and to his expectations for the future. Because the nurse practitioner will be dealing frequently with patients who are chronically ill, she should not be surprised to learn in her first encounter with each new patient that his symptoms are of long duration. It is to be expected, however, that the nature or severity of a given symptom may change through time and it may be assumed that some such symptom change or an alteration of the patient's life situation or a change in his attitude toward his symptoms has led him to seek help at this time.

One way to discern what is unique about the patient's present circumstances is to ask him: "What is it about this problem that has brought you here *today*?" or "How does the pain you're having today differ from that you had last month, when you did not seek medical attention?"

Careful identification of the patient's present needs and expectations will enable the nurse practitioner to establish correct priorities among several actions that could and perhaps should be undertaken on the patient's behalf. By concentrating on current facts and feelings, the practitioner can identify which specific information about the patient's illness, probable diagnostic tests, and possible treatment measures should be given during this first interchange. Such selectivity is advisable because the patient's anxiety level tends to be high during his first meeting with a new care giver. The greater an individual's anxiety level, the more difficulty he will have in attending to events occurring in his environment. The patient will not be able to comprehend and react appropriately to a large volume of new information about his illness given during his initial interview with the practitioner. By carefully determining which of many worries about his condition occupies the foreground of his attention during this contact with the health care system, the nurse practitioner can better coordinate her interests and efforts with the patient's wishes and intentions.

The patient should be asked to relate current facts and feelings to past events in order that the nurse may understand the natural history of his illness and may evaluate his success in handling previous crises. Through such historical investigation the practitioner may discover that the patient's present illness is a complication of an earlier illness, that the present illness has little or no relationship to previous bouts of similar symptoms, or that the patient's disappointment with previous treatment for the same or a different illness has caused him to procrastinate in seeking treatment for this episode.

By helping the patient to relate present facts and feelings to his future expectations, the practitioner can help the patient to commit himself to striving toward health. It can be assumed that the ill person who presents himself for medical care is in a state of crisis. It is known that persons in crisis can be easily influenced to learn new methods of coping with problems. By helping the patient to understand the probable outcome of his present condition, given each of several possible courses of action, the practitioner enables the patient to make realistic and informed choices concerning available treatments. In exploring the relationships among his present condition, possible actions, and probable outcomes, the patient comes to see his disease, treatment, and recovery not as magical and totally unpredictable occurrences but as events which are susceptible to logical explanation and control. The latter conception of health and disease affords the patient a more hopeful view of his future, suggesting as it does that his problem can be investigated, understood, and ameliorated through rational interventions by himself and his care givers.

USE SUPPORTIVE PHRASEOLOGY

Throughout the interview, the nurse practitioner should be careful to phrase her comments and questions so that the patient will find the subliminal messages in her communications non-judgmental, non-threatening, and emotionally supportive. For instance, when asking the patient about a particular aspect of his medical history, the nurse should say, "Tell me how you've relieved this pain in the past" rather than, "Explain what you've done to relieve your pain in the past." The phrase "Tell me" suggests a certain equality between nurse and patient and is more likely to be construed as an invitation to discussion. The word "Explain" sounds imperative and can be interpreted by the patient as a demand that he somehow justify his actions to the nurse.

When the patient's undirected narration regarding a particular symptom has not provided all the information that the practitioner desires on the point in question, it is better to say, "Can you describe your coughing in more detail?" than to fire a volley of questions that invite monosyllabic answers and discourage the patient's volunteering of useful information.

If the nurse is puzzled about some part of the patient's history, it is better to say, "I'm not sure that I follow that last point. Would you go over it again?" rather than to say, "I don't understand that." In the former response, the nurse takes upon herself the responsibility for failure in communication; in the latter, she risks estranging the patient because, above all, the person who seeks medical care hopes to be understood. Under these circumstances an even better response might be, "I want to be perfectly clear about what you've just told me. Please tell me again what happened." This response makes it clear that the patient's need to be understood is paralleled by the nurse's wish to understand.

Although her questions should not limit the patient's responses, the nurse should phrase her requests so that she does not seek too much information through one question. For instance, "How does your appetite today compare with your appetite a year ago?" would be a better exploratory comment than "Tell me about your previous health," because the former question indicates the general category of information being sought and guides the patient in organizing his thoughts for an informative response.

SELECT TERMS CAREFULLY

In order to obtain an accurate medical history, the nurse practitioner must take pains to speak in terms the patient can understand. The nurse will probably instinctively not use polysyllabic medical terms, such as "cholelithiasis" or "thrombocytopenic purpura," which she herself normally does not use frequently. She may, however, in rephrasing the patient's complaint, unconsciously substitute some commonly used medical term, such as "cystitis" or "thrombosis" or "ulcer" for the patient's reference to a "bladder infection," a "clot in my brain," or a "draining sore on my leg." If the patient is unfamiliar with a medical term used by the nurse, he may be frightened by it, assuming that the nurse has identified an additional and more serious disorder than the one for which he sought treatment. Or he may infer that the nurse's use of the term in her conversation with him indicates that most lay persons would understand it. Believing that, the patient would probably not confess his unfamiliarity with the word, but might attempt to conceal it by changing the subject or by lapsing into silence. The patient's misunderstanding of a medical term used by the nurse might also lead him to give erroneous information in that he might, in his confusion, agree to having a symptom which he had not, in fact, experienced.

On the other hand, in her efforts to be understood by the patient, the nurse should not immediately lapse into the vernacular in describing body functions, secretions, and excretions. Previous experience with illness or with hospitals may have enabled the patient to acquire an extensive vocabulary of medical terms. An interest in reading scientific or medical literature may have

8 CHAPTER 1

had a similar effect. The patient who himself uses correct medical terminology in describing his disease and its symptoms might interpret the nurse's use of less precise language as a tendency on her part to patronize him.

The nurse practitioner can best judge the patient's medical language proficiency by noting, during the early part of the interview, which physiological and pathological terms he uses to describe his current complaint, the history of his present illness, and his medical history to date.

VALIDATE THE ACCURACY OF INFORMATION EXCHANGED

Effective communication between individuals is very difficult to achieve, and the nurse practitioner should not assume that the patient understands everything that she says to him, nor that she has understood all of his communications to her. Rather, at frequent intervals throughout the interview, the nurse should validate the data which she has derived from the patient's story and should evaluate the patient's perception of the information given him.

At the time of the patient's first interview with the practitioner, his anxiety level will probably be very high, because he is operating under a great deal of uncertainty concerning the significance of his symptoms, the security which he will be able to find in this new milieu, the probable length of his illness, and its future effects on himself and his family. Because the patient's anxiety may block his perception of facts given him by the nurse, she may have to repeat information or directions several times, and to highlight crucial points with examples or demonstrations.

Throughout the interview, the nurse should also check the patient's perception of the meaning of his symptoms, the cause of his illness, and the probable consequences of his disability. A useful way to do this is to rephrase the patient's comments periodically throughout the discussion. Hearing another describe his situation in his own terms often helps the patient put these events in the proper time sequence and perspective. After each rephrasing the nurse should ask questions such as, "And what was your reaction to this?" or "And what did you make of that?" or "And how did you feel at that time?" If rapport has been established between the two, such questions will probably elicit a clear description of the feelings generated in him by the events in question.

In evaluating the patient's perception of his situation, the nurse should try to learn what aspect of his illness and symptoms is of greatest importance to him. This information may help to predict how the patient will respond to illness, to treatment, and to persons in his environment. If to him the most important aspect of his leg ulcer is its unaesthetic appearance, then he may resist watching or helping with topical treatments of the lesion. He may even, in his reluctance to look at the ulcer, neglect needed dressing changes or clinic visits.

VERIFY THE TOPIC UNDER DISCUSSION

Since it is advisable, especially during early portions of the interview, to let the patient direct the flow of conversation, and since in following his own thought associations the patient will not present different categories of information in the same sequence in which the practitioner orders that information in the patient's chart or in her own mind, the practitioner should check repeatedly to be sure that she and the patient are speaking about the same issue. If such checking is not done, the nurse may spend a great deal of time questioning the patient about the onset and nature of a particular symptom which she believes the patient to be currently suffering only to learn that the symptom under discussion is not current but associated with an earlier illness that the patient associates, correctly or incorrectly, with his present problem.

To ensure that such misunderstandings do not occur, the nurse should frequently clarify time relationships in the patient's story with such questions as, "Now that happened when?" or "When did this symptom develop in reference to the other problems you've been telling me about?" or "Was this before or after the operation?"

If at some point the nurse doubts that she and patient are addressing exactly the same issue, she might seek clarification with some such comment as, "Let's see if we're talking about the same thing. As I understand it, you've been losing some weight over a twelve month period, but your greatest weight loss, about twelve pounds, has occurred in the last six weeks. Is that correct?"

Staying on the same subject as the patient does not mean that the practitioner should avoid commenting on the relationship of the material under discussion to information revealed in an earlier part of the history. There can be great educational benefit to the patient in the nurse's demonstration of a possible connection between the current problems and a previous illness. For instance, "So this present episode of diarrhea began abruptly two weeks ago, following administration of an oral antibiotic. But you did have a two day bout of the same watery diarrhea and griping last year when you were travelling in Mexico?"

GIVE INFORMATION, WITHHOLD ADVICE AND OPINION

While taking the patient's medical history it is sometimes helpful for the nurse practitioner to give information to the patient, but she should not give him advice on the handling of problems. This principle is often ignored because both patient and practitioner assume that the nurse has greater knowledge of disease and treatment than does the patient. However, if the patient is to take an active part in his own care, he should begin making as many decisions as possible concerning treatment procedures and modification of life situations to accommodate his illness and treatment. The proper aim in caring for any patient is to assist him to achieve the greatest possible degree of self-determination in the least possible time. Advising the patient what he should do to improve his situation encourages unhealthy dependence upon others by implying that he is incapable of directing his own affairs. If, on the other hand, the nurse gives the patient the information needed to select the best among several available treatment regimens or the most satisfactory of several possible modifications of his home or work routines, and then encourages the patient to select the best course of action, the practitioner confirms the patient as an intelligent, capable, independent agent who is responsible for his own future welfare.

Usually there are differences of age, sex, race, education, occupation, health, and/or cultural background between the practitioner and patient. These differences make it impossible for the nurse to understand fully either the patient's life situation or his peculiarly individualistic response to illness. Since the nurse's opinions about the patient's circumstances will not exactly match his, and since the patient's opinions are most worthy of consideration in the diagnosis and treatment situation, she risks offending him and jeopardizing the mutual trust that is so essential to the success of their relationship if she attempts to direct his activities in line with her own rather than his opinions of his situation. For instance, if in responding to a female patient's statement that she is unmarried and pregnant, the practitioner indicates by word or facial expression any moral condemnation of the patient, that judgment by the nurse and the resentment which it creates in the patient will hamper further communication between them. Likewise, if the nurse makes a slighting comment about the patient's physician or displays an attitude of doubt or surprise concerning his previous treatment, she may not only destroy the patient's confidence in a valuable ally, but also erode his trust in all health professionals.

The relationship of the nurse practitioner to the patient during the medical history interview resembles that of counselor to client. The nurse's demonstration of unconditional positive regard for the patient as he presents himself for help will make it easier for him to describe his troubles and to explore his attitudes and expectations concerning health care. If the patient has to some extent been unable to accept the fact of his illness or the resultant changes in body structure and function, the nurse's positive regard for him in the face of these symptoms and disabilities will help reconcile him to his altered body and social role.

CONSIDER THE EFFECTS OF INTERPERSONAL DISTANCE

If at some point during the interview the practitioner feels that the patient may be distorting or withholding information, she should consider the emotional distance between herself and the patient, and its influence on their communication. As mentioned earlier, if as the patient discusses a particular issue he perceives the nurse's manner toward him to be critical, disparaging, or condescending, he may defend himself by withdrawing from the interchange. While most patients under these circumstances would not go so far as to interrupt the interview and leave the room, many would change the subject, fall silent, or display avoidance behavior. Movements by the patient which increase the physical distance between himself and the nurse are frequently the first clue to an interviewing error on her part.

The practitioner should first note what subject was being discussed when the patient moved away from her. Then she should look back to see what she had been saying, doing, or thinking just before the patient's movement. For instance, had she just attempted to restate the patient's opinion concerning an important matter, or reflected the patient's feelings about a troublesome event, or asked a question to obtain additional personal information? Perhaps she has completely misunderstood the patient's opinion, or verbalized a feeling which the patient is not yet willing to accept, or asked for information which the patient is not willing to reveal. If it appears to the nurse that the patient's withdrawal is the result of her failure to understand him or to provide adequate emotional support, she may, by sensitively exploring the problem area still further, re-establish rapport with the patient.

Some patients enjoy, even need, close physical contact with an understanding and helpful person when under stress. A patient of this type may be greatly comforted by a reassuring touch on his shoulder or hand. Such a gesture by the nurse practitioner when she realizes that she has misunderstood the patient or has unwittingly offended him may reduce the emotional distance between them and re-establish rapport. On the other hand, a few patients will be made very anxious by physical closeness to another. If the nurse were to touch a patient of this type in an effort to reassure him, she might alienate the patient to the point that he would stop volunteering any useful information.

It would be impossible, on first meeting the patient, to be certain whether he relishes or abhors personal closeness; however, most persons communicate by subtle bodily movements a desire for physical contact with another and such movements are perceived at a subliminal level. Therefore, a good rule of thumb for the nurse practitioner to follow would be: if the patient is distressed and the nurse feels an inclination to touch him in a reassuring gesture, she should do so. If she has a question as to the advisability of touching him, she should not.

CONCLUDE WITH SUPPORT

Finally, the practitioner should end the history-taking interview with an attitude of support for the patient. One way to accomplish this is to summarize the information given by the patient concerning his chief complaint, previous health history, family health history, and personal data. The nurse's reiteration of the signal points in the patient's history is comforting to him because it indicates that the nurse has understood him and is conscientious enough about her responsibilities to summarize the data for verification.

After the nurse's summary of salient points and the patient's correction of any misunderstandings that may have occurred, the nurse should again shift the burden of responsibility for the interview to the patient with the question, "Is there anything else which you would like to tell me?" This question should not be employed to prolong the interview unduly, but to give the patient an opportunity to bring forth any information which he has forgotten or was unable to interject at an earlier point in the interview. The data given in response to this question, even if offered in an off-hand manner, is often extremely valuable in planning effective patient management.

Before taking leave of the patient, the nurse practitioner should give him an idea of what action she will now take on his behalf; what tests she will order, what consultations she will seek, what medications and treatments she will prescribe. At the same time, she should indicate when she will next meet with the patient and what, if anything, the patient is to do before that meeting. For instance, is he to come to the hospital for a chest x-ray; is he to consult the social worker for help in resolving financial problems; is he to bring a urine specimen to the laboratory? Again, since the patient's high anxiety level will make it difficult for him to assimilate large quantities of unfamiliar new material, it would be better to give him written rather than oral directions.

BIBLIOGRAPHY: TECHNIQUES OF HEALTH INTERVIEWING

Balint, Enid, and Norell, J. S., Eds.: *Six Minutes For The Patient.* London, Tavistock, 1973.

Bernstein, Lewis, Berstein, Rosalyn, and Dana, Richard: *Interviewing, A Guide for Health Professionals.* 2nd ed. New York, Appleton-Century-Crofts, 1974.

Bird, Brian: *Talking With Patients.* 2nd ed. Philadelphia, J. B. Lippincott, 1973.

Enelow, Allen, and Swisher, Scott: *Interviewing and Patient Care.* New York, Oxford University Press, 1972.

Engel, George, and Morgan, William: *Interviewing the Patient.* Philadelphia, W. B. Saunders Co., 1973.

Francis, V., Korsch, B., and Morris, M.: Gaps in doctor-patient communication. *New Eng. J. Med.* 280:535–540, March, 1969.

Kadushin, Alfred: *The Social Work Interview.* New York, Columbia University Press, 1972.

Knapp, Mark. *Nonverbal Communication in Human Interaction.* New York, Holt, Rinehart and Winston, 1972.

Vander Zanden, James, and Vander Zanden, Marion: The interview. *Nursing Outlook* 11:743–745, October, 1963.

2
THE CONTENT OF THE PATIENT'S MEDICAL HISTORY

The patient's medical history is a detailed and structured account of all the events in his life that must be taken into account in order to provide for his present and future health needs. A complete and accurate medical history serves several purposes. It provides information from which to diagnose the patient's illness and upon which to build a plan of treatment. It yields data regarding development of the patient's present illness that may be used as legal evidence in a liability or malpractice suit. It supplies information which may be used in filing the patient's insurance claims. The medical history may also serve as valuable source material for scientific research and for educating different types of health workers.

A considerable body of information is needed about a patient in order to diagnose his illness and plan treatment which is realistically adapted to his circumstances. Physical discomfort and anxiety might make it difficult for a patient to relate his medical history completely, logically, and clearly. Therefore, the nurse practitioner must, throughout the interview, gently but firmly guide the patient's conversation toward those items of information needed to clarify his problems. In order to provide such direction, the nurse practitioner should have firmly in mind a detailed outline of the various categories of information to be explored in analyzing health problems, together with key questions which will elicit significant information in each category.

To some degree the length of the medical history which should be obtained for a particular patient depends upon the nature of the patient's illness; that is, a less detailed medical history will be needed to treat a patient with an acute skin irritation than one with a chronic gastrointestinal disorder. A carefully constructed and detailed medical history is often of greater importance than either a physical examination or laboratory tests in the diagnosis and treatment of chronic illness. Hence, nurse practitioners will need to take detailed medical histories on the chronically ill patients to whom they give care.

The outline of content to be included in a patient's medical history does not vary much from one physician to another or from one nurse practitioner to another, since logic and the natural history of illnesses dictate what information should be accumulated, and human psychology determines the general sequence in which the several categories of needed information should be pursued. The nurse practitioner should memorize the standardized medical history content outline and follow it conscientiously in order not to ignore information of potential value in patient care, and in order not to waste her own or the patient's time in rambling, unproductive conversation about his problems.

The information to be included in the patient's medical history includes the following categories. In general, the interview should be guided to obtain the information in the sequence shown.

1. Identifying data
2. Informant
3. Chief complaint
4. Present illness
   a. Chronology
   b. Symptoms
   c. Significant negative findings
5. Family history
6. Personal history
   a. Marital status
   b. Educational information
   c. Occupational information
   d. Habits
   e. Review of a typical day
7. Past medical history
8. Review of systems
   a. General
   b. Skin
   c. Head
   d. Eyes
   e. Nose and sinuses
   f. Mouth, pharynx, larynx
   g. Neck
   h. Respiratory system
   i. Cardiovascular system
   j. Gastrointestinal system
   k. Urinary system
   l. Genital system
   m. Musculoskeletal system
   n. Nervous system
   o. Endocrine system
   p. Psychological status

IDENTIFYING DATA

In many office, clinic, or hospital situations, an attendant, clerk, or nurse will have recorded the patient's identifying data on the chart before he is introduced to the nurse practitioner. In beginning the health interview, the practitioner should review the identifying data with the patient to double check accuracy of the record. Identifying data should include the patient's name, sex, age, birthdate, place of birth, race, nationality, marital status, address, current occupation, and usual occupation.

The medical record should include the patient's family name, first name, and middle name. A woman's given name and maiden name should be obtained as well as her husband's full name to insure that her record is not confused with that of another patient of the same last name.

The patient's birth date should be obtained as a check against the accuracy of his stated age. A discrepancy between the two may signal a defect in the patient's memory or a desire to misrepresent his age, and either of these observations would give the nurse a hint of possible later problems in patient management.

The patient's place of birth may yield clues to his cultural background or to diseases to which he might have been exposed in infancy and childhood. For instance, a black man giving Liberia as his place of birth and schooling might be expected to have a different attitude toward himself and his relationship to a white nurse practitioner than would a black man who had been born and reared in Mississippi. A Latino patient who had been born in southern rural Mexico would probably have been exposed to amebiasis in childhood, while a Latino born in southern California would be less likely to have had the same exposure.

The patient's race is occasionally of diagnostic significance. Sickle cell anemia is thought to occur only in persons of the Negro race. Pernicious anemia is rare in Orientals.

The patient's nationality or national origin should be included in the medical record as another indicator of his cultural background. Learning that the patient is an Italian who has only recently immigrated to the United States, the nurse could expect that he would probably have difficulty adhering to a low carbohydrate diet.

The nurse practitioner should determine the patient's marital status in order to know whether he has economic dependents who would suffer if he became unable to work. The patient's marital status may also provide a clue to his rehabilitation potential. The patient who is married and has a teen-age child living at home would probably receive greater emotional support and physical assistance from close associates than would a bachelor living alone in an apartment house. Marital status may occasionally have epidemiologic significance. If the patient should later be diagnosed as having venereal disease, tuberculosis, another contagious disease, or drug addiction, it would be advisable for the nurse practitioner to check the patient's spouse for the same disease.

In determining the patient's address, the practitioner can estimate, to some degree, his socioeconomic status and can gauge how difficult it will be for the patient to make clinic visits or for the patient's relatives to visit him in the hospital. The ghetto dweller will usually have less money to spend for health care than the suburban dweller. The patient who cannot drive and who lives many miles from the clinic would be likely to miss his clinic appointments in bad weather.

Learning the patient's usual occupation will help the practitioner to assess his economic status. If he has recently changed jobs, the nurse can judge the degree to which illness has decreased his strength or impaired his motor and mental function.

INFORMANT

It will be helpful to others who will use the patient's medical record for the nurse practitioner to indicate the informant for the medical history (patient, spouse, relative, friend) and to evaluate the accuracy of the account. If later developments cause the practitioner or the physician to question some aspect of the medical history, it would help to know that the original account of the patient's problem was given by his daughter-in-law, with whom he did not live but whom he happened to be visiting when illness struck. It would be important too, for the nurse to note in the record that during the interview, the patient seemed confused, drowsy, preoccupied, or anxious, since any of these conditions would decrease his mental acuity and could jeopardize the accuracy of the record.

CHIEF COMPLAINT

After checking the accuracy of the identifying data and indicating from whom the historical data were obtained, the practitioner should ascertain the patient's chief complaint. Here it is desirable to list only one symptom or problem. However, many patients, particularly those with chronic diseases, will have several symptoms. It will, therefore, be necessary for the nurse to identify which of the patient's many complaints is most troublesome to him at the present time. Careful clarification of this point is needed, because the patient who is chronically ill may have experienced symptoms of poor health for several weeks or months. The nurse must assume that there has been some change either in the symptoms themselves, in the patient's perception of those symptoms, or in the patient's life situation that has caused him to seek help now for a problem with which he has been confronted for some time.

In identifying the patient's chief complaint, it is important that the nurse not impose her own opinions upon the patient. Because she has greater knowledge than he of pathophysiology and often can better interpret the significance and probable course of a given symptom, she might not agree with him in estimating the relative importance of his several complaints.

The nurse can elicit the patient's chief complaint by making an open-ended, non-directive request such as, "Tell me about your problem." and then allowing the patient to describe the problem in his own way. The object, at this point in the interview, is for the patient to talk openly about his problem, revealing his observations, concerns, and expectations. The nurse should not interrupt him to ask for specific information but should encourage him to talk freely by giving him her undivided attention and by nodding or echoing a key word when the patient hesitates in his presentation. If the patient outlines his current situation completely without identifying its single, most troublesome aspect, the nurse should help him to do this by asking something like, "And of all this, the most troublesome is . . . ?" or "And so you are most distressed about the . . . ?"

Once identified, the chief complaint should be recorded in the patient's own words, that is, as a symptom rather than a diagnosis, unless his manner of describing the complaint is misleading or downright vulgar. By using the patient's terminology, the nurse avoids two types of errors. First, she will not mistakenly apply a former physician's or nurse practitioner's diagnosis of a prior illness to the patient's present problem. Second, she will not limit her consideration of all possible explanations for his problem by directing her thinking from the beginning toward one particular diagnosis. Of course, at the beginning of their conversation, if the nurse practitioner has not established enough rapport with the patient to win his trust, the complaint with which he introduces his history may not be his primary concern, but merely a justification for seeking help. If the nurse's conduct of the interview finally convinces the patient of her acceptance and support, he will eventually talk about the symptom he is most worried about.

In order to encourage the patient to speak freely and at some length about his chief concern, the nurse should not take notes while he is talking. She should sit quietly, in a relaxed fashion, listening carefully to his comments until she is satisfied that he has identified the problem for which he seeks attention. When that is clear, the practitioner should record the chief complaint in a word or phrase, using the patient's terminology. Even though the nurse may later diagnose a more serious disorder than the one pointed to by the chief complaint, and even though she successfully treats the more serious disorder, the patient will be dissatisfied with his care, however well planned and executed, if no effort is made to alleviate his chief complaint.

HISTORY OF PRESENT ILLNESS

Once the chief complaint has been recorded, the nurse should investigate the history of the patient's present illness. Information about how and when this illness began, how it affected him, what he did about it, and what resulted from these efforts will amplify the chief complaint and clarify its relationship to other symptoms and events. Once again, as she begins to investigate the history of the present illness, the nurse should encourage the patient to do most of the talking and should introduce questions only after the patient has first explored the subject without direction. The purpose of the nurse's direct questioning should not be to extract information from the patient but to clarify and expand information which he has already freely given.

The nurse should introduce the topic by asking, "What is your usual state of health?" in order to obtain a standard against which to compare the effects of the current illness. Then she should request a full history of the present episode with the following comment: "Now tell me as much as you can about the development of this problem from the time that it began until now." The objective here is to obtain a complete chronology of events relating to the present illness including treatment received, responses to treatment, subsidence or disappearance of symptoms, changes in symptoms, relation of symptoms to activities, and degree of discomfort or disability experienced. Probably the patient will describe his illness in terms of its subjective and objective characteristics. From her knowledge of the natural history of illnesses, the nurse will be aware of groups of symptoms which tend to occur in association with each other in specific diseases.

After the patient has sketched out the general sequence of symptom development, indicating significant time relationships, the nurse should ask direct questions to obtain additional information of two types. First, she should determine whether the patient has experienced any of the symptoms usually associated with each of the symptoms he has mentioned (nausea as well as vomiting, burning on urination as well as urinary frequency). Second, she should analyze each of the symptoms of his present illness in regard to duration, onset, character, and course. To obtain the first type of information, a simple straightforward question will suffice. "You mentioned that you have been having blurred vision. Do you ever see double?" or, "You say you become short of breath on walking up a flight of stairs. Do you ever wake up at night because you have trouble breathing?"

In analyzing each of the patient's symptoms, the nurse should begin by determining how long before the present date the symptom first appeared. If the symptom has been remittent, the record should indicate when it first appeared, for how long, and how often it has disappeared between initial onset and the present. If the patient has had the symptom for some time, he may have difficulty remembering the exact date on which it first appeared, subsided, or reappeared. With guidance from the nurse, he may be able to relate symptom development to some holiday or important family event and pinpoint exact time relationships in that way.

After the duration of the symptom has been established, the onset of the symptom should be investigated. Here the nurse should look for a precipitating event, asking questions such as, "On the occasion that you first experienced this pain, what were you doing?" "Where were you?", "Who was with you?", "What happened first?", "Show me where the pain began", How rapidly did it develop?", "How severe was it at first?", "Did it change in intensity with the passage of time?" Answers to these questions will reveal whether onset of the symptom was sudden or gradual, which information will be useful in determining the nature of the underlying pathophysiology. For instance, dyspnea develops more rapidly in bacterial pneumonia than in bronchogenic carcinoma. Weakness develops more slowly in pernicious anemia than in anemia due to internal hemorrhage. A description of the circumstances surrounding symptom onset may reveal predisposing or precipitating factors. If the patient was shovelling snow or running to catch a bus when the symptom first occurred, perhaps it has been caused by muscular exertion. If he was arguing with his wife or attending his father's funeral when the symptom first appeared, perhaps it is provoked by emotional stress. If he was grooming a dog or cleaning a damp basement when he first noted the symptom, maybe it was evoked by an allergen. If he was entering a walk-in freezer when the symptom occurred, maybe it was precipitated by cold exposure.

Another way to identify precipitating causes for a symptom is to ask a direct question. "Is there anything you do that seems to precipitate an attack?" An equally useful piece of information, factors that alleviate the symptom, can be obtained by asking, "What do you do to relieve the attack?" Often through deductive reasoning or blind trial and error, a patient does discover some means of alleviating a troublesome symptom. Knowledge of such empirical remedies can help the practitioner diagnose the patient's illness.

Analysis of each symptom also involves consideration of its characteristics; that is, its quality, location, intensity, periodicity, and related symptoms.

A nurse practitioner might obtain information about the quality of a symptom by asking, "What does the pain feel like?", "How would you describe the discomfort?", "What is the consistency of these diarrheal stools?", "What kind of headache?", "What kind of rash?", "What type of change in color?"

In describing the quality of a given symptom, the patient will frequently use helpfully descriptive words or phrases as "gnawing" pain, "burning" pain, "grinding" pain, "stabbing" pain, "vise-like" pain, "pinching" sensation, "fluttery" sensation, hands "like ice," red "as fire," "buzzing sound," or "metallic taste." Sometimes, however, the patient will use phraseology, the meaning of which is not immediately apparent to the nurse, either because it is not specifically descriptive, since different people may use the same term to mean more than one thing, or because the expression is a slang term peculiar to one subcultural group. Some potentially confusing phrases are "a catch in my side," "winded," "off my feed," "all done in," "a falling out," "dragging my feet," "trouble with my water," "a noise in my head," "nervous," "seeing things," "feeling lousy." The nurse should clarify the meaning of such phrases by asking, "What do you mean by that?" or "I don't follow, could you tell me more about that?"

In investigating the location of a symptom, the nurse should determine both where the symptom begins and whether, and to what point, it migrates. It helps to ask the patient to "point with your finger to where the pain is." If the patient can do so, it may be possible to identify the site of underlying pathology promptly and accurately, thereby considerably narrowing the range of possible diagnoses to be considered. If, instead, the patient locates his pain by placing his entire hand over the part or waves his hand over a large body area, the nurse can infer either that the pathological tissue change is widespread or that nerve supply to a large area has somehow been affected by the disease process. The nurse can determine whether and in what manner the pain radiates or migrates with questions like these, "Does this pain ever move from the place where it starts?" "To what other parts does it go?" "How long does it take to spread from the first location to other locations?"

Intensity or severity of each symptom is another characteristic that should be analyzed. The nurse can solicit this information by direct questioning, "How severe is the itching?" or by asking the patient to compare the discomfort to some standard that both can agree on, as, "Would you say this pain is more or less severe than labor pain?" She may determine severity of symptoms by asking for quantification, "How much sputum do you raise in one paroxysm of coughing?" or "How much blood was there, a few flecks, a teaspoonful, an ounce, or . . .?"

Another way to judge the severity of a symptom is to determine what influence it has on the patient's normal activities. One might ask, "When you feel this pain, what do you do?" or, "When you get this pain, are you able to continue with whatever you're doing?" or, "But you didn't cut short your visit, did you?" or, "But you are still working?" or "Has this frequency of urination had any effect on your work or social life?" or "Give me a rundown of your activities on a normal day." In relating his daily routines, the patient will frequently reveal how the present illness has altered his life by contrasting his present activities with those before appearance of his symptoms. "I go to bed right after supper now, but I used to stay up to hear the ten o'clock news." "I take the bus to work now, even though it takes longer. I can't stand the 'El' stairs any more." "Lately I've eaten six or seven small meals a day instead of three big ones. I can't eat as much now that my stomach is swollen."

The practitioner should determine whether any of the patient's symptoms displays a pattern of periodicity. For instance, is the nausea related in some way to eating, drinking, or changes in position? Is the swelling related to changes in position, menstrual period, or intake of fluids? Is the joint pain better or worse during pregnancy? During which season is the dyspepsia most troublesome? How is the fatigue related to daily work routines? The nurse can obtain useful information along this line with such questions as, "Are these attacks more common in cold weather or warm weather?", "Is there any particular time of the day when this sweating is most apt to occur?" or, "How does eating affect the pain?" By thus seeking patterns of symptom recurrence, the nurse may uncover evidence which identifies the most probable of several possible causes for the symptom.

Finally, analysis of a symptom includes consideration of any other symptoms that are associated with it. She might ask, "Are there any other symptoms that usually occur along with this?" or, "And when you feel this discomfort, what else happens?" or, "Have you noticed anything else?" or, "Is there anything else about all this that bothers you?" In response to questioning, the patient might reveal another symptom, which he is not particularly concerned about but which, in conjunction with the first, has diagnostic significance. Perhaps, whenever he experiences dyspnea, he also develops a non-productive cough. Perhaps, following some episodes of palpitation, he has brief fainting spells. Maybe, in addition to swelling of his calf, he has noted that dorsiflexion of his foot causes calf pain.

Significant negative findings should also be recorded in the history. From experience, the nurse will have learned which symptom clusters tend to reflect particular changes in tissue structure or function. In analyzing each of the patient's symptoms, the nurse should question whether he has also experienced the other symptoms that tend to occur in conjunction with it in familiar disease conditions. For instance, the patient reports that he has been vomiting: the nurse should enquire whether or not he has experienced nausea. The patient complains of exertional dyspnea: the nurse should ask whether or not he has had nocturnal dyspnea. The patient has noted clay-colored stools: the nurse should determine whether or not he has experienced sharp right upper quadrant pain or fatty food intolerance. The patient complains of nocturia: the nurse should find out whether he has also noticed urinary hesitancy, dribbling, frequency, or diminution of stream. In recording secondary symptoms that tend to be associated with a principal symptom, the nurse should indicate the time relationships between the two; that is, she should determine exactly how long after nausea is experienced vomiting usually occurs or how frequently a spell of palpitations is followed by a syncopal attack.

As part of the History of Present Illness, the nurse practitioner should determine what treatment the patient has been given for his current illness, who prescribed it, and what the effects of treatments have been. A suitable question here would be, "And what has, so far, been done for this pain?" or, "What has been done to relieve the pain?" If the patient's answer does not state the person who treated him, the nurse may ask, "Who gave you this pain medication?" or, "Who advised you to apply warm soaks?" or, "Who dressed the 'sore' on your leg?" If the patient's answer doesn't reveal the result of treatment, the nurse might ask, "What effect did the medicine have?" or, "After you applied warm soaks, how did the leg look and feel?"

As the last item under Present Illness, the nurse should ask the patient what he thinks is the cause for his current problem. This is a useful question, because the patient may have empirically identified some of the etiologic and precipitating factors underlying his symptoms but not shared his observations with the nurse in the early stages of the interview. On the other hand, if the patient's notion of disease causation is totally erroneous, the nurse must know what he thinks in order to understand his feelings about his situation so that she may correct his misunderstandings.

Occasionally the nurse will have difficulty deciding whether to record a particular problem under History of Present Illness or Past Medical History. A good rule of thumb to follow is this: If the problem is one for which the patient is currently receiving medication, treatment, or follow-up care, include it in the record of Present Illness. If the problem is one for which the patient is not now experiencing symptoms or receiving care, include it in the History of Past Illnesses.

FAMILY HEALTH HISTORY

After exploring the history of the patient's present illness, it is logical to investigate the health of his next of kin. Such information is helpful because some diseases have a familial incidence, being caused in part by hereditary factors or constitutional weakness. For instance, a genetic predisposition has been found to exist for diabetes mellitus, essential hypertension, and carcinoma of the breast.

As she concludes the section on History of the Present Illness and begins inquiry into the Family History, the nurse should signal her change in viewpoint with a transitional comment so that the patient will not be confused or offended by the change of subject. If this is not done, the patient may interpret the nurse's shift from concentration on his problems to concentration on his relative's problems as a lack of genuine interest in his concerns. A clarifying statement might be, "Now that I know pretty well what your previous health has been, I'd like to learn something about the health of your nearest relatives, since that information may help me to understand your present problems." Then the present age and state of health or the age at death and the cause of death should be obtained for each of the patient's parents, grandparents, sisters, brothers, children, aunts, uncles, and cousins. The spouse's age and state of health should also be noted. These data can most easily and clearly be recorded in tabular fashion. High incidence of a particular disease will be immediately apparent from such a table. The patient should then be asked whether any one of his blood relatives has had heart disease, stroke, rheumatic fever, arthritis, anemia, bleeding tendency, diabetes, hay fever, asthma, skin allergies, tuberculosis, cancer, or emotional illness.

If, as sometimes happens, the patient does not know the official cause of death of one of his relatives, the nurse should enquire about the symptoms and treatment for this relative's last illness; the information received may allow her to guess at the diagnosis or to identify the organ system most affected. If one or both of the patient's parents died of heart disease, it is easy to understand why it would be especially frightening to him to develop chest pain, dyspnea, palpitations, or dependent edema. In general, those diseases known to have been fatal to one's close relatives are viewed as potential threats to one's own life. This is so much so that even when the patient's illness is completely different from any which has beset his parents he may feel compelled to look for similarities between his own symptoms and those associated with his mother's or father's terminal illness.

PERSONAL HISTORY

After the Family History is completed, the practitioner should shift the focus of the interview back to the patient for investigation of his Personal History. If the interview has been skillfully executed thus far, the patient will have developed enough trust in the nurse's abilities and motivations to talk comfortably with her about personal matters. The nurse could begin by asking, "Are you married?" and, if he is, enquire as to his wife's age and state of health. Many patients would be offended if the nurse were to ask, "Are you happily married?", but the nurse will probably be able to discern the patient's attitude toward his spouse and his marital relationship from his tone of voice, facial expression, and choice of words in discussing the mate's age and state of health. If the patient is not now married, the nurse should determine whether he ever has been, and whether that union ended in separation, divorce, or death of the partner. If the spouse is dead, the nurse should find out the cause and date of death, and the patient's reaction to this loss.

Next, the practitioner should determine the age and state of health of any children the patient may have. If any of his children is deceased, the nurse should investigate the date and cause of death, together with the patient's reactions to his son's or daughter's demise. In talking about the serious illness or death of a close family member, the patient may reveal anxieties and expectations relating to his own present illness that he was unable to express during the initial description of his symptoms.

In order to round out her view of the patient in his usual life role, the nurse should determine both his educational background and his occupational history. Since, in our society, higher social status is accorded those with collegiate education than those without, persons with a high-school education or less may be reluctant to talk about past schooling. If in his Past History, Family History, or Marital History, the patient has not described his formal schooling, the nurse should ask what kind of work he does, since his occupation may automatically reveal the amount and type of his educational preparation. If the answer to this question does not reveal the patient's educational background, the nurse may ask directly, "How far did you go in your schooling?" The nurse should determine not only what job the patient now holds, but also how long he has held that position and what jobs he has held in the past. If the patient has changed jobs or occupations recently, the nurse should question him to determine the reason for the change. Perhaps waning strength or loss of function due to illness has caused him to lose his previous job or to seek one that is less demanding. If the patient has not recently changed jobs but is employed at a lower occupational level than his formal education would have prepared him for, the nurse may find an explanation for the disparity in his general energy level, the amount of his ambition, or his skill in interpersonal relations.

After determining the patient's occupation, the nurse should ask exactly what duties he is expected to carry out on his job. This information will be useful later in deciding when the patient can be allowed to return to work, or whether he must change jobs or request a modification of work routines to accommodate lowered energy levels or increasing disability.

The patient's military history, if any, should be included as part of the Personal History. The location of his overseas assignment may be of diagnostic significance, since some infectious diseases are endemic to certain countries. The work he performed while in service may have provided him an alternative occupation, should his illness make it necessary for him to change jobs. The fact that he was given a medical discharge from the service would indicate that more information is needed about his health status during his service career.

The nurse should investigate the patient's use of alcohol, tobacco, drugs, coffee, tea, and soft drinks. Patients who are allowed to generalize often minimize the amount of their drinking, smoking, and drug use. Therefore, the nurse should seek quantification of use by asking not, "How much do you drink?", which can be answered "Moderately," but rather, "How many bottles of beer (or highballs or glasses of wine) do you drink each day?" and "How many cigarettes do you smoke each work day?" "On Saturday or Sunday?" Likewise, on finding that the patient takes aspirin for headache, the nurse should ask, "How many aspirin pills do you take to relieve a headache?" Because people are frequently unaware of just how much coffee or tea they do drink, the nurse can get more reliable information by asking not, "How much coffee do you drink each day?" but "Think of a normal work day. Now run through the day and tell me at which points you usually drink coffee and how many cups you drink on each occasion." For some patients it will be important to discover which soft drinks were imbibed and in what quantity, since Coca-Cola contains significant amounts of potassium ion and Pepsi-Cola contains significant amounts of sodium ion.

Another aspect of the patient's personal life about which the nurse should gather information is his social and recreational activities. The nurse might ask, "What are your hobbies or recreational pastimes?" "Do you attend any church, club, or other group gatherings on a regular basis?" Such information can be useful in selecting suitable recreational or occupational therapy activities for the patient or in identifying possible sources of emotional and financial support for the patient within the community.

The patient's financial status should also be included in his Personal History. His occupation may reveal something about his earning power but, in order to judge how great a financial threat his present illness may be, the nurse should know whether the patient owns or is buying his home, whether he has savings, whether he has health insurance, and whether he has any unusual expenses, such as for the college education of his children. The patient may volunteer some financial information while talking of his current symptoms, his past illnesses, his family members, or his job, but the nurse will probably have to question him directly concerning certain financial matters. If the patient understands that the nurse seeks this information in order to make the best possible plan for his care, he will probably not be offended by her questions. She might phrase her questions thus: "I realize that you may be concerned about the cost of hospitalization and treatment for your illness. Do you have health insurance?" and, "Are there any pressing family expenses that will be difficult for you to meet if you should be unable to work for a while?" or, "If your illness has given rise to some financial problems, I can make arrangements for you to talk with a social worker who can help you to locate financial assistance."

Finally, as a means of summarizing the patient's Personal History, the nurse should ask him to recount in some detail his activities throughout a typical day. She might solicit the desired information by saying, "In order that I may get a clear picture of what your life is like, take a normal day and tell me everything that you do from the time you get up in the morning until you go to bed at night." While she is taking the Personal History, the nurse should be trying to draw for herself a personal profile of the patient which will indicate what kind of a person he is, what strengths and weaknesses he has, how intelligent, open, and self-disciplined he is, and what support he can draw from his environment. All this information will help her to predict how well the patient will cooperate with his prescribed treatment regime and will suggest how best to provide him with needed health teaching.

PAST MEDICAL HISTORY

The purpose for the Past Medical History is to provide a backdrop of information about the patient's previous health against which to interpret the significance of his present symptoms. Many chronic diseases develop as a late stage of a previously acute illness that has undergone serial recurrences and complications. For instance, rheumatic cardiovalvular disease may develop as a complication of repeated episodes of acute rheumatic fever. Hypertensive heart disease may follow years of untreated or inadequately treated hypertension. Further, the effects of certain disease processes are so far reaching that the disease may present at one point as a disturbance in one organ system, be treated successfully or unsuccessfully, and present at a later time as a disturbance in another organ system. For example, diabetes mellitus may first be diagnosed as a result of a patient's developing keto-acidosis in conjunction with acute pneumonia. The same patient may, after years of satisfactory diabetic management with diet regulation and insulin administration, develop symptoms of diabetic gangrene of the toe. By reviewing the patient's past health, the nurse practitioner may learn of a previous episode of ill health which, together with his current symptoms, suggests a diagnosis for the current illness.

Even if the patient's present illness is in no way related to any of his previous illnesses, his Past Medical History can provide very useful information. The manner in which the patient has responded, both physiologically and psychologically, to illness in the past is a useful indicator of how he will probably respond to this current illness. If, in the past, he has weathered acute infections, major surgery, or serious injury, has responded promptly to treatment and recovered without serious setbacks, complications, or sequelae, and if his general level of health is about the same now as before, the nurse may expect him to withstand current stresses successfully. Further, if the patient's previous experience with illness and treatment was positive, he will tend to expect a favorable outcome from current therapy and will be well motivated to cooperate with the treatment program.

Sometimes after a patient has talked about his present illness at some length, he will, as a natural extension of that topic, begin to talk about his previous illnesses and hospitalizations. Usually, however, he will not voluntarily describe *all* of his previous episodes of ill health. His memory will have to be jogged in order to recall certain disorders. Direct questioning will be needed to elicit certain information that he finds insignificant, confusing, or anxiety provoking. Therefore, the nurse will not be able to use here the nondirect method of interviewing that was suggested for obtaining the history of the Present Illness. Rather, a series of direct questions will be needed to elicit the needed information.

The past history should include information about all previous episodes of illness, injury, and surgical procedures. In order not to neglect any important aspect of the patient's previous health, the nurse should base her questioning on a prearranged outline, such as:

1. General level of former health
2. Childhood diseases
3. Immunizations
4. Allergies
5. Medical diseases
6. Surgical operations
7. Traumatic injuries
8. Psychiatric illnesses
9. Obstetrical history
10. Previous hospitalizations

The nurse may explore the patient's previous health level by asking, "How has your health been in the past?" or, "How would you describe your health before this present illness began?" The patient's answer to this question must be interpreted in the light of his general reaction to his present problem: that is, if the nurse observes a tendency in the patient to deny or minimize symptoms in the present illness, then a response from him that his previous health was "pretty good" should be weighed accordingly. On the other hand, if in attempting to specify his chief complaint, the patient mentions many, vague, unrelated, and relatively inconsequential complaints, his description of his previous health as "terrible," "poor," or "very bad" would need further clarification. In both instances the nurse should question the patient further. "What do you mean by 'pretty good'?" or, "' terrible' in the sense that you had what kinds of problems?" As a standard against which to evaluate the patient's previous health level, the practitioner should determine whether the patient has been employed, what kind of work he has done, what hobbies and pastimes he has engaged in, and how much rest he has required. Information along these lines will enable the nurse to judge whether the patient has been in relatively good health or poor health prior to this episode.

Incidence of the following childhood diseases should be recorded: measles, mumps, chicken pox, whooping cough, scarlet fever, diphtheria, poliomyelitis, rheumatic fever, tonsillitis. Here, the nurse should seek the dates for each disease, a description of the patient's symptoms in each illness, the treatment which was received, and any complications that resulted from the disease. Information concerning symptoms and treatment will enable the practitioner to judge whether the disease in question was correctly diagnosed and whether the patient's memory for the event is accurate.

The nurse should inquire whether and when the patient has had inoculations or vaccinations against diphtheria, pertussis, tetanus, smallpox, typhoid fever, poliomyelitis, measles, influenza, or other infectious diseases. If the patient has not been immunized against tetanus and has recently suffered a potentially infected deep puncture wound, he should be given tetanus antitoxin. If he has been immunized against the disease, he should be given a booster dose of toxoid. Again, if the patient has not been immunized against a disease to which he is unusually susceptible or which constitutes, for him, a severe health risk, the nurse should provide the necessary vaccination or inoculation as part of his current care. Thus, the pregnant woman who has not been immunized against rubella and has been exposed to the disease should be given gamma globulin. The person planning a trip to underdeveloped tropical countries should be vaccinated against typhoid fever. The older patient with severe emphysema or diabetes mellitus who is especially susceptible to respiratory infections should, perhaps, be immunized against influenza to protect him against pneumonia as a complication of influenza. The nurse should also ask whether, following any immunization procedure, the patient has experienced a hypersensitivity reaction. If the patient has once suffered a chill, fever, arthralgia, myalgia, or vomiting following typhoid immunization but should be revaccinated now because he has taken a job as a hospital orderly, it would probably be desirable to skin test him first to determine his present reactivity to the vaccine and, if he is strongly reactive, to give less than the usual dosage of vaccine. If the patient has been immunized for cholera, typhus, yellow fever, or other disease against which citizens of this country are not routinely protected, the nurse should inquire why the immunization was done. A history of recent overseas travel may suggest possible diagnoses for the present illness.

The Past History should include a list of all substances to which the patient is allergic. In addition to asking, "Are you allergic to anything? Any chemicals?", it may be helpful to ask "Have you ever had asthma? Hay fever? Attacks of wheezing? Hives? Have you ever had trouble with watering of your eyes or skin rashes?" If the patient reports that he is allergic to a certain food, animal dander, or pollen, the nurse should ask when, how, and by whom it was determined that he was allergic to the subject in question, since without specific hypersensitivity testing, the identification of a particular allergen may have been largely presumptive. The nurse should specifically inquire whether the patient has demonstrated allergy to aspirin, penicillin, or iodine-containing compounds, since all three frequently produce hypersensitivity reactions and the nurse may wish to use aspirin or penicillin to treat the patient or may order a diagnostic test utilizing an iodine-containing dye. If the patient gives a history of allergic illness, the nurse should learn when the disease first appeared, how it was treated, how it responded to treatment, and the dates of any recurrences.

In investigating the patient's history of medical and surgical illnesses, the nurse might start by asking, "What is the sickest that you have ever been?" or, "What illnesses have you had for which you were given medications?" It may be necessary to prod the patient's memory by asking such other questions as "Have you ever had a high fever? Chills? Convulsions?", "What acute infectious diseases have you had?" "Have you ever been hospitalized?"

The nurse should bear in mind that the patient may be confused or misinformed as to the diagnosis of a previous ailment. Therefore, if a patient should state that he had had pneumonia some years before, the nurse should question him in some detail about the symptoms he experienced, the diagnostic tests that were performed, the treatment he was given, and the course of the disease in order to make an educated guess as to whether the disease was pneumonia, what type of pneumonia it was, and what about the patient's condition and/or activities had caused him to develop pneumonia. Once the nature of each of the patient's previous ailments has been clearly established, it should be possible to identify a pattern of illness. Perhaps he has had a series of severe pulmonary infections, or allergic manifestations in several organ systems, or numerous traumatic injuries, or repeated urinary infections, or several congenital anomalies. By recognizing some pattern or theme in the patient's previous episodes of ill health, the nurse may find clues to the diagnosis of his present problem or may be able to anticipate possible complications of illness, treatment, and hospitalization. The patient with a history of several severe respiratory infections would be especially vulnerable to postoperative pneumonia.

The nurse should ask the patient, "Have you had any surgical operations?" and then list these in chronological order, indicating for each the date, type of procedure, surgeon's name and address, hospital at which surgery was done, and effects of the operation. Knowledge that the patient has had a particular surgical procedure may automatically eliminate certain diagnoses or suggest the possibility of certain others. The patient with periumbilical pain who has previously had an appendectomy is not now suffering from acute appendicitis. The patient with postprandial weakness, palpitation, nausea, distention and diarrhea who has had a gastrectomy is probably experiencing the "dumping syndrome" caused by a too rapid emptying of the stomach.

Sometimes a patient will have a mistaken impression of the exact type of operation he has had, either because the surgeon did not take time to explain the procedure to him in detail or because he could not understand the explanation given him. Therefore, the nurse should not accept without questioning a patient's statement that he has had his stomach removed, but should verify that information by asking what symptoms the patient had before surgery, what medical treatment he had been given before surgery, why the decision was made to operate, what type of postoperative course he experienced, and what the effects of surgery had been. After learning all this, the practitioner can better evaluate the accuracy of the patient's report of his operation. The nurse should record the surgeon's name and address and the hospital in which each operation was performed so that she may later obtain detailed and accurate information about the operation, should that information be needed.

The Past Medical History should include a record of any injuries the patient has ever experienced. The fact that a patient had months before suffered severe blows to the head in a robbery attempt should be considered when diagnosing focal convulsions. The fact that a patient has suffered a head injury in an automobile accident would be significant in diagnosing symptoms of sensorimotor loss in the extremities. The nurse should begin her investigation in this category by asking, "Have you ever had a severe injury or accident?" "A head injury?" "Broken bones?" "Severe bruises?" "Burns?" "Any cuts that required stitches?" and "Were you ever in an automobile accident?" "Have you ever been shot, stabbed, or beaten up?" If the patient gives a history of injury, the nurse should determine the date and place the injury occurred, name of the attending physician, name of the hospital in which treatment was given, type of injury, symptoms, treatment received, length of hospitalization, and any resulting disability.

In obtaining the patient's Past Medical History, the practitioner should seek information about mental and emotional as well as physical illness. Because of the stigma associated with emotional illness, patients usually do not volunteer information about illnesses of this type. The practitioner should question each patient about his previous mental health, and can facilitate discussion of the topic by using a direct, matter-of-fact approach, initiating the inquiry with, "Have you ever had a nervous breakdown?" "Severe nervousness?" "Depression?" "Crying spells?" "Emotional problems?" "Do you describe yourself or does anyone else describe you as an emotional person?" If the patient admits to having had emotional difficulties, the nurse should question him further to determine when the problem occurred, what precipitated it, what symptoms the patient experienced, how, where, and by whom the patient was treated, how he responded to treatment, and whether the patient continues to suffer emotional discomfort. The Psychiatric History yields information about how the patient has handled stress in the past, and may alert the nurse to aspects of the patient's present situation which he may find particularly threatening.

For the woman patient, the Past Medical History should include an Obstetrical History. The nurse should record the patient's age at menarche; the frequency, duration, and volume of menstrual flow; the number of previous pregnancies and live births; the types of delivery for each; any complications of pregnancy, labor, delivery, or puerperium; age at menopause; and the quality of sex life. Sometimes the Obstetrical History is directly related to the present illness, as in the case of a multiparous woman who seeks medical attention for a cystocele or a rectocele. On other occasions, some aspect of the Obstetrical History may be indirectly related to a current problem, as in the case of a patient with chronic pyelonephritis whose initial episode of acute pyelonephritis occurred some years before in conjunction with an otherwise uncomplicated pregnancy. In exploring the patient's Obstetrical History as well as her Surgical History, the nurse should ask whether the patient has ever had blood transfusions, and if so, when, why, how many, and whether there were any untoward reactions. A transfusion would be important in a patient with symptoms of liver dysfunction, and a previous transfusion reaction should alert the nurse to possible trouble if the patient should require transfusion as treatment for the present illness.

REVIEW OF SYSTEMS

As a final step in obtaining the patient's medical history, the nurse practitioner should determine which symptoms or disorders of each physiological body system the patient is now experiencing or ever has experienced. The purpose of such a review of symptoms by body systems is to check on the completeness of information given in the History of Present Illness and to amplify both the History of the Present Illness and History of Past Illnesses. A patient may fail to volunteer information about a diagnostically significant symptom during early portions of the health interview, because he either has forgotten the symptom or accords it little importance.

In order to determine the patient's experience with the entire scope of symptoms of possible significance to his diagnosis and treatment, the nurse should question him concerning all of the symptoms and disorders commonly associated with each body system. A logical way to organize symptoms referable to each system would be to seek information first about pain or discomfort in the organs of the system, second about functional disturbances of the system, third about illnesses involving the system, and finally about diagnostic tests used to identify malfunctioning of the system. Since the absence of a particular symptom may have as great a diagnostic significance as the presence of another, the practitioner should take pains to record significant negative as well as positive findings. Further, the patient's chief complaint and the history of his present illness will often cause certain of his present and past symptoms to be of special significance, while others, in the context of his present problems, will be relatively unimportant. The nurse should, accordingly, list the unimportant symptoms briefly and simply and should develop in more detail those symptoms and disorders that relate directly to the present illness. Each symptom or dysfunction claimed by the patient should be described as to date, time, and circumstances of onset; duration; severity; frequency; and influencing factors.

So that she may be certain that no significant present or past finding is overlooked in the System Review, the nurse should organize both the systems and symptoms and disorders associated with each into some logical sequence, commit this outline to memory, and follow the outline faithfully in questioning the patient about present and past findings. A logical order to follow is to inquire first about general symptoms, then skin symptoms, then symptoms of each physiologic system encountered as one progresses from the crown of the head to the soles of the feet. Following is an outline illustrating a suggested sequence for obtaining detailed and helpful information from a Review of Systems:

1. *General symptoms:* weakness; fatigue; fever, chills, profuse perspiration; night sweats; weight changes.

2. *Skin:* pruritus; color changes; changes in texture; changes in temperature; excessive moisture; unusual dryness; bruises; petechiae; changes in

birthmarks or moles; changes in the amount, color, texture, or distribution of body hair; brittleness, ridging, or pitting of nails; rashes; hives; infections; delayed healing of a wound; skin tests; injections; vaccinations; immunizations; desensitizations.

3. *Head and face:* headache (location, character, severity, duration); facial pain (location, character, severity, duration); vertigo; syncope; seizures; trauma (location, type, severity).

4. *Eyes:* pain; photophobia; itching; burning; blindness; diplopia; excessive lacrimation; visual acuity; recent changes in acuity; glasses worn; date of last refraction; infection; glaucoma; cataract; foreign bodies; operations.

5. *Ears:* earache; itching; discharge; tinnitus; acuity of hearing; infections; foreign bodies; operations.

6. *Nose and sinuses:* sinus pain; epistaxis; nasal obstruction; nasal discharge; postnasal drip; sneezing; change in sense of smell; frequent colds; allergic rhinitis; foreign bodies; operations.

7. *Mouth, pharynx, and larynx:* sore tongue; tender gums; toothache; mucosal erosions; bleeding gums; tooth abscesses, tooth extractions; dentures; excessive or deficient salivation; changes in sense of taste; sore throat; difficulty in swallowing; hoarseness; infections; operations.

8. *Neck:* pain; stiffness; swelling; distended veins; lesions; enlarged nodes; operations.

9. *Endocrine system:* goiter; tremor; weakness; increased or decreased sweating; heat or cold intolerance; dryness of skin or hair; changes in skin pigmentation; exophthalmos; unusual growth pattern; unusual gain in weight or height; change in hair distribution; change in glove or shoe size; change in body configuration; voice change; impotence; polyuria; polydipsia, polyphagia; fatigue; hormone therapy, tests for infertility or sterility, basal metabolism test, urine testing for sugar and acetone.

10. *Breasts:* pain, lumps; swelling; discharge; changes in contour; changes in nipples, gynecomastia, mammography, operations.

11. *Respiratory system:* pain associated with breathing; pleuritic pain; dyspnea; rales; cough; sputum; wheezing; hemoptysis; night sweats; chest colds; pneumonia; bronchitis; asthma, bronchiectasis; tuberculosis; date of most recent tuberculin test and chest x-ray; operations.

12. *Cardiovascular system:* chest pain on exertion (location, radiation, severity, frequency); palpitations; exertional dyspnea; nocturnal dyspnea; orthopnea; cyanosis; syncope; fatigue; murmur; leg cramps; varicosities; cold extremities; rheumatic fever; hypertension; heart attack; heart medication; date of most recent ECG.

13. *Blood:* anemia (type and treatment); bleeding tendency; enlarged, tender, or suppurative nodes; transfusions; transfusion reaction; date of last blood count.

14. *Gastrointestinal system:* heartburn, epigastric pain; abdominal pain; anal itching or burning; increased thirst; increased or decreased appetite; food intolerances; dysphagia; eructations; indigestion; jaundice; colic; flatulence; tarry stools; blood in stools; constipation; diarrhea; tenesmus; change in bowel habits; use of laxatives; antidiarrhetics; ulcer; hepatitis; cirrhosis; gall bladder disease; appendicitis; colitis; hemorrhoids; dates of upper or lower GI series; gall bladder studies; proctoscopy; operations.

15. *Urinary system:* flank pain; dysuria; polyuria; nocturia; oliguria;

anuria; hesitancy; dribbling; diminution of stream; retention; incontinence; enuresis; hematuria; cloudy urine; genital sores; syphilis; gonorrhea; renal or bladder infection; renal or bladder stones; kidney, ureter, bladder x-rays; operations.

16. *Reproductive system* (male): Testicular pain; change in size of scrotum; penile lesion or discharge; positive serology; potency; sexual habits.

Reproductive system (female): Menstrual history: age at menarche; regularity and frequency of menstruation; duration and amount of flow (number of pads per day); date of last period; dysmenorrhea; amenorrhea; menorrhagia; metrorrhagia; vaginal discharge; vulvar itching; abscesses; lesions; venereal disease and treatment; contraceptive drugs and devices.

Obstetrical history: number of pregnancies; number of live births; number of abortions; complications during pregnancy; complications of labor and delivery; operations.

Menopause: age at menopause; fatigue; hot flashes; irritability; depression; changes in frequency and character of flow; date of final menstrual period; post-menopausal bleeding; operations.

17. *Musculo-skeletal system:* pain in extremities; pain in neck or back; joint stiffness; joint swelling; joint discoloration; joint crepitation; limitation of joint motion; strains or sprains; flat feet; deformities; arthritis; gout; osteomyelitis; fractures; dislocations; amputations; x-rays of head, spine, ribs, or extremities, operations.

18. *Nervous system:* headache; vertigo; syncope; memory loss; amnesia; unconsciousness; nervousness; hallucinations; nightmares; insomnia; depression; changes in emotional state; ataxia; tremor; muscle weakness; muscle atrophy; limitation of motion; paralysis; convulsions; aphasia; speech difficulty; pain; numbness; paresthesias; visual disturbances; disturbances of smell.

SUMMARY

Following the detailed Review of Systems, the nurse should summarize the patient's medical history by providing a brief review of the major facts revealed in each category of the history. Thus, the summary for a particular patient might read as follows: This 68 year old married Caucasian male complains of exertional dyspnea beginning nine months ago following a severe "chest cold" and increasing steadily in severity to the point where, presently, he must sit down for several minutes to "catch my breath" after ascending one flight of stairs. The patient is a semiretired farmer, who now raises chickens for a living and has been in good health all his life except for an appendectomy at the age of 35 and a chronic "smoker's cough" of several years' duration. The patient's father and mother both died of heart trouble, his father at 77 years of age and his mother at 78 years. His two siblings both suffer heart trouble and high blood pressure. The patient and his wife own a 150 acre farm, and their only child, a man of 40, lives with them and farms for them. The patient drinks approximately two bottles of beer each Saturday, smokes two packs of cigarettes each day, and takes two aspirin to relieve a headache every month or so. So far, the patient has managed to live on his Social Security payments without dipping into his savings. Review of systems revealed that, in addition to exertional dyspnea, the patient has experienced occasional precordial pain with exertion, nocturnal dyspnea, nocturia, and hesitancy in starting the urinary stream. The patient seems hopeful that treatment can relieve his symptoms but wishes to avoid hospitalization because "my wife is the nervous type and doesn't like to be separated from me."

BIBLIOGRAPHY: CONTENT OF THE PATIENT'S MEDICAL HISTORY

Aegidius: The critical negative. *Canad. Med. Assoc. J.* 107:598, October 7, 1972.

Burnside, J.: *Adams' Physical Diagnosis.* 15th ed. Baltimore, Williams & Wilkins Co., 1974.

DeGroot, A. E., et al: Technics, problems, and gains in interviewing next of kin. *Ohio State Med. J.* 69:189–194, March, 1973.

Hochstein, Elliot, and Rubin, A.: *Physical Diagnosis.* New York, The McGraw-Hill Book Co., 1964.

Hopkins, Henry: *Leopold's Principles and Methods of Physical Diagnosis.* 3rd ed. Philadelphia, W. B. Saunders Co., 1965.

Judge, Richard, and Zuidema, George: *Physical Diagnosis: A Physiologic Approach to the Clinical Examination.* 2nd ed. Boston, Little, Brown and Co., 1968.

Kampmeier, Rudolph, and Blake, Thomas: *Physical Examination in Health and Disease.* 4th ed. Philadelphia, F. A. Davis Co., 1970.

Leaverton, L. E.: Is your patient history adequate? *J. Iowa Med. Soc.* 62:601, November, 1972.

McPhetridge, L. Mae: Nursing history: One means to personalize care. *Amer. J. Nurs.* 68:68–75, January, 1968.

Morgan, William, and Engle, George: *The Clinical Approach to the Patient.* Philadelphia, W. B. Saunders Co., 1969.

Prior, John, and Silberstein, Jack: *Physical Diagnosis.* 4th ed. St. Louis, The C. V. Mosby Co., 1973.

Small, Iver Ed.: *Introduction to the Clinical History.* 2nd ed. Flushing, New York, Medical Examination Publishing Co., 1971.

Stern, Thomas: *Clinical Examination.* Chicago, Year Book Medical Publishers, 1964.

3
THE PHYSICAL EXAMINATION

Section I. Overview

GENERAL PROCEDURE FOR EXAMINATION

In examining the patient physically the nurse practitioner will need to use her senses of sight, touch, hearing, and smell to acquire information about the structure and function of various body parts.

The examination should be conducted in a well lighted, well heated room, and the patient should be prepared for the examination by being completely undressed, by being protectively draped, and by being given an explanation of the purpose and general procedure for the examination. Disrobing the patient and providing good lighting will make it easier for the nurse to make accurate observations. A warm room and skillful draping will protect the patient from chilling. An explanation of the procedure and thoughtful draping will minimize patient embarrassment.

To minimize patient discomfort and to conserve time and energy for both patient and nurse, the practitioner should examine all structures in a particular body region before progressing to the next. That is, when examining the chest she should investigate breasts, axillary nodes, rib cage, lower respiratory tree, heart, and great vessels (elements of four different body systems). In like manner, when examining the abdomen she should investigate stomach, liver, spleen, bowel, abdominal aorta, uterus, bladder, and inguinal nodes (elements of four different systems).

Physical findings should not be recorded in the same sequence in which they were elicited since, in order to diagnose the patient's illness, each important physical finding must be interpreted relative to the functional efficiency of one body system or another. For example, all findings from all body regions which reflect cardiovascular functioning should be recorded in the same part of the record. Thus, distended neck veins, dyspnea, cardiac murmurs, hepatomegaly, splenomegaly, ascites, and pedal edema should all be recorded in the same section of the record, even though they were detected in several different body regions and at different times during the examination. All findings should be recorded as accurately as possible; quantifying data and descriptive terms should be provided when possible.

A workable procedure for conducting the examination is as follows: Place the patient in a sitting position while examining the head, neck, back, and chest. Place the patient in a recumbent position while examining the breasts, axillae, heart, lungs, abdomen, genitalia, and extremities. Finally, perform pelvic and rectal examinations.

In general, four methods of inquiry are used in physical examination. Generally, too, in investigating each body part the practitioner should employ these four methods in the following sequence: observation (or inspection), palpation, percussion, and auscultation.

The Method of Observation

Observation, as a tool of physical examination, consists of much more than simply looking at a part. Rather, observation implies careful and systematic inspection according to a pre-established plan designed to ensure the greatest possible objectivity and awareness on the part of the examiner. By following a prearranged routine in conducting the examination and by forcing oneself to break down observation of each part into several small steps, each treating a different aspect of that part, the practitioner can decrease the possibility of overlooking a significant finding. For instance, oversights can be minimized if in examining the head the nurse trains herself to follow a fixed and logical routine: first, observe the size, shape, position, and degree of motion of the total head; then, observe the scalp for scars or signs of trauma; then, examine the mastoid processes and external ears; then, observe the facial area from forehead to chin, checking each part in turn for contour, symmetry, movement, color, and texture.

The Method of Palpation

Palpation consists of feeling a part in order to learn something of its structure or function. Palpation of some structures, such as the eye, is best carried out through the use of light touch. For other structures, like the liver, spleen, or kidney, firm, deep pressure will be needed to palpate the organ. Usually the tips of the fingers are used for palpation, since the concentration of nerve endings in the fingertips makes them highly sensitive to touch. However, the palm or the lateral aspect of the hand is more sensitive than the fingertips in detecting vibrations, as from a bruit, and the dorsum of the hand is more sensitive than the fingertips in detecting skin temperature changes.

Since extreme pressure against the fingertips tends to decrease touch perception, the strong pressure which must be exerted to palpate deep-lying structures such as the liver and kidney may blunt the sensitivity of the examining fingers. To offset this difficulty, it is advisable to use two hands to palpate deep structures: place one hand over the other, relax the lower hand completely, and then apply pressure with the upper hand to guide the lower hand firmly over the surface of the structure to be explored.

Ballottement, a special type of palpation, may be used to detect the presence of fluid in a body cavity or to determine the presence of masses buried under large quantities of fluid. Ballottement operates upon two physical principles: first, pressure applied to a fluid-filled container is transmitted equally in all directions throughout the fluid; and second, when force is applied to a container enclosing both fluid and solid components, the fluid will be displaced more rapidly than the solid. To detect the presence of ascites, the patient is placed in supine position and, while a second nurse exerts firm pressure on the midline of the abdomen with the edge of her hand, the examiner places the palm and extended fingers of one hand along one flank and then with the other hand exerts a light blow to the opposite flank. If fluid is present in the peritoneal cavity, a fluid wave initiated by the blow will be transmitted across the abdomen, and detected by the examiner's hand on the opposite flank. The pressure of the assisting nurse's hand on the midline of the abdomen will block transmission of the impulse through the abdominal wall.

When using palpation the nurse should warm her hands thoroughly (the hands should be washed before the examination, anyway, for aseptic and aesthetic reasons) before placing them on the patient's skin so that the patient does not respond to cold discomfort by withdrawing from or tensing against the examiner's probing fingers. The nurse can facilitate patient comfort, too, by palpating tissues as gently as possible even though, on occasion, it may be necessary to cause the patient some discomfort in order to adequately examine the part in question. In such an instance, the nurse should indicate her awareness of the patient's discomfort, explain why further examination is necessary even in the face of pain and, if the occasion seems to warrant it, interrupt the examination briefly to allow the patient respite from distress.

As in the case of observation, the practitioner will, with continued practice in palpation, become familiar with normal variations in the size, density, contour, and texture of different tissues and organs so that she may correctly identify those pathological structures that are accessible to her examining fingers.

The Method of Percussion

Percussion consists of tapping the body surface to produce sound and touch vibrations in underlying tissues that will reveal the character of those tissues. The technique is based on the principle that media of different densities distort sound waves in different degrees, so that blows of equal strength over tissues of different densities produce sounds of differing pitch and intensity.

Generally, a blow over very dense tissue produces a dull or flat sound; a blow over tissue of little density produces a tympanic or drumlike sound. Thus, percussion over gas-filled lung, stomach, or bowel will produce tympany; a blow over compact heart, liver, or spleen will produce dullness.

The technique of percussion consists of placing one hand on the patient, with only the middle finger firmly pressed against the skin, and then directly striking the first phalanx of the middle finger of that hand with the flexed finger of the other hand (Fig. 1). After contacting the extended finger (pleximeter) of the hand on the patient using a flicking motion from a flexed wrist, the striking fingertip (plexor) is quickly withdrawn in order to avoid damping sound transmission.

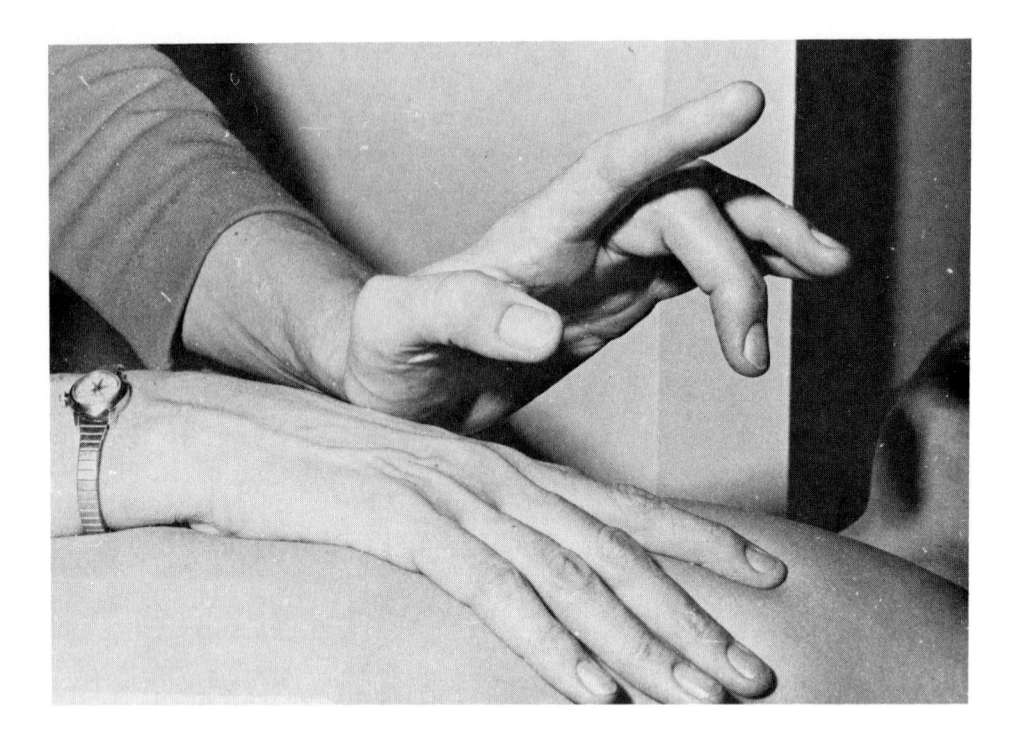

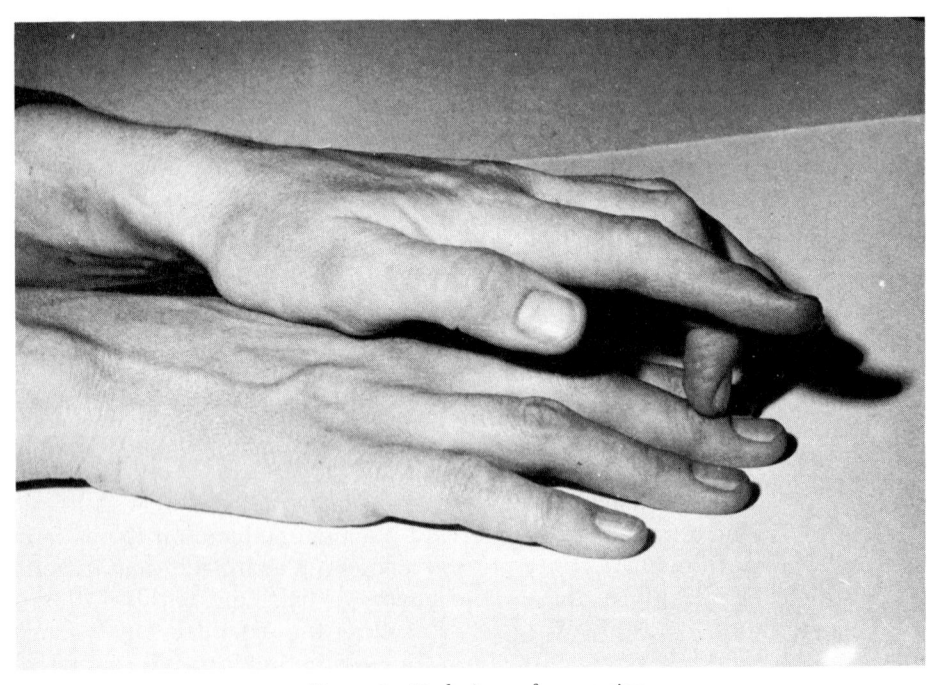

Figure 1. Technique of percussion.

Since the value of percussion as a diagnostic technique depends upon the examiner's interpretation of the sounds produced, the room in which the examination is conducted should be quiet enough that the practitioner can detect even slight changes in sound pitch and intensity. Further, since the change in sound from resonance to dullness is easier to perceive than the reverse, in percussion the nurse should always move from an area of more resonance to an area of less, as from lung to liver rather than from liver to lung.

The Method of Auscultation

Auscultation consists of listening to sounds produced by the functioning of various organs, especially the heart, blood vessels, lungs, stomach, and intestines. Auscultation can be performed by applying the ear directly to the body surface, but usually a stethoscope is used to amplify body sounds and conduct them in an aesthetic fashion to the examiner's ear, while at the same time reducing extraneous noise. The practitioner should use a stethoscope equipped with both a bell and a diaphragm, as the former is best suited for perception of low-pitched sounds and the latter for high-pitched sounds. For maximal sound transmission, the stethoscope tubing should be thick-walled and approximately 12 inches in length, and the ear pieces should be small enough to fit snugly in the ear without slipping so far into the auditory canal that they occlude sound passage entirely.

Because the diagnostically significant sounds produced by body organs are of relatively low intensity, the room in which auscultation is performed should be as quiet as possible. To prevent patient discomfort, the nurse should warm the stethoscope chestpiece in her hand before applying either bell or diaphragm to the patient's skin. In order to pick up visceral sounds, the diaphragm should be positioned in full contact with the body wall. The bell should be placed very lightly against the body wall since, if pressure is exerted, the skin which is stretched beneath the bell will act as a diaphragm, interfering with transmission of low pitched sounds. The nurse should prevent anything from rubbing against the tubing of the stethoscope, and should refrain from moving the chestpiece against the skin, as either motion will produce external noises capable of obscuring significant sounds and confusing the examiner.

Auscultation of a given part, like observation, palpation, or percussion, should follow a regular routine so that the part is thoroughly examined, and so that perception of an unusual sound at one point does not distract the examiner from listening at other significant points.

Preliminary Survey and Vital Signs

As the practitioner commences the examination she should help the patient to a comfortable sitting position and put him at ease with a remark such as, "This examination will take about thirty minutes. Don't hesitate to ask any questions which occur to you as we proceed. Shall we begin?"

At the beginning of the examination the nurse should determine and record the patient's height, weight, temperature, heart rate (radial pulse and apical rate), respiratory rate, and blood pressure (in both arms, and in both sitting and recumbent positions). Most patients will have had their height, weight, and vital signs measured in previous encounters with health workers. By thus starting the physical examination with a familiar routine the nurse emphasizes that this procedure is an integral part of the patient's total health care and allows him time to adjust to her intrusion of his personal space bubble before greater physical exposure and more intimate handling occur.

Throughout the time when she is determining the patient's measurements and taking his vital signs and after these findings have been recorded, the nurse should be observing the patient to determine his sex, race, apparent age, body build, state of nutrition, gait, posture, specific malformations, motor activity, apparent intelligence, and emotional state, and any abnormal findings such as pallor, flushing, cyanosis, jaundice, diaphoresis, noisy respirations, voice abnormality, speech problems, tremors, tics, or unpleasant body odors. If the examination is conducted in a clinic, the nurse should observe whether the patient required help to get to the clinic or to enter the examining room. If the examination is conducted in the patient's hospital room or his home, the nurse should observe his immediate environment for clues to his condition. An unemptied urinal, bed pan, or emesis basin should be examined to determine the quantity, color, consistency, odor, and presence of blood in urine, stool, vomitus, or sputum. An unfinished tray may reveal lack of appetite. If a Levin tube, tracheostomy tube, or chest tube is in place, the character and amount of drainage or secretions should be noted. If intravenous fluids are running, the nurse should observe the nature of the fluid being administered and note whether any drugs have been added to the solution. If intake-output records are kept at the bedside, the nurse should check the volume of fluid movement into and out of the patient within the past 24 hours. If a respirator is running, she should estimate the rate and depth of the patient's ventilation and note whether or not oxygen is being administered. Finally, she should observe whether the patient has been restrained, whether bed siderails have been applied, and whether he is using additional pillows or bedcovers.

As a part of the general overall survey, the practitioner should examine the patient's skin. She should observe the texture and turgor of the skin; its color and temperature; the amount, character, and distribution of hair; the color, shape, and angle of the nails. She should look for surgical or traumatic scars and note the description, size, and location of any skin lesions (macules, papules, pustules, vesicles, nodules, blebs, crusts, scales, moles, warts, xanthomas, petechiae, ecchymoses, purpura, tumors, or ulcers).

Section II. Examination of the Head and Neck

In examination of the head, observation and palpation will be the chief means of inquiry, with percussion and auscultation being used only infrequently. The practitioner should systematize the examination by turning her attention first to the head as a whole, then to the hair and scalp, and finally to the face, from forehead to chin.

First, the nurse should observe the size, shape, symmetry, and degree of movement of the skull. An abnormally small head usually will be associated with mental retardation. An abnormally large head may occur as a result of hydrocephalus or acromegaly. An abnormally elongated skull is sometimes seen in sickle cell anemia. Cervical osteoarthritis or torticollis can limit movement of the head.

Next, the nurse should palpate the skull to locate any lumps, depressions, or areas of tenderness. Palpation should proceed from the frontal to the occipital region, using a rotary motion of the fingertips and working from the center to the lateral aspects of the cranium. Since small irregularities of the skull may be missed in examining patients with thick hair, the nurse should ask the patient whether he has noted any lumps or depressions. The location, size, and consistency of any masses should be carefully noted and each mass explored to see whether it is fixed or movable, and whether it fluctuates on palpation.

The size, position, color, and symmetry of the ears should be noted. Elongated ear lobes are often seen in patients with pernicious anemia. Distortion of the external ear may result from repeated mechanical trauma, as from numerous boxing injuries. Collections of urate crystals are sometimes deposited in the helix of the ear in patients with gout. The ear lobes are usually deep red in the patient with polycythemia vera.

Next the color, texture, and amount of the hair should be noted. Dryness and brittleness of the hair is common in the aged and in myxedema. Fine, silky hair is characteristic of hyperthyroidism. Alopecia may occur in secondary syphilis, following severe emotional stress, or following administration of cytotoxic drugs for treatment of malignancy. The scalp should be examined for lacerations and lesions. A smooth, round lesion attached to the overlying skin but not to underlying bone is probably a sebaceous cyst or wen. Crusts and flakes may indicate eczema, seborrheic dermatitis or contact dermatitis from a hair dye or spray.

EXAMINATION OF THE FACE

When examining the face the nurse should first note the patient's expression as a possible indicator of his response to illness and to the situation in which he finds himself. The nurse's social and professional experience will have prepared her to interpret expressions of anxiety, hostility, pain, depression, embarrassment, fear, resignation, and disinterest. However, stoical or overcontrolled patients may successfully mask their feelings from all but the most observant nurse. Facial expression may reveal the true feelings of such a patient only after he has developed sufficient rapport with the examiner to relax and let down his guard.

Certain facial expressions are pathognomonic of particular diseases. Risus sardonicus, a grotesque, grinning expression due to spasm of facial muscles, is seen in tetanus. A flat, expressionless, masklike facies with occasional drooling is characteristic of paralysis agitans. A wide-eyed, startled expression is apt to develop in the hyperthyroid patient with exophthalmos. The deaf patient often presents a faintly confused or quizzical expression. The patient with poor vision may wear a perpetual frown or squint. Patients with malignant and chronic wasting disease often wear an expression of exhaustion or defeat. Manic depressive patients may appear angry, excited, or dejected, depending upon the phase of their illness.

While studying the patient's facial expression the nurse should note the symmetry and proportion of facial structures. Probably the two sides of the face are never exactly alike, but marked differences between the two might indicate trauma, inflammatory processes, or neoplastic growth. Following a cerebrovascular accident one side of the face may sag as a result of paresis or paralysis of the facial muscles.

Some diseases will change the proportionate size of certain facial structures. In acromegaly the supraorbital ridges, the malar prominences and the mandible increase in thickness to a greater extent than other facial structures. Thickening of the cranium, most pronounced in the frontal and occipital regions, occurs in osteitis deformans.

When examining the face the practitioner has an excellent opportunity to observe the color of the patient's skin. In light-skinned persons, especially, severe anemia produces marked facial pallor. In pernicious anemia the pallor is of a faint yellow tinge as a result of increased serum bilirubin levels. Bright yellow jaundice is seen in hepatitis when the level of serum bilirubin exceeds a critical level. Jaundice with a slightly greenish tinge is characteristic of obstructive jaundice, such as that resulting from obstruction of the hepatic or common bile ducts. In hypertension the face is often flushed. In polycythemia the face typically exhibits a bluish-red coloration. The tissue oxygen lack resulting from cardiac failure or chronic lung disease may cause cyanosis, which is most noticeable in the tip of the nose, the cheeks, and the lips. In carbon monoxide poisoning the tissues are typically bright pink in color. Many tuberculous patients exhibit flushing over the malar eminence. Facial skin may show increased pigmentation in hyperthyroidism and Addison's disease. Brownish discoloration of the forehead, cheeks, and nose often occurs in pregnancy and may persist following delivery. A "butterfly rash" in the form of a reddish discoloration over the bridge of the nose and both cheeks is sometimes seen in lupus erythematosus.

Circumscribed red or brown discolorations, hemangiomas or "birthmarks," may occur on the face. Because of their cosmetic significance, these discolorations may have social or emotional effects upon the patient, but they are usually medically insignificant.

The texture of the facial skin may have diagnostic significance. In myxedema the skin is coarse, dry, and inelastic, may appear edematous, but does not pit on pressure. In hyperthyroidism the skin is thin and velvety smooth. In chronic eczema the skin is usually thickened and scaling. In acne vulgaris the skin may be thickened and scarred following healing of pustules. In aged persons the skin is thin and fragile, and subcutaneous blood vessels are readily visible.

The state of hydration of the facial tissues should be evaluated. The patient who is dehydrated owing to excessive vomiting or prolonged diarrhea will develop dry, wrinkled skin, sunken cheeks, and sunken eyeballs. The face of the patient in chronic renal failure with fluid retention is pale and puffy. In early renal failure facial edema is most marked in the soft periorbital tissues. As failure persists or progresses, facial edema becomes generalized and is usually bilateral unless the patient habitually lies on one side, in which case the dependent tissues may become more waterlogged than those on the other side.

Transitory localized swelling of the periorbital tissues, the lip, or the earlobe occurs in angioneurotic edema, an allergic response to certain foods, drugs, and bacterial proteins.

While observing the color and texture of the facial skin the practitioner should note whether superficial blood vessels are visible. The chronic alcoholic patient may develop permanently dilated small blood vessels over the nose, cheeks, and chin. The pregnant patient and the cirrhotic patient may have spider nevi or dilated, pulsatile arterioles, as a result of increased estrogen levels.

While observing facial skin color and texture the nurse should also note the presence of excessive sweating or the absence of sweating. Increased perspiration may occur in acute anxiety, in severe pain, in acute septicemia, in the crisis stage of pneumonia, in pregnancy, and in hyperthyroidism. Occasionally, as a result of interruption of impulses through portions of the sympathetic nervous system, there may be localized inhibition of sweating.

Adequate light is required to evaluate the patient's skin color accurately. Full daylight, particularly from a north window, is the best light source; but, when this is not available, properly filtered light from a high intensity bulb should be used. In appraising subtle changes in skin color the nurse may need to tilt the patient's head this way and that to focus available light on various facial planes. While thus manipulating the patient's head the nurse can investigate the mobility of the head. Normally it should be possible to flex the patient's head forward until his chin rests upon his sternum, and to rotate his head in a 90 degree turn to both the right and the left. Limitation of head flexion may indicate cervical arthritis. Limitation of head rotation may result from cervical muscle contracture or cervical arthritis.

Occasionally the nurse will observe abnormal head movements. A tic or spasmodic contraction of certain muscles of the face or neck which gives rise to facial grimaces is a nervous habit that typically increases in frequency or force when the patient is under tension. In the patient with cerebral palsy, involuntary muscle spasms may cause repeated grimacing and slow continuous, purposeless rolling of the head. In aged patients, severe cerebral arteriosclerosis may so injure the basal ganglia as to produce muscular tremor of the lips and tongue. Tremor of the lips and tongue may occur in chronic alcoholism and thyrotoxicosis.

The amount, character, and distribution of facial hair may provide clues to the patient's diagnosis. In the male with advanced cirrhosis the beard may be scant or absent as a result of the liver's inability to detoxify estrogens. There may be increased growth of facial hair in females with Cushing's syndrome. During pregnancy there is often an increase in the amount of fine hair over both the face and body. Thinning and loss of hair in the outer half of the eyebrows may be seen in myxedema.

When examining the face the nurse may encounter lesions of different types. Lipomas or fatty tumors may occur in subcutaneous tissues of the face as well as in other body areas. They are soft, discrete, and freely movable under the skin and over deeper structures. Basal cell and squamous cell carcinomas typically develop on the nose, lips, cheek, forehead, or temple. These lesions may be ulcerated or raised above the surface of surrounding tissue.

Cheilosis or fissures at the angle of the mouth may develop in riboflavin or niacin deficiency. Herpes simplex, or fever blisters, often appear on the lips or on the nostril during acute febrile diseases. Chancres, the painless, indurated ulcers of primary syphilis, may develop on the lip. In acute and subacute bacterial endocarditis, petechiae may appear on the mucosa of the lips as a result of embolic obstruction of small blood vessels.

Facial tissues are frequently the site of infectious processes. Folliculitis, a simple infection of hair follicles resulting in the formation of numerous small erythematous nodules, is especially likely to occur in the bearded areas. Furunculosis, an extensive follicular or sebaceous gland infection in which there is destruction of subcutaneous tissue, is most common in diabetics and in persons weakened by wasting disease.

Warts and moles frequently occur on the skin of the face. They should be examined for signs of chronic irritation, since such lesions can undergo malignant degeneration.

EXAMINATION OF THE EYE

When examining the eye the nurse should first appraise its position within the bony orbit. Typically, in Caucasians the eyeball does not protrude forward from the socket as far as the supraorbital ridge of the frontal bone, although in Negroes such a finding would not be abnormal. Unusual protuberance of the eyeballs, or exophthalmos, may occur in hyperthyroidism. Enophthalmos, the condition in which the eye is sunken into the skull, may result from loss of retrobulbar fat in chronic wasting disease.

Normally when the eyelids are closed they should meet completely, when the lids are opened the pupil and most of the iris should be uncovered, and when the lids are opened wide a small strip of sclera should be visible between iris and lid margin. Drooping of the upper lid, or ptosis, may result from injury to the oculomotor nerve or dysfunction of cervical sympathetic nerves. Ptosis of both lids may be seen in myasthenia gravis. Inability to close the lids completely may result from injury to the facial nerve or from severe exophthalmos.

In the hyperthyroid patient with exophthalmos the upper lid appears to be retracted in that the lid slit is wider than usual. Further, even when the eye is not intentionally opened wide, a small strip of sclera is visible between the iris and lid. When the exophthalmic patient is directed to look downward, the lid moves down tardily and in brief jerks.

Visual acuity can best be tested by using a Snellen Chart (Fig. 2). For this test the patient should be seated in a chair placed 20 feet in front of the chart. The nurse should then have the patient cover one eye at a time and direct him to read the letters aloud from the top of the chart down. Record the last row in which the patient was able to accurately interpret the majority of the letters. The numeral corresponding to this line on the chart is used as the lower figure in designating the patient's visual acuity. The upper figure is the distance the patient was seated from the chart (usually 20, unless the patient is unable to see even the top letter at a distance of 20 feet, in which case his chair may be moved closer to the chart and the upper figure lowered accordingly). Record the visual acuity measurement for each eye, as: O.D. (right eye) 20/20;

THE PHYSICAL EXAMINATION 43

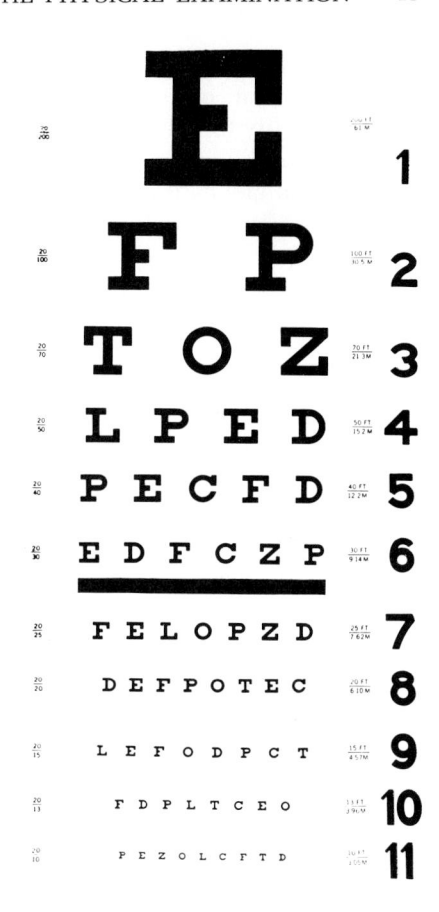

Figure 2. Snellen Chart. (Courtesy American Optical Company.)

O.S. (left eye) 20/30. Also record whether or not corrective glasses were worn during the examination.

Evaluation of eyeball movements will yield information about the third, fourth, and sixth cranial nerves. Strabismus, or deviation of one eye so that its visual axis no longer parallels that of the other eye, may be due to neurologic disease or errors in refraction. To test for strabismus the nurse, holding a flashlight, should stand directly in front of the patient and instruct him to look directly at the light. If the patient is able to fixate both eyes on the light, the nurse will observe that the reflections of the flashlight beam overlie the centers of the pupils of both eyes. If only one eye is able to fixate, the light reflection will overlie the pupil of the fixating eye, but will be located over some portion of the deviated eye other than the pupil.

Nystagmus, an involuntary rhythmic back-and-forth movement of the eye in a lateral or vertical direction, may occur in normal persons with severe myopia or ocular fatigue or may be due to such neurological diseases as multiple sclerosis or encephalitis.

To test the range of ocular motion the nurse should stand in front of the patient, immobilize his head by holding his chin with her left hand, and direct him to focus on her right index finger as she holds it at the east, west, northeast, southwest, northwest and southeast compass points at the periphery of his vision. Inability to move the eye through full range of motion may be due to weakness of extraocular muscles or to lesions of either the oculomotor, trochlear, or abducens nerve.

The ability to converge, or turn the eyes inward to focus on a near object, can be tested by asking the patient to follow with his eyes the nurse's index finger as she moves it from a point 18 inches in front of his face to the bridge of his nose. Patients with exophthalmia will be unable to converge.

The eyelids may be edematous in nephritis and nephrosis. A stye or hordeolum is a suppurative inflammation of a sebaceous gland on the lid margin. In diabetes mellitus and in hypercholesterolemia, flat or slightly raised xanthelasmic plaques may develop on the inner aspect of the upper eyelid as a result of disordered fat metabolism.

Ectropion, or eversion of the lid, and entropion, or inversion of the lid, are especially likely to occur in aged persons. Conjunctival irritation and infection are likely to occur in either condition. Inflammation of the eyelids from weeping, eyestrain, irritants, or infection will be characterized by redness, soreness, and crusting of the lid margins.

Excessive tearing may result from emotional stress or as a reflex response to severe pain. Unusual dryness of the conjunctiva may be due to lack of vitamin A or to chronic conjunctivitis.

The bulbar conjunctiva can be examined by holding the eyelids apart with the fingers while the patient directs his gaze up, down, to the left, and to the right. To examine the palpebral conjunctiva of the lower lid the nurse should pull down the skin of the lower lid while the patient gazes upward. The palpebral conjunctiva of the upper lid can be examined by directing the patient to look down, grasping the lashes of the upper lid and pulling the lid downward and forward, exerting pressure with an applicator one centimeter above the lid margin, then everting the lid over the applicator. Normally, a few small blood vessels will be visible in the conjunctiva. If the conjunctiva is inflamed, these vessels will be dilated and engorged and the entire conjunctiva may appear reddened. In anemia and in edema of the eyelids, the normally pink palpebral conjunctiva may appear unusually pale. In bacterial endocarditis conjunctival petechiae may be found. Physical injury or severe coughing may cause conjunctival hemorrhage, with production of an irregular, bright red patch of varying size, which will be resorbed only after several days. The sclera, normally bluish white in color, may become slightly lemon yellow in pernicious anemia, bright yellow in hepatitis, and greenish yellow in obstructive jaundice in the same way that the facial skin may be discolored by bile pigments in these diseases.

The normal cornea is clear and smooth. A scratch or ulceration of the cornea due to trauma from a foreign body can be seen by examination with a hand lens. Scarring following healing of a corneal ulcer may be revealed as a focal irregular opacity in the otherwise clear cornea. Arcus senilis, a gray ring lying just within the outer border of the cornea, represents a normal degenerative change when seen in an aged patient. In a younger person it may indicate disordered lipid metabolism.

The color of the iris in both eyes should be noted. Although rarely the color of the two may differ in the normal person, pigmentation changes in one eye may result from glaucoma or such inflammatory diseases as syphilis, gonorrhea, tuberculosis, or rheumatic fever. Normally, there should be no break in the continuity of the iris except for the centrally located pupil. Irregularity of the iris may be the result of surgical treatment for glaucoma or inflammatory change.

Normally the pupils are round, regular in outline, equal in size if equally illuminated, and will constrict if additional light is directed toward them. Marked irregularity of the pupil may result from iritis and consequent adhesions of the iris to the anterior lens surface. Inequality in the size of the pupils may be a congenital abnormality or may be due to head injury, cerebrovascular accident, or damage to cervical sympathetic or cranial nerves.

Myopic persons tend to have larger pupils than those with normal vision, and patients with hyperopia tend to have smaller pupils than those with normal vision. Dilated pupils may be noted in persons who are anxious and in patients who are taking such parasympathetic depressants as atropine. Pupillary dilation is also seen in coma, in the second and fourth stages of anesthesia, and in paralysis of the oculomotor nerve. Abnormally constricted pupils may be seen in morphine addicts and in glaucoma patients who are being treated with parasympathetic stimulants.

Normally the pupil should respond quickly to light changes, constricting when exposed to light, dilating when surroundings are darkened. Further, when light is directed from the side onto only one eye, not only that pupil but also the one of the opposite eye should constrict, though to a slightly less degree (Fig. 3). Normally, too, the pupil should constrict when the gaze is fixed on a near object, and should dilate when fixed on a far object. Argyll Robertson pupil, a constricted pupil which does not react to light, is typically seen in tabes dorsalis, a neurological manifestation of tertiary syphilis. To test

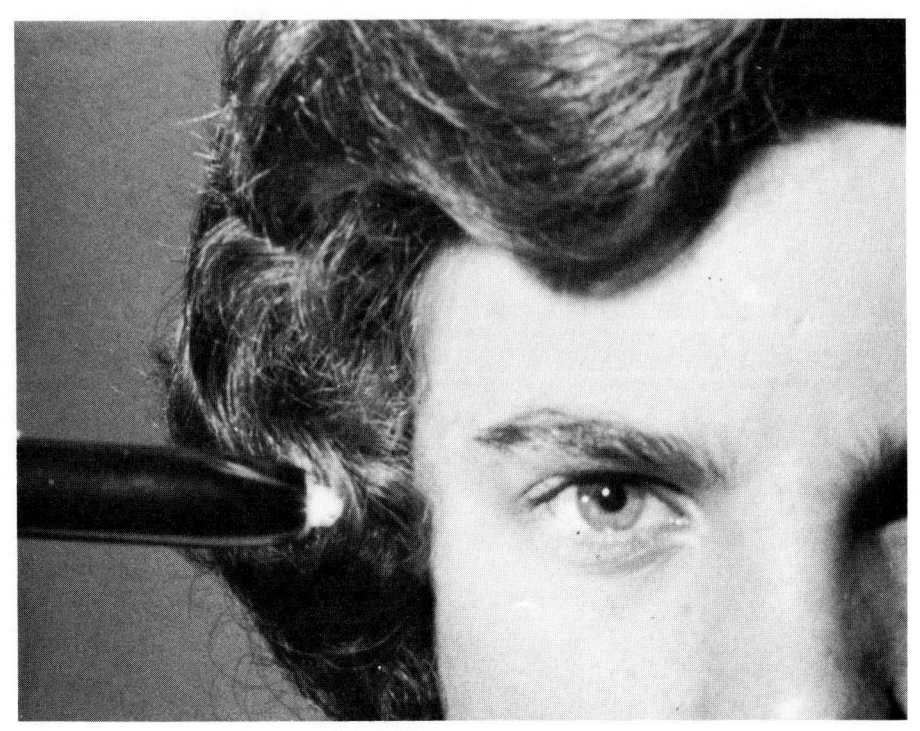

Figure 3. Testing for pupillary light reflex.

the pupillary light reflex the nurse should stand or sit facing the patient, instruct the patient to direct his gaze straight ahead to a distant point, and then direct a light from the side onto first one eye and then the other. Constriction of the pupil being illuminated constitutes a *direct* reaction to light. Constriction of the opposite pupil, which has received no increase in light, is a *consensual* pupillary reaction. To test the pupillary response to accommodation, note the change in pupillary size when the patient is directed to read written material held, first, at some distance from his face and, then, just in front of his nose.

When examining the pupillary opening the practitioner will at the same time be observing the lens of the eye, which is normally transparent. Cataract, or opacity of the lens, is apt to develop in patients with diabetes or direct trauma to the eye.

Ophthalmoscopic Examination of the Eye

The nurse should inform the patient that the room needs to be darkened during the ophthalmoscopic examination and then should decrease the light in the room by turning off the overhead lights, closing blinds, or pulling shades. In examining the patient's right eye the nurse should stand on the patient's right side, hold the ophthalmoscope in her right hand, and look through the scope with her right eye. Likewise, in examining the patient's left eye, the nurse should stand on the patient's left side, hold the ophthalmo-

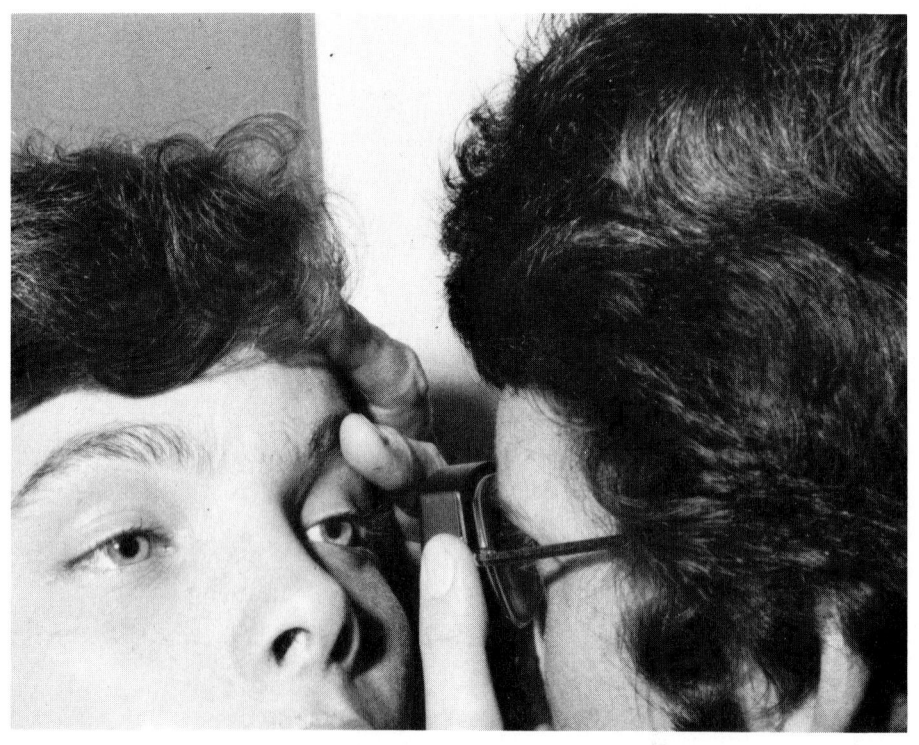

Figure 4. Ophthalmoscopic examination.

scope in her left hand, and look through the instrument with her left eye. To inspect the patient's right eye the nurse should turn on the ophthalmoscope light, set the 0 lens in place, and direct the patient to fix his gaze on some object over the nurse's shoulder and across the room. The nurse should then use her left hand to steady the patient's head and lift his right upper eyelid. Holding the ophthalmoscope directly in front of her own eye and standing slightly to the patient's right side, the nurse should direct the light beam in a slight medial direction through the patient's pupil. The nurse should then slowly move her head closer to the patient's eye. At a distance of about one foot, the pupil will reflect a bright red glow or "red reflex" if the cornea, aqueous, lens, and vitreous are all clear. An opacity in any of these media will create the appearance of black defects in the red reflex. After checking for the red reflex the nurse should move her head still closer to the patient until, finally, the nurse's forehead rests upon the dorsum of her own left hand as it rests on the patient's forehead. At this point, with the 0 lens still in place, if both the nurse and the patient have normal vision, the patient's fundus should be visible. If the fundic structures are blurred the practitioner should substitute positive or negative lenses until the retinal vessels can be seen in sharp outline. In order to visualize the fundus properly the nurse should resist accommodating by imagining that she is focusing on a distant point rather than on a structure which is located only a few inches in front of her own eye.

Funduscopic examination should begin with inspection of the optic disc or nerve head and end with inspection of the macula. The disc, which is normally round or vertically oval and of a paler pink than the surrounding retinal tissue, is located slightly to the nasal side of the center of the retina. By directing the ophthalmoscope light beam into the eye from a point 15 degrees lateral to the patient's line of vision, the nurse can focus on the optic disc. If the disc is not immediately visible, follow the course of a retinal vessel to locate it. Normally the disc is flat or slightly depressed centrally (physiological cupping) and has sharp edges (Fig. 5). Occasionally, black pigment depos-

Figure 5. The normal fundus with physiologic cupping of the disc. (From Adler, F. H.: *Gifford's Textbook of Ophthalmology*. 4th ed. Philadelphia, W. B. Saunders Co., 1947.)

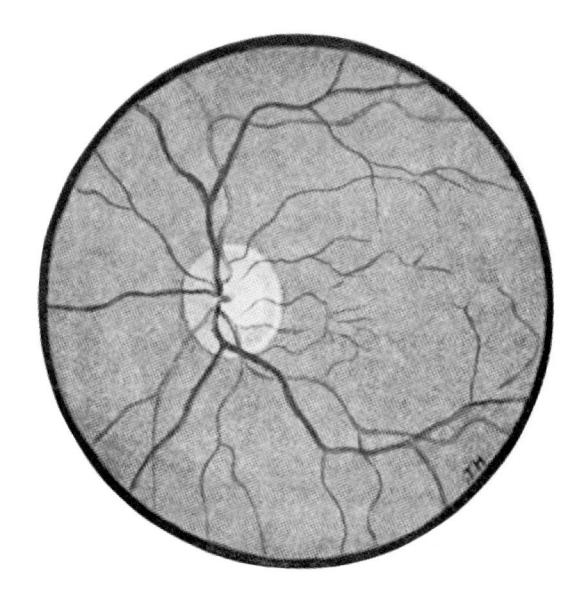

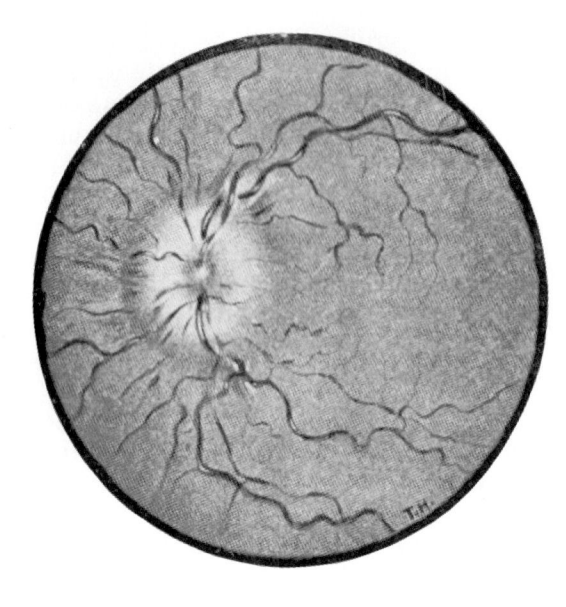

Figure 6. Early stage of choked disc, showing blurring of the nasal half, dilated veins and a few small hemorrhages just off the disc. (From Adler, F. H.: *Textbook of Ophthalmology.* 7th ed. Philadelphia, W. B. Saunders Co., 1962.)

its or a margin of white nerve sheath may wholly or partly encircle the disc, but these findings are without medical significance.

Edema of the optic nerve head, or papilledema, indicates an increase in intracranial pressure and is characterized by dilation of the small blood vessels supplying the disc, elevation of the disc, and blurring of the disc margin (Fig. 6).

In glaucoma, increased intraocular pressure causes cupping or deep excavation of the optic disc (Fig. 7). Glaucomatous cupping of the disc differs from physiological cupping in that, in the former, the entire disc is depressed and there is no rim of normal disc tissue at the periphery of the nerve head. With death of the optic nerve, the tiny blood vessels that normally supply the

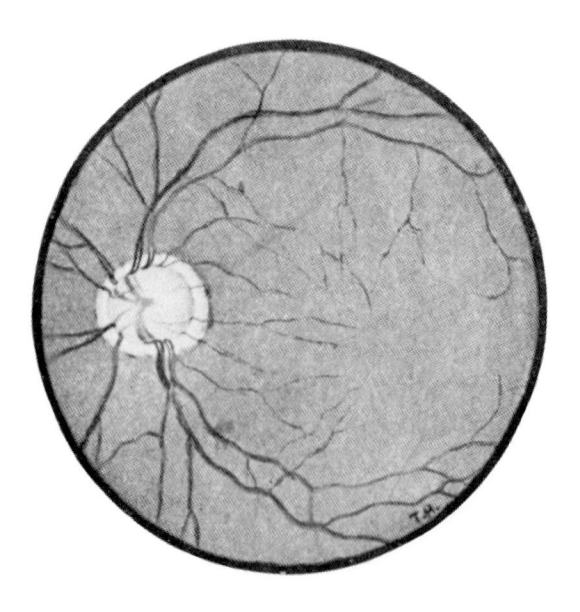

Figure 7. Cupping of the disc in chronic glaucoma. (From Adler, F. H.: *Gifford's Textbook of Ophthalmology.* 4th ed. Philadelphia, W. B. Saunders Co., 1947.)

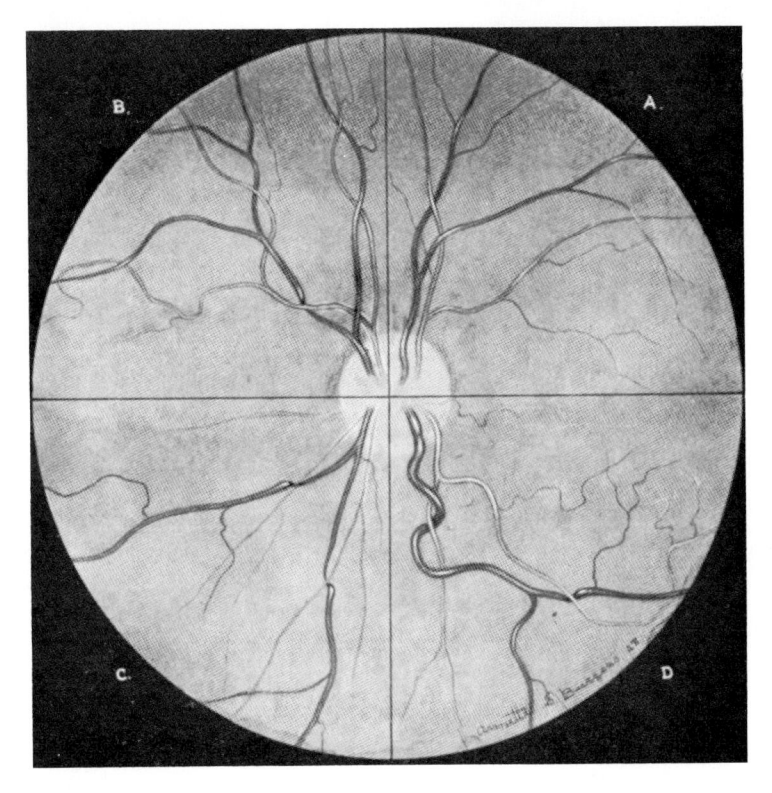

Figure 8. Retinal arteriosclerosis. *A*, Normal fundus; *B*, senile arteriosclerosis without hypertension; *C*, retinal arteriosclerosis with hypertension; *D*, retinal arteriosclerosis, showing copper-wire arteries. (After Friedenwald, courtesy of the Wilmer Institute.)

disc disappear, giving the disc a dead white rather than the normal creamy pink color.

Veins and arteries enter and leave the disc in four sets—an artery and vein pair radiating from the disc in each of the upper nasal, lower nasal, lower temporal, and upper temporal directions. Each of these vessel pairs should be inspected from the disc to the periphery. The arteries are narrower and of a brighter red color than the veins, and demonstrate a narrow white stripe of reflected light along their course. Normally, both arteries and veins spread out to the retinal periphery in softly curving lines without sudden sharp changes in direction. Generally, arteries and veins interweave somewhat in their course to the periphery but, under normal circumstances, veins are not indented by overcrossing arteries. The appearance of venous pinching or nicking at such crossings is suggestive of arteriolar sclerosis, as is an increase in intensity of the arteriolar light reflex (copper-wire or silver-wire appearance).

In hypertension there are, characteristically, narrowing of retinal arterioles, points of local vascular constriction, increased light reflex, and, if vessels are ruptured, flame-shaped hemorrhages.

In diabetes mellitus, retinopathy may include vascular changes characteristic of arteriolar sclerosis as well as microaneurysms, small round hemorrhages, and yellow and waxy exudates. It is customary in describing retinal hemorrhages and exudates to indicate the location, size, and appearance of the abnormality. For instance, the practitioner might record the finding of an

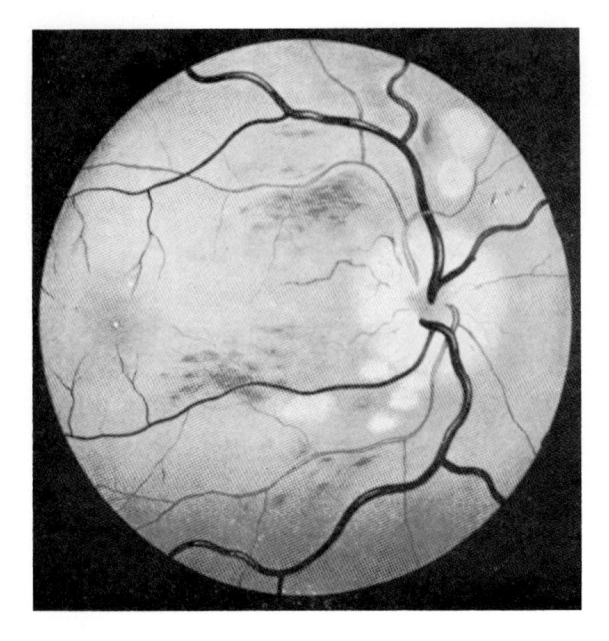

Figure 9. Grade IV hypertensive changes, with no sclerosis. In addition to extreme narrowing of the arteries, note flame-shaped hemorrhages, cotton-wool patches and edema of disc. (Courtesy of H. G. Scheie, M.D., in Adler, F. H.: *Textbook of Ophthalmology.* 7th ed. Philadelphia, W. B. Saunders Co., 1962.)

irregular hemorrhage of approximately one disc diameter (D.D.) in size, at the 10 o'clock position.

After all four vessel pairs have been inspected, the nurse should examine the retina between the vessels either by asking the patient to focus in the six cardinal directions or by moving her head and the ophthalmoscope to focus on all four quadrants of the fundus while the patient maintains his fixed forward gaze.

Finally, the macula and its central depression, the fovea centralis, should

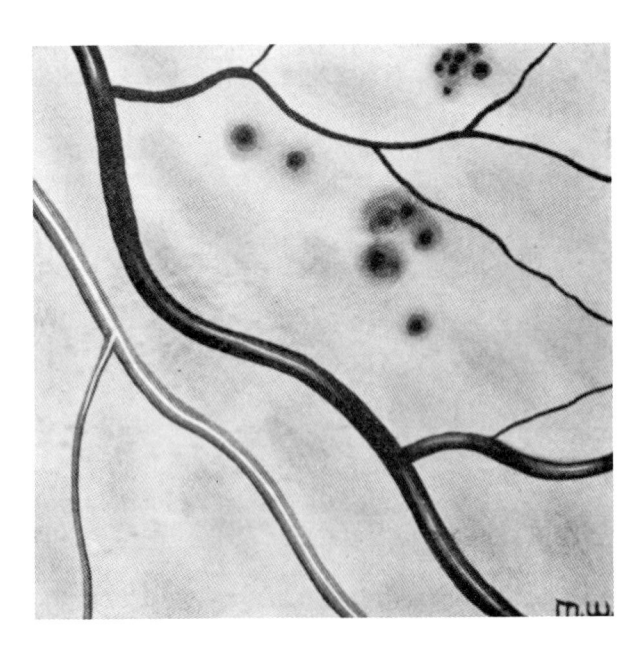

Figure 10. Round hemorrhages in deep layers of the retina. (From Adler, F. H.: *Textbook of Ophthalmology.* 7th ed. Philadelphia, W. B. Saunders Co., 1962.)

be examined. The macula is an avascular area, slightly darker in color than the surrounding retina, which is located two disc diameters from the disc toward the temporal side. If difficulty is encountered in locating the macula, the nurse may direct the patient to look directly at the ophthalmoscope light. When he does so, the macula will be in the nurse's direct line of vision.

EXAMINATION OF THE EAR

With the otoscope held in one hand, the nurse should pull the patient's auricle slightly upward, backward, and outward with the other in order to open the meatus, and then should insert the otoscope speculum into the auditory canal in a slightly anterior direction. Debris or cerumen may have to be removed with a cotton-tipped applicator in order that the tympanum or eardrum can be visualized. Redness and excoriation of the walls of the external auditory canal may result from infection, which is commonly caused by yeasts or fungi. If the canal is not obstructed by debris the drum can easily be visualized when the patient's head is bent toward the opposite shoulder. The normal eardrum is shiny and pearly gray in color and the membrane is so situated that the upper posterior portion of the drum is closer to the examiner than is the lower anterior portion. The eardrum may be pink when inflamed and white if there is purulent material in the middle ear. Normally, the drum is slightly concave and so thin that the short process, the handle, and the tip of the malleus, one of the bones of the middle ear, are visible through the membrane. A triangular light reflex in the shape of an upright cone reflects downward and antericrly from the tip of the malleus when the drum is in normal position and in good condition. These landmarks may be obscured if pus accumulates in the middle ear in otitis media and causes the drum to bulge outward. If middle ear infection is suspected the mastoid process should be palpated for tenderness.

Hearing loss may be of three types: conductive, perceptive, and mixed. Conductive losses may result from obstruction of the external auditory canal, perforation of the eardrum, loss of mobility of ossicles of the middle ear, or fluid accumulations in the middle ear. Perceptive losses result from disorders of the inner ear, the auditory nerve, or the brain. Mixed losses result from a combination of middle ear and neurological disorders.

A rough test should be made of the patient's hearing ability in each ear by masking his opposite ear (rotate one finger in the auditory meatus) while whispering a question to which the patient must indicate understanding by a verbal answer. If the room is quiet the patient with normal hearing will be able to correctly interpret a quiet whisper at a distance of two feet from his ear. If a hearing defect exists the nurse can differentiate conduction from neural loss with the aid of the tuning fork (Fig. 11). To accomplish the Rinne's test the tuning fork is set in motion and placed on the mastoid process (Figure 12). When the patient indicates that he can no longer hear the sounds (conducted through bone), the tuning fork is held, as shown in Figure 13, a few inches in front of the ear. The patient is then asked to indicate whether or not the tuning fork vibrations (conducted through air) can still be heard. The patient with conduction deafness will hear more clearly when the tuning fork vibrations are transmitted through bone than through air. The patient with

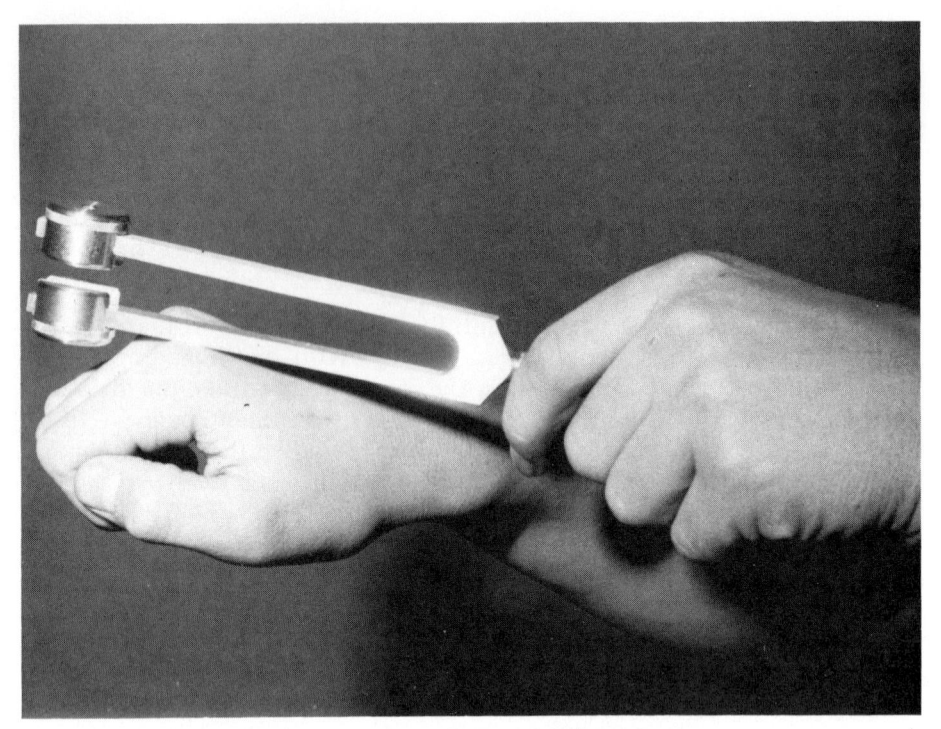

Figure 11. Setting the tuning fork into motion.

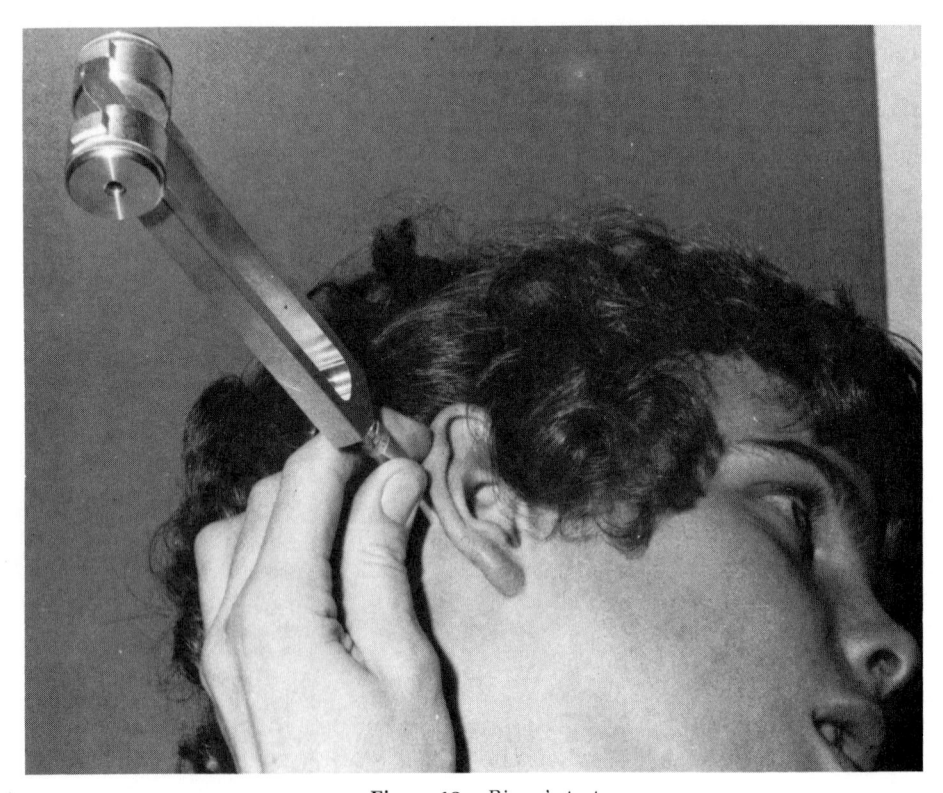

Figure 12. Rinne's test.

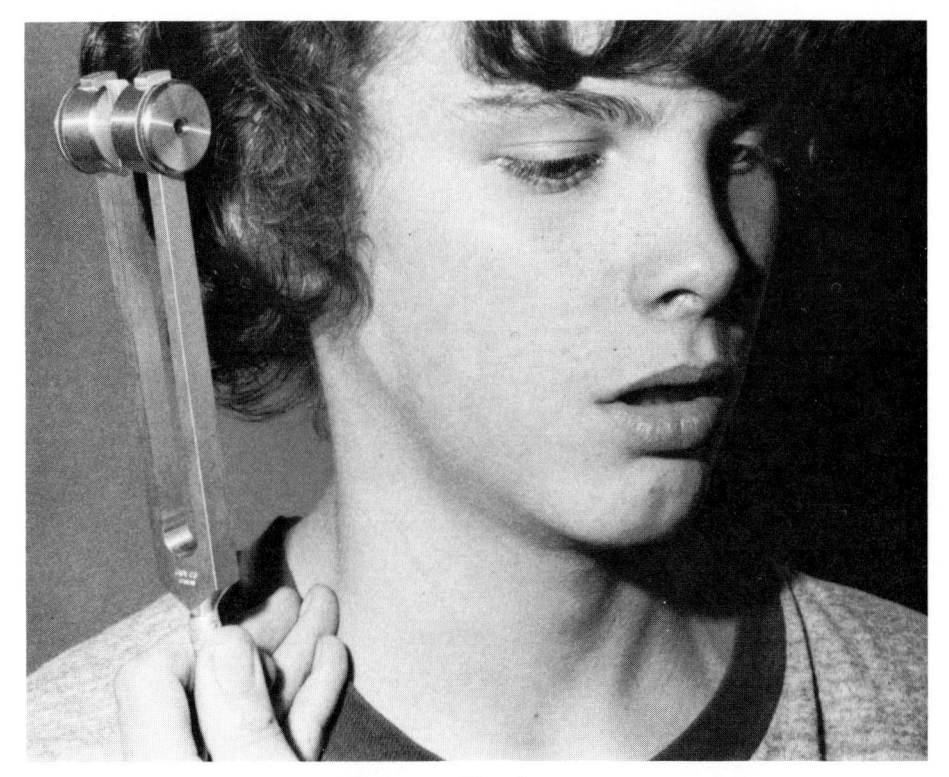

Figure 13. Rinne's test.

neural deafness will not hear the sound well through either means. To conduct the Weber test the tuning fork is set into motion and placed against the midline of the upper forehead (Fig. 14). If the patient has normal hearing the sound will be heard equally in both ears. The sound will be loudest in the deaf ear in conduction deafness, loudest in the normal ear in neural deafness.

Following the examination of the ears, the speculum should be set aside for later cleansing, the instrument head should be changed, and the examination of the nose should be done using a nasal speculum.

EXAMINATION OF THE NOSE

The external nose should be examined for deformity or asymmetry. Extreme flattening or lateral deviation of the nose may be the effect of an old fracture of the nasal cartilage. Saddle nose, or marked depression of the nasal bridge, is suggestive of congenital syphilis. A thin nose with narrowed nasal passages is characteristically seen in the patient with chronically enlarged adenoids who habitually breathes through his mouth.

In patients with acute allergic or infectious rhinitis, the tip of the nose and rims of the nostrils may be reddened from frequent nose-blowing. In chronic alcoholics and in persons suffering constant exposure to the elements, the small blood vessels of the nose and cheeks often become permanently dilated and engorged. In chronic acne rosacea, there may be overgrowth of

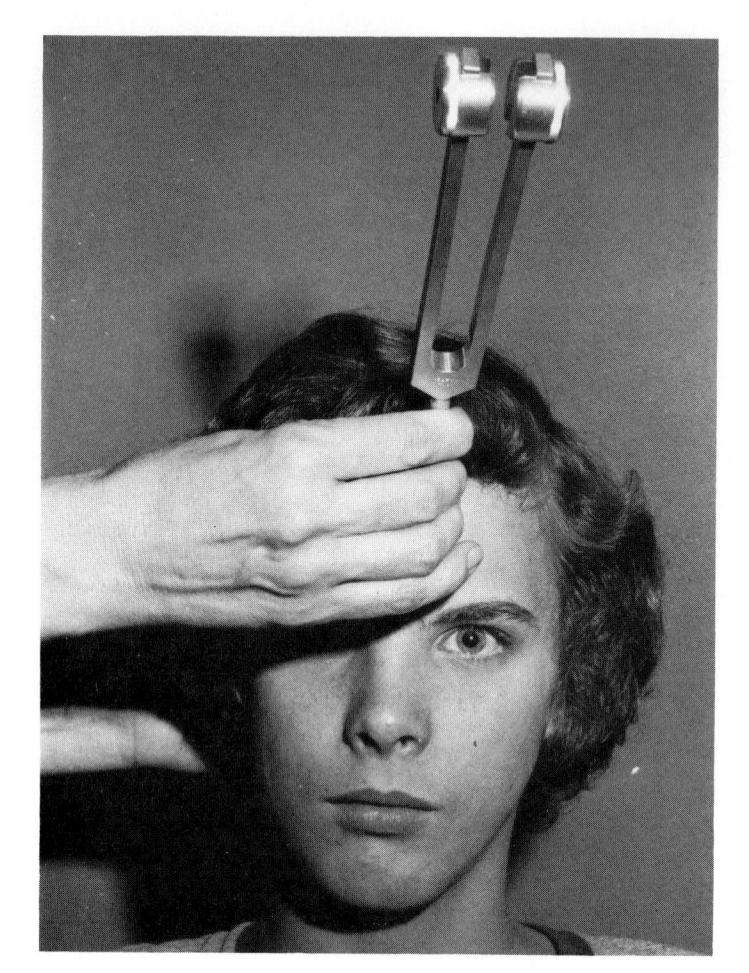

Figure 14. Weber's test.

skin, hypertrophy of sebaceous glands, and dilation of pores, giving rise to a bulbous and discolored nose.

The practitioner should use a nasal speculum and a small flashlight to examine the nasal passages. The patient's head should be tilted slightly backward and the tip of the nose pushed gently upward to examine the nasal vestibule. Infection of hair follicles in this area may give rise to small furuncles. The septum should be inspected for position and perforations. While it is common for the septum to incline slightly toward one side or the other, a marked septal deviation may be the result of a former nasal fracture. If a marked deviation is seen, the patient should be instructed to sniff while first one and then the other of his nostrils is blocked, in order to determine whether his septal deviation is of such magnitude as to obstruct air passage through either nostril. Perforation of the bony septum, which may be best visualized by shining a flashlight beam into one nostril and then observing a reflected spot of bright light in the opposite nostril, is frequently due to syphilis.

The mucous membrane lining the nasal passages is normally pink in color. The mucosa will be reddened and edematous in viral rhinitis and pale and boggy in allergic rhinitis. A copious thin, watery discharge may be evident in allergic rhinitis or in the early stages of the common cold. In later stages of the common cold or in chronic sinus infection, nasal discharge tends to be less copious, thicker, and may be purulent in character and offensive in odor.

Kiesselbach's area on the anterior portion of the nasal septum just a short distance above the floor of the nose, in which there is a large network of capillaries, should be examined carefully, as it is the area from which epistaxis often occurs in hypertension, uremia, and nasal trauma. Patients with chronic allergic rhinitis may develop nasal polyps, which appear as pale, globular, gelatinous masses attached to the mucosa overlying the turbinates, the lower and middle of which bones may be seen high on the lateral wall of the nasal passages.

The paranasal sinuses frequently are the site of acute or chronic inflammation. Sinus infection may produce redness and swelling of the overlying tissues; that is, over the eyebrow in frontal sinusitis, or over the malar eminence in maxillary sinusitis. Sometimes inflammation of sinus tissues will produce no outward change in the patient's appearance, but pressure over the infected cavity will produce pain. To detect involvement of the frontal sinus, the nurse should exert pressure on the bony ridge just below and behind the eyebrow (Fig. 15). To test the condition of the maxillary sinus, firm pressure should be exerted over the malar eminence. To investigate the

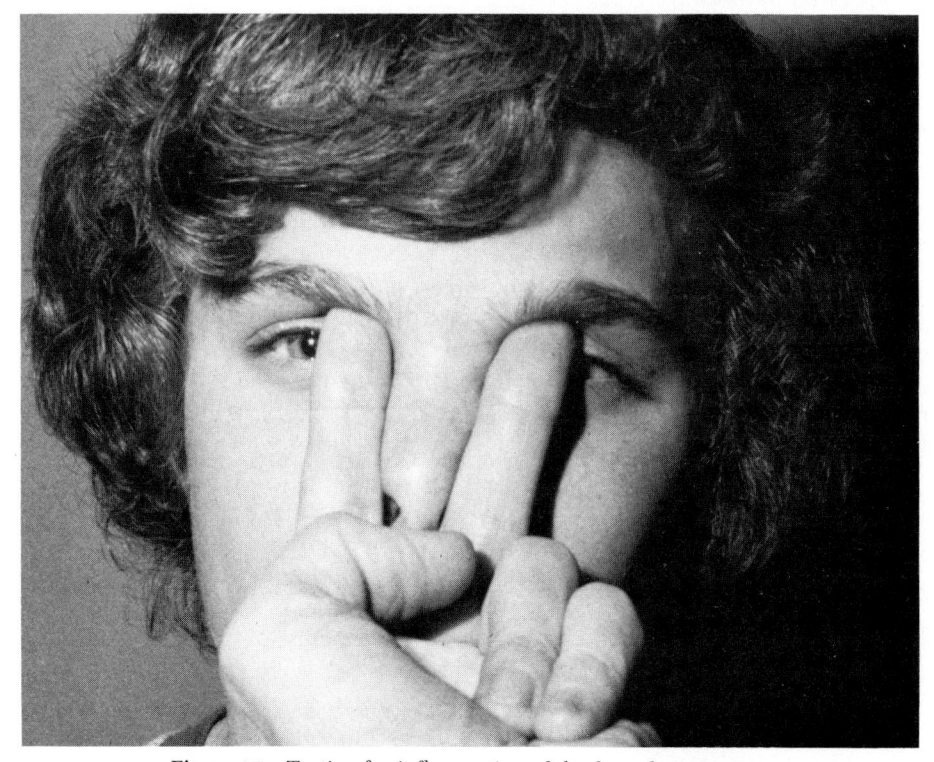

Figure 15. Testing for inflammation of the frontal sinuses.

ethmoid sinus, pressure should be placed on the side of the nasal bone. Since pressure exerted on even healthy bone will usually produce some discomfort, it will be helpful to apply the same amount of pressure bilaterally in order to determine whether greater discomfort is perceived over one sinus than another, a finding which is suggestive of sinusitis.

EXAMINATION OF THE MOUTH

When examining the mouth, a tongue depressor should be used to retract the lips and cheeks in order to facilitate proper visualization of all structures.

If the patient has dentures or dental bridges, the nurse should check the "fit" of these prostheses and then have the patient remove them before further examination is undertaken. The number, location, color, and condition of the patient's own teeth should be noted. Normally, there are 32 teeth in the adult mouth. If teeth are missing, the nurse should question the reason for their removal. Although tooth color varies somewhat from one person to another, severe tooth discoloration may suggest inadequate oral hygiene. Excessive tea drinking and cigarette smoking will discolor tooth enamel, but stains of this type are removed by the mechanical cleansing techniques included by most dentists as part of the routine annual dental checkup. Persons who have lived in an area where the water has high fluorine content are apt to develop pitting and brown discoloration of the teeth. Following death of a tooth, or removal of its nerve supply, a tooth tends to darken. Carious areas are often black in color. Short, peg-shaped teeth that are notched on the bite surface result from congenital syphilis.

Malposition of teeth is a common finding. The third molars may erupt at an angle because there is insufficient room in the dental arch for proper placement. If a malpositioned tooth exerts pressure against adjacent teeth it may cause pain. If a malpositioned tooth overrides another, it may create a pocket in which food debris tends to collect and putrefy. Without treatment dental caries or decay and cavitation will lead to breakage of teeth, with formation of sharp fragments which can be chronically irritating to the tongue and buccal mucosa. Extractions necessitated by tooth decay leave gaps in the line of teeth into which adjacent teeth may wander; this movement may result in misalignment of teeth on the opposing ridge by upsetting bite balance.

With increasing age, the gums tend to gradually recede from the teeth, exposing an increasing amount of tooth root. If oral hygiene is poor, tartar, a composite of calcium salts, is deposited at the base of the teeth, just below the gum line, further irritating the gingival tissue and creating pockets in which food particles lodge and bacteria multiply.

Eventually a full blown infection develops, in which frank pus can be expressed from the juncture of gum and tooth. Finally, the increasingly exposed tooth weakens in the socket, becomes abscessed, and must be removed. An abscessed tooth is usually painful when struck, as a result of extension of the inflammatory process to underlying jawbone and periosteum.

Vitamin C deficiency causes the gum tissue to become reddened, friable, and hemorrhagic. In the epileptic prolonged use of diphenylhydantoin often causes marked generalized gingival hypertrophy. In chronic lead poisoning a blue-black line may be found along the margin of the gums. In Addison's disease the gums may evidence the same melanotic discoloration as occurs in the skin. In secondary syphilis grayish white slightly elevated mucous patches may occur on the gingival or buccal mucosa. Removal of the thin gray exudate or membrane with a tongue blade reveals a painless superficial erosion that teems with spirochetes.

The buccal mucosa may, like the lips, show pallor in anemia, yellow discoloration in jaundice, a dusky blue cast in chronic circulatory disorders, and melanotic discoloration in Addison's disease. In the early stages of measles small blue-white spots surrounded by a red areola (Koplik's spots) may be found in the buccal mucosa in the posterior portion of the mouth. Leukoplakia, a premalignant lesion, may appear as a gray-white, indurated plaque on the buccal surface overlying a jagged tooth fragment. In subacute bacterial endocarditis, petechiae may be seen on the buccal mucosa. In thrombocytopenia, purpuric spots may be seen throughout the oral mucosa.

When examining the mouth, the openings of the salivary ducts should be identified. The opening of Stensen's duct, which drains the parotid gland, lies opposite the upper second molar teeth. The opening of Wharton's duct, which drains the mandibular gland, lies in the floor of the mouth to the side of the frenum linguae. Inflammation of a salivary gland may cause reddening of the duct orifice. Obstruction of a salivary duct will be followed by swelling of the gland and distortion of normal structure.

The tongue should be examined for size, color, surface characteristics, and movement. An unusually large tongue is often seen in acromegaly, cretinism, and mongolism. There may be localized swelling of the tongue due to infection or tumor formation. An unusually small tongue is seen in malnutrition and paralysis of the hypoglossal nerve.

There may be marked pallor of the tongue in severe anemia, and marked reddening in either riboflavin or niacin deficiency. The tongue may be covered with a white coating if the patient has had diminished food intake or has poor oral hygiene. In thrush, infection by Candida albicans produces numerous small white patches on the upper surface of the tongue. Infection by Aspergillus niger, which may occur as a consequence of prolonged use of broad spectrum antibiotics, will produce a black hairy-looking tongue, owing to the presence of a mass of mycelia.

The papillae normally visible on the upper surface and sides of the tongue may be diminished or absent in pernicious anemia, riboflavin deficiency, and niacin deficiency. Superficial transverse fissures on the upper surface of the tongue may be considered normal. Deep longitudinal fissures, on the other hand, are characteristic of syphilis. In "geographic tongue," a condition of unknown cause, areas of atrophic epithelium alternate with areas of hypertrophic epithelium, creating a maplike appearance. Typically, these areas of atrophy and hypertrophy shift from day to day.

Numerous pathological lesions may appear on the tongue. The syphilitic chancre, a painless, indurated ulcer, may occur on the tongue when the mouth is the portal of entry for the infection. Mucous patches of secondary syphilis may develop on either the superior or inferior surface of the tongue. Leukoplakia, a flat, gray-white premalignant lesion, may occur on the tongue as well as on the lip or the buccal mucosa. The tongue may also be the site of malignant tumor, usually a firm, painful ulcer, occurring at a point of chronic irritation from a snagged tooth or an ill-fitting dental bridge and increasing slowly in size.

Tremor of the tongue may be noted in chronic alcoholism and thyrotoxicosis. Lateral deviation of the tongue on protrusion may be seen in patients with cerebrovascular accident, and paralysis of the hypoglossal nerve. In myasthenia gravis the patient may not be able to protrude the tongue several times in rapid succession, as a result of easy fatigability of muscle.

The anterior or bony palate normally is smooth and covered with transverse mucosal folds. In cleft palate, a developmental abnormality, failure of the palatal arch to close results in direct communication between the mouth and nasal cavity. Perforation of either the hard or the soft palate may result from gummatous destruction of tissue in tertiary syphilis.

If, at any point in the oral examination, it should be necessary to palpate any lesion or tissue, the nurse should apply a rubber glove from which all glove powder has been washed and should maintain the mouth in the open position with a mouth gag unless she is convinced that the patient is alert and controlled enough not to close his jaws on her hand.

As part of the physical examination the nurse should attempt to elicit the gag reflex by stroking the posterior portion of the tongue or the posterior pharynx with an applicator or tongue blade. The normal gag reflex includes elevation of the soft palate, gagging, and grimacing. Absence of the gag reflex may indicate a lesion of either the glossopharyngeal or vagus nerve.

The tonsils, which lie on either side of the rear of the mouth at the opening of the pharynx, become reddened and swollen when infected. In acute tonsillitis purulent exudate may be seen in the crypts scattered over the tonsillar surface, and the soft palate may be noticeably hypermic. If the infectious process extends outside the tonsillar capsule to involve surrounding tissues a peritonsillar abscess develops that may spread to the point that a bulge can be seen in the soft palate on the same side.

A tongue blade and flashlight should be used to examine the oropharynx. Maximum visibility of the part can be achieved by directing the patient to open his mouth without protruding his tongue, then using a tongue blade to apply gentle pressure downward and forward on the anterior two thirds of the tongue.

Bacterial infection of the pharyngeal wall will cause the mucosa to be edematous and hyperemic. A localized swelling of the wall may indicate a retropharyngeal abscess. While normally there is a thin layer of clear mucus covering pharyngeal mucosa, infections of the nose and sinuses may lead to the appearance of copious mucopurulent secretions in the posterior oropharynx.

While examining the mouth and oropharynx the practitioner will have occasion to note the odor of the patient's breath. Offensive breath odor may be due to poor hygiene, pyorrhea alveolaris, purulent tonsillitis, purulent sinusitis, lung abscess, or bronchiectasis. A sweet or flowery breath odor can be detected in uncontrolled diabetes mellitus. An ammoniacal breath odor is often noted in the uremic patient.

EXAMINATION OF THE NECK

Once the practitioner is familiar with the surface landmarks and the underlying anatomy, examination of the neck is relatively easy because the neck is so small that no structure lies far from the body surface.

With the patient seated comfortably, his hands resting in his lap, and his head tilted back slightly, the nurse should first inspect the neck for symmetry, unusual swellings, pulsations, and degree of motion. In evaluating symmetry the nurse should inspect first one side and then the other in the following areas: under the angle of the jaw, under the chin, in the anterior triangle of the neck (anterior and superior to the sternocleidomastoid muscle), in the posterior triangle of the neck (posterior and inferior to the sternocleidomastoid muscle), and in the supraclavicular area.

In parotitis, swelling of the parotid gland may be obvious not only in front of and behind the ear but also in the region of the neck immediately below the ear. In mumps, palpation will reveal that the swollen gland is firm and quite tender to touch. Enlargement of the tail of the parotid gland causes the earlobe to be displaced laterally. The parotid gland may also be swollen because its duct is obstructed by a stone, which may be palpable as a small hard mass in the buccal tissue opposite the upper second molar tooth. An enlarged submandibular salivary gland is felt as a firm, slightly moveable circular mass below the mandible and in front of the ear. Enlarged sublingual salivary glands may be felt under the chin.

After examining the surface contours of the neck, the nurse should palpate the neck structures, beginning in the subauricular area, proceeding to the back of the neck, then to the inferior triangle, the supraclavicular region, and finally the anterior triangle. Palpation of tissues in each region will be facilitated by relaxation of muscles in the region; therefore, the head should be extended when the back of the neck is being palpated. In order to investigate anterior structures the patient's chin should be turned away from and the head tilted toward the side being palpated.

Normally, the cervical lymph nodes are not palpable unless the patient is extremely thin, in which case the nodes may be felt as small, freely moveable masses. In order to palpate lymph nodes the nurse should use gentle pressure of the palmar surfaces of the middle three fingertips in a to-and-fro motion over the skin in front of the ear (preauricular nodes), behind the auricle (postauricular nodes), under the occipital ridge (suboccipital nodes), under the ridge of the mandible (submandibular nodes), under the chin (submental nodes), along the side of the sternocleidomastoid muscles (cervical nodes), along either side of the trachea (cervical nodes), and in the supraclavicular fossae (supraclavicular nodes). When palpable nodes are found the nurse should note and later record the exact location of the node, its diameter in centimeters, its consistency, its degree of mobility, and tenderness, if present. Enlarged subauricular glands may signify an infection of the external ear; large suboccipital glands may indicate a scalp infection or infestation; swollen submandibular or submental glands may accompany an infection of the mouth; enlarged glands in the anterior triangle may occur in upper respiratory infection; a large supraclavicular gland may herald a gastric or pulmonary malignancy; and enlarged glands in several sites may indicate leukemia or lymphoma.

When moving the patient's head into various positions for the purpose of palpating lymph nodes, the nurse can also investigate the condition of cervical muscles and bones. Limitation of head and neck movement may result from cervical arthritis, cervical muscle spasm, or meningeal irritation. Spastic neck muscles will be taut and tender to palpation. Torticollis, which may be the result of congenital shortening or inflammatory injury to the sternocleidomastoid muscle, results in permanent tilting of the head to one side and underdevelopment of tissue on the dependent side of the face. In severe dyspnea due to respiratory obstruction, the sternocleidomastoid and scalene muscles, or accessory muscles of respiration, may be seen to contract forcibly on inspiration.

Normally, the external jugular vein, which runs from the angle of the jaw diagonally across the sternocleidomastoid muscle to the suprasternal notch, is not distended when the patient is in the sitting position. In congestive heart failure or superior vena cava obstruction, increased venous pressure may cause jugular distention in the upright position. With the patient in recumbent position and his head turned slightly to the opposite side, pulsations of the deep jugular vein, which are transmitted backward from the right atrium, normally can be seen through tissues medial to the sternocleidomastoid when a flashlight beam is directed tangentially to the neck.

The carotid artery emerges from behind the sternoclavicular joint and ascends the neck obliquely alongside the internal jugular vein toward the angle of the mandible (Fig. 16). Carotid pulsations normally can be observed through the tissues of the neck only in a very thin patient, but can be palpated from the sternal notch to the angle of the jaw by rolling the fingertips over the medial border of the sternocleidomastoid muscle. The amplitude of carotid pulsations on one side should be compared with that on the other, but both

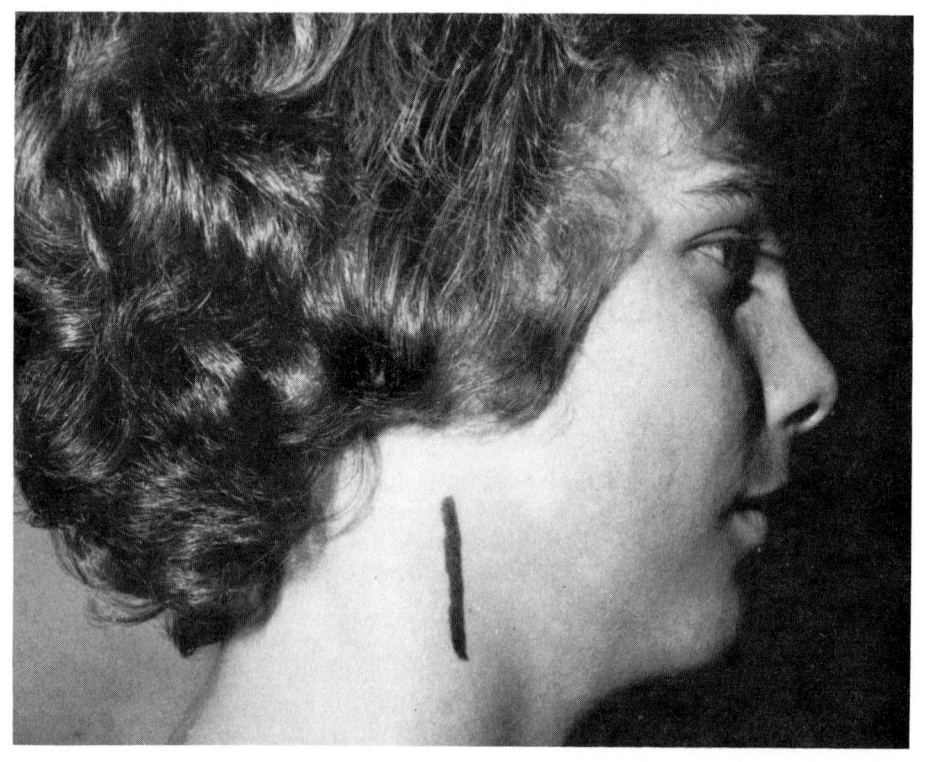

Figure 16. Location of the carotid artery.

carotids should not be palpated at the same time, lest brain circulation be unduly interfered with. Unusually forceful carotid pulsations may be found in aortic valve insufficiency, hyperthyroidism, and hypertension. A carotid aneurysm will often produce a visible enlargement with expansile pulsations occurring with each heart beat.

By applying the stethoscope bell lightly over the vessel, auscultation of a carotid artery narrowed by arteriosclerosis or tumor will often reveal a systolic bruit.

Both larynx and trachea normally lie in the midline of the neck. In thin persons and in males the thyroid cartilage of the larynx is easily seen midway between the chin and the sternal notch. The position of the trachea can be checked by placing the patient in a forward-facing position and then inserting the index finger into the sternal notch to contact the trachea. The finger is then rolled off the trachea to the right and to the left, and the distance between the trachea and manubrium on either side is noted (Fig. 17). Deviation of the trachea from the midline may be due either to a space-occupying lesion of the neck or to an intrathoracic mass.

Normally, the thyroid gland, which is attached to the trachea below the larynx, is not visible except in an extremely thin person. To palpate the thyroid, the practitioner should stand behind the patient, extend the neck slightly, and use the fingertips of both hands to locate the isthmus of the gland, which traverses the trachea just below the cricoid cartilage and the two

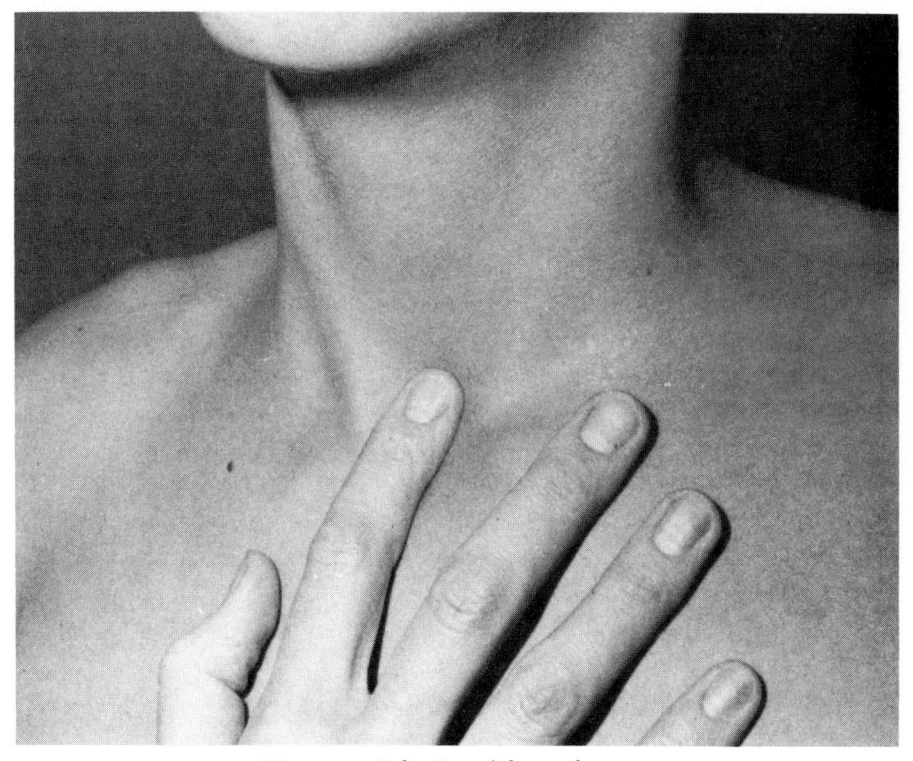

Figure 17. Palpation of the trachea.

pyramidal lateral lobes, which lie on either side of the trachea and are partially covered by the sternocleidomastoid muscles. With her fingers resting on the thyroid tissue, the nurse should ask the patient to swallow; this action will cause the thyroid gland to move upward through the examining fingers (Fig. 18). Since other subcutaneous soft tissues do not move during swallowing, the nurse can determine the size and consistency of the thyroid and the presence of any nodules as the gland moves against her fingers. In order to examine the lateral lobes fully, the nurse should insert the index and middle finger of each hand between the medial border of the sternocleidomastoid muscle and the cricoid cartilage and palpate the lateral lobe of the thyroid with a light rotary motion. It is advisable also to palpate one lateral lobe at a time, in each instance inclining the head slightly toward the side being examined to relax the sternocleidmastoid muscle.

In thyrotoxicosis the thyroid gland is usually enlarged bilaterally, soft in consistency, and of increased vascularity. Auscultation over a greatly enlarged thyrotoxic gland may reveal a systolic bruit, which results from increased blood flow through the tissue. Occasionally a thrill may also be detected over such a greatly enlarged and hypervascular gland.

In simple or endemic goiter due to insufficient iodine intake the gland may be soft or firm in consistency, and show slight diffuse enlargement, but there are no signs of toxicity since the metabolic rate is normal or slightly depressed.

A single, hard thyroid nodule is characteristic of thyroid carcinoma. With continued growth, a malignant tumor eventually breaks through the thyroid

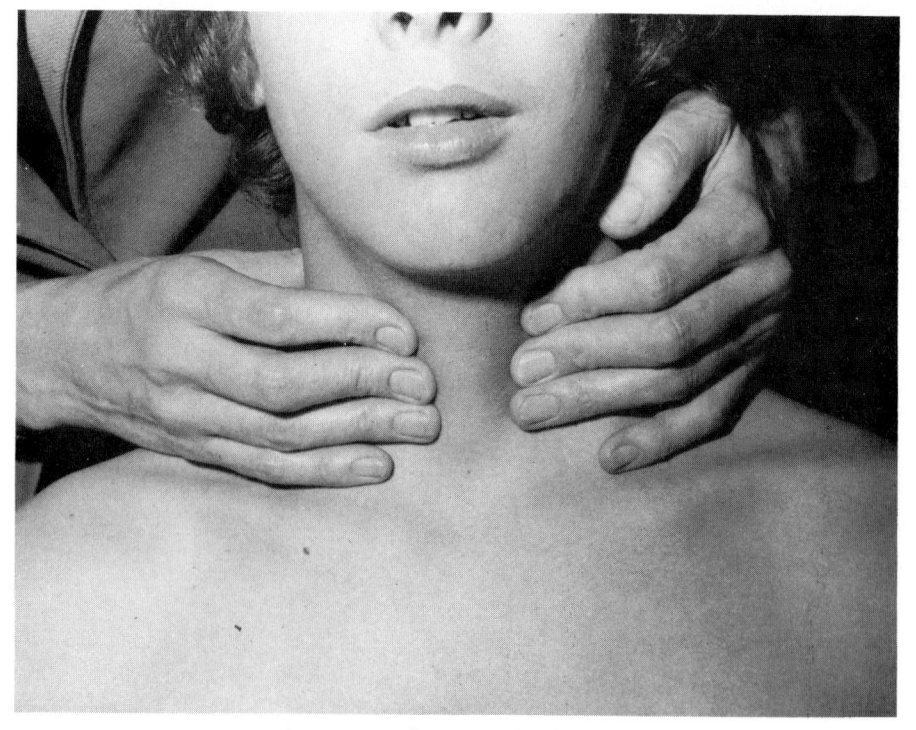

Figure 18. Palpation of the thyroid gland.

capsule, attaches the gland to surrounding tissue, and metastasizes to cervical lymph nodes.

The parathyroid glands are imbedded in thyroid tissue, two on each of the lateral thyroid lobes, and are normally not palpable.

Section III. Examination of the Thorax

EXAMINATION OF THE BREASTS

The practitioner should examine the breasts of both men and women patients, since men as well as women can develop breast infections, cysts, and malignancies. In preparation for the examination the patient should be disrobed to the waist. A towel should be used to drape the breasts before and after the actual examination. Breast examination should begin with the patient in sitting position with her arms hanging loosely at her sides and with both breasts exposed so that each can be compared with the other (Fig. 19). The size, shape, color, surface contour, skin characteristics, and symmetry of the breasts should be noted. Although it is not unusual to find some difference in the size of the two breasts, questioning will usually reveal that the size difference has been present since puberty and represents a developmental irregularity. A recent increase in the size of one breast, on the other hand, suggests inflammatory or neoplastic disease. During pregnancy the breasts become enlarged and the areolae become wider and more deeply pigmented. Usually this enlargement of the areolae will persist following delivery.

The two nipples should be located at the same level and should protrude forward slightly from the breast surface. Occasionally one or both nipples may be inverted or turned inward, and this phenomenon must be differentiated

Figure 19. Inspection of the breasts with arms at the sides. (From Hopkins, H. V.: *Leopold's Principles and Methods of Physical Diagnosis*. 3rd ed. Philadelphia, W. B. Saunders Co., 1965.)

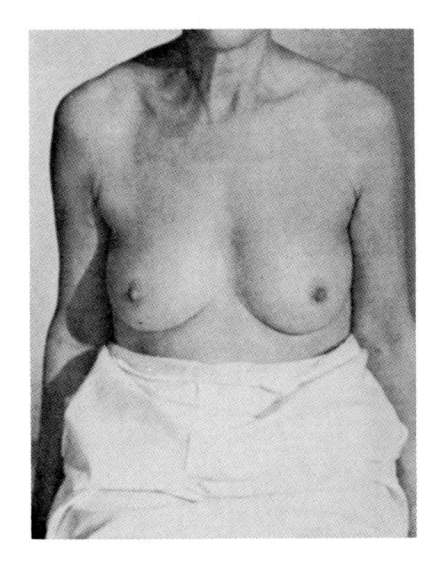

from retraction or drawing in of the nipple due to disease of breast tissue. Questioning will reveal that, in nipple inversion, the abnormality has been present since puberty; in retraction, the change in nipple contour and direction is recent. In carcinoma, the nipple is usually deflected so as to point in the direction of the breast lesion. A nipple fissure or crack in the postpartum patient is usually related to infectious mastitis or breast abscess. Enlargement of one breast or bulging of the surface contour may suggest an underlying abscess. Unilateral ulceration of the nipple is suggestive of a malignant dermatosis of the nipple area. The presence of discharge, crusting, or blood on the nipple is indicative of disease of the ductile system. Clear, yellow, or green discharge may be seen in chronic cystic mastitis. Bloody drainage is most commonly due to benign intraductile papilloma.

The skin of the breast should be observed for edema, color changes, and retraction signs. Edema of the breast causes the hair follicles to become more noticeable as the tissue between them swells, giving rise to tissue which has an "orange peel" or "pigskin" appearance. This sign may be found in either inflammatory or malignant breast disease. Reddening of the skin of the breast suggests underlying inflammation. In advanced adenocarcinoma of the breast the overlying skin may be markedly pigmented. Retraction signs, in the form of dimpling, depression, or unusual shadow formation, can result from post-inflammatory scarring, but are more commonly due to malignant tumor. If asymmetry, surface swellings, and retraction signs are not visible when the patient sits erect with her arms at her sides, the breasts should again be inspected when she raises her arms above her head, rests her hands on the practitioner's shoulders and leans forward slightly, and places her hands on her hips and presses them toward the midline (Figs. 20–22). Through any of these maneuvers it may become obvious that the tissues of one breast do not move upward or outward as freely as those of the other, which would suggest that breast tissue is fixed to tissues of the anterior chest wall.

With the patient still in the sitting position, the practitioner should begin breast palpation by exerting gentle traction on the nipple to determine

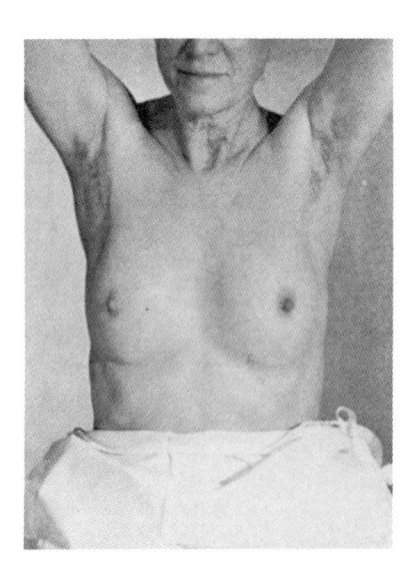

Figure 20. Inspection of the breasts with the arms raised above the head. (From Hopkins, H. V.: *Leopold's Principles and Methods of Physical Diagnosis.* 3rd ed. Philadelphia, W. B. Saunders Co., 1965.)

THE PHYSICAL EXAMINATION 65

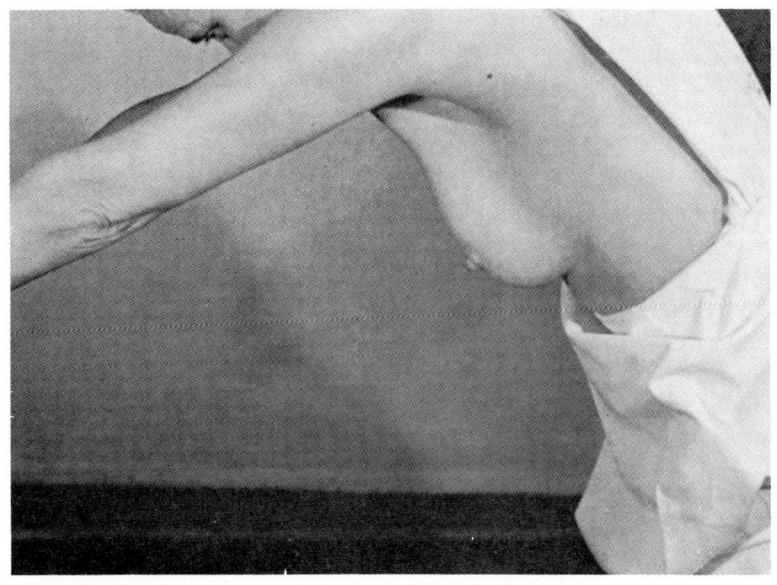

Figure 21. Inspection as the patient leans forward. The relative mobility of each breast should be noted and any inequality recorded. (From Hopkins, H. V.: *Leopold's Principles and Methods of Physical Diagnosis.* 3rd ed., Philadelphia, W. B. Saunders Co., 1965.)

whether or not it is adherent to underlying tissue. Then the remainder of the breast tissue should be palpated, using the palmar aspects of the fingers in a rotary motion, beginning in the upper outer quadrant and moving systematically in a clockwise fashion. Palpation must be done in such a way that breast tissue is compressed against the chest wall directly and not over an un-

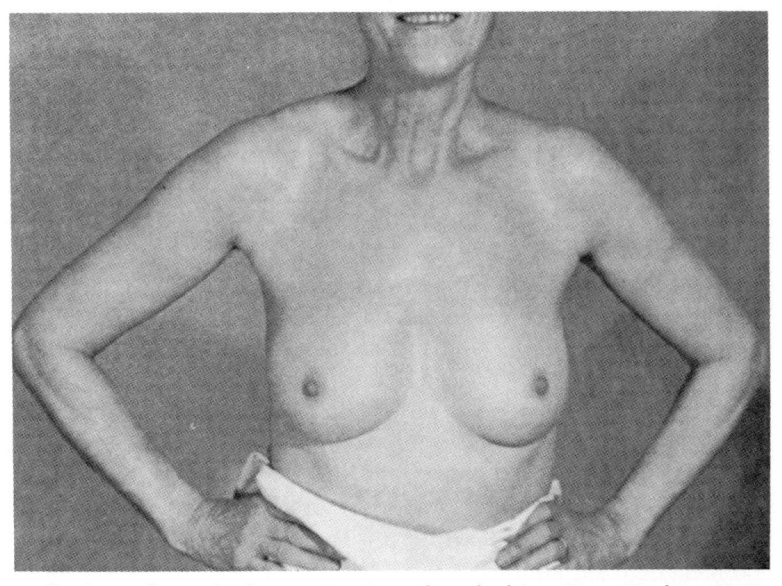

Figure 22. Tensing the pectoral muscles by pressing inward on the hips. (From Hopkins, H. V.: *Leopold's Principles and Methods of Physical Diagnosis.* 3rd ed., Philadelphia, W. B. Saunders Co., 1965.)

derlying double fold of skin, since in the latter situation it would be difficult to differentiate a mass within breast tissue from the increased resistance afforded by the skin interposed between the breast and the chest wall.

After the breast has been palpated with the patient in the sitting position, palpation should be repeated with the patient in the supine position. If the breasts are large or pendulous, a small pillow or folded towel should be placed behind the ipsilateral scapula, thus shifting the breast tissue and causing it to lie more evenly on the chest wall. The four quadrants of the breast should again be palpated in clockwise progression, using a gentle rotary motion of the palmar aspects of the fingers and moving, in each quadrant, from the periphery toward the areola. The patient's arm should be elevated above her head while the inner half of the breast is palpated and should lie at her side when the outer half of the breast is palpated. While the subareolar area is palpated, the practitioner should note the movement and elasticity of the nipple, which normally responds to manipulation by changing shape, as a result of the presence of erectile tissue. A gentle rolling or stripping motion is used to milk from the ducts any unusual drainage or discharge.

In palpating the breast, the practitioner should be aware that a strip of breast tissue extends from the upper outer quadrant of the breast upward toward the axilla. This "tail" of breast tissue and the axillary and supraclavicular lymph nodes must be palpated as part of the breast examination. In examining the patient's axilla for enlarged nodes, the practitioner should use one hand to palpate the tissues of the axilla while supporting the weight of the patient's ipsilateral arm with her hand. While using her fingertips to palpate the tissues of the lateral, thoracic, anterior, and posterior walls of the axilla, the practitioner should move the patient's arm through full range of motion in order to insure that an enlarged node does not escape detection by being hidden under muscular or fatty tissue (Fig. 23A and B). Enlarged supraclavicular nodes should be sought by rolling the fingertips into the depression just above the collar bone.

There is considerable variation in the consistency of normal breast tissue. In the young adult female, breast tissue is usually soft and fairly homogeneous in character. In post-menopausal women the breast tissue may feel nodular or stringy as a result of ductile tortuosity secondary to loss of fat and other involutional changes. In each woman the consistency of breast tissue varies somewhat with the various phases of the menstrual cycle. Typically, the breasts become engorged and tender, with an accentuation of their lobular architecture, just before menstruation and decongest rapidly following menstruation. Therefore, the best time to examine the breasts is the week following menstruation, since the breast lobules will be least prominent and least likely to obscure a pathological mass in the breast.

If the patient has complained of tenderness or a mass in one breast the practitioner should palpate the opposite breast first in order to have a standard of "normal" breast consistency against which to evaluate the consistency of the diseased breast and also to insure that a significant finding in the presumably uninvolved breast is not overlooked in the practitioner's concern about recognized abnormality in the other.

When a breast mass is palpated, its size, shape, consistency, surface characteristics, sensitivity, and attachment to underlying or overlying tissues

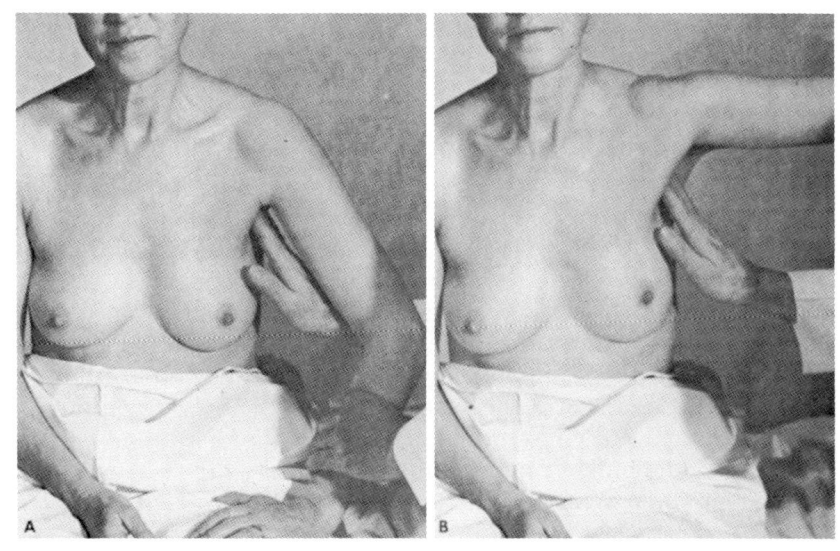

Figure 23. Palpation for axillary lymph nodes. This is done with the arm at the side (A) and with the arm raised (B) to tense the axillary fascia. (From Hopkins, H. V.: *Leopold's Principles and Methods of Physical Diagnosis.* 3rd ed. Philadelphia, W. B. Saunders Co., 1965.)

should be noted. In recording the location of a breast mass, the practitioner may consider that the breast represents a clock face and then locate the lesion as being, for instance, 2.5 centimeters from the nipple on the one o'clock axis. The size of the mass in all three dimensions should be carefully specified in order to determine at a later date whether there has been any increase or decrease in size of the mass.

Carcinoma of the breast is most common in the upper outer quadrant of the breast or in the subareolar area. A malignant breast tumor is typically hard, irregular in outline, and non-tender; because it tends to become fixed to superior and inferior tissues, it often produces indentation of overlying skin and limits movement of the breast upon the chest wall.

At some time in her care of each female patient the practitioner should teach the patient to examine her own breasts, using the techniques described here, and should advise that self-examination of the breasts be carried out routinely following each menstrual period.

Breast examination of the male patient may reveal hypertrophy of breast tissue or gynecomastia as a result of hormonal imbalance in portal cirrhosis or estrogen therapy for prostatic carcinoma. Very rarely, carcinoma of the breast occurs in males.

EXAMINATION OF THE LUNGS

When examining the thorax the practitioner should refer to commonly accepted landmarks in order to locate specific chest structures and to chart significant findings. It is customary to relate physical findings in the posterior thorax to the midvertebral line, midscapular line, posterior axillary line, and first thoracic vertebra. The midvertebral line is a vertical line that overlies the vertebral spines; the midscapular line is a vertical line that intersects the lower tip of the scapula when the arms lie alongside the lateral chest wall; the posterior axillary line is a vertical line that is continuous with the posterior axillary fold.

The commonly used reference points in the anterior thorax are the midsternal line, the right and left sternal border, the suprasternal notch, the supraclavicular fossa, the angle of Louis, the mid-clavicular line, and the anterior axillary line (Fig. 24). The midsternal line is a vertical line that extends through the center of the sternum and the xiphoid process. The suprasternal notch is the soft tissue depression immediately above the manubrium; the supraclavicular fossa is the depressed area immediately above the clavicle. The angle of Louis is the horizontal ridge at the junction of the manubrium and gladiolus, at which point the costal cartilage of the second rib is attached to the sternum. The mid-clavicular line is a line that drops perpendicularly from the middle of the clavicle; and the anterior axillary line is a vertical line that is continuous with the anterior axillary fold.

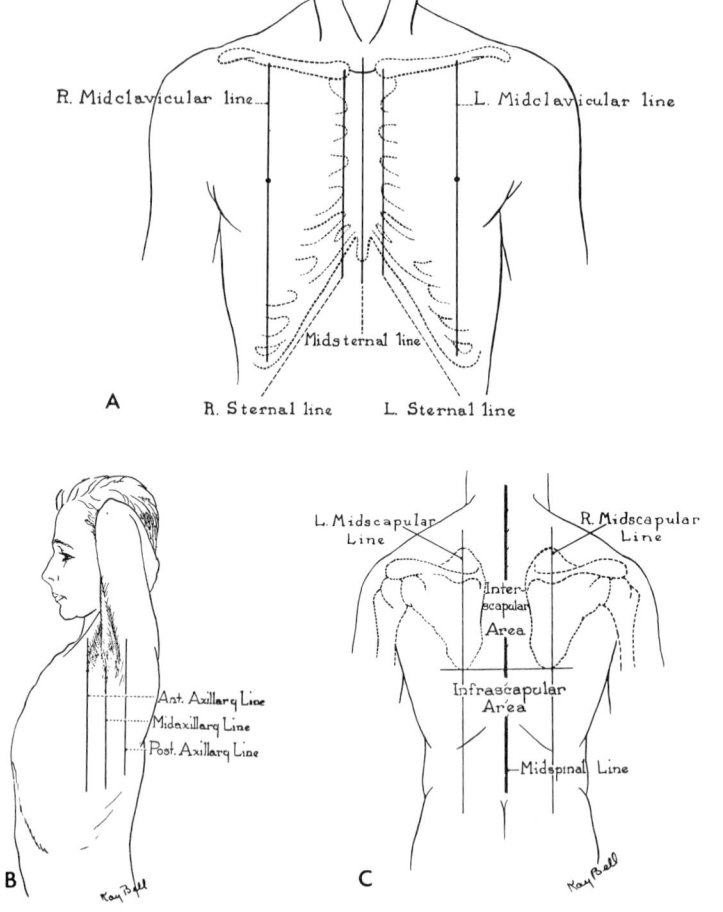

Figure 24. Reference lines on the chest wall: A, anterior view; B, axillary view; C, posterior view. (From Delp, M. H., and Manning, R. T. (Eds.): *Major's Physical Diagnosis.* 8th ed. Philadelphia, W. B. Saunders Co., 1975.)

Inspection

The practitioner should use inspection, palpation, percussion, and auscultation in examining the chest. With the patient in the sitting position, inspection should be used to determine the size, shape, surface contour, and symmetry of the chest cavity. In the normal adult the chest is symmetrical; it is oval in cross section, with a greater lateral than anteroposterior diameter, and the ribs extend slightly farther forward than does the sternum. The ribs course forward from the spine at roughly a 45 degree angle, progressing downward and outward to the lateral chest wall, then angling upward across the anterior chest to their attachment with costal cartilage and with the sternum. The lower costal cartilages join the sternum at a 90 degree angle, which widens somewhat with inspiration. The intercostal spaces are normally flat or slightly depressed.

Chest asymmetry of minor degree is not significant. That is, very often one shoulder is slightly higher than the other, and one usually sees slightly greater muscle development on the side of the dominant hand. Marked asymmetry of the chest may be seen in patients with scoliosis or with large aortic aneurysms. There is a marked increase in the anteroposterior diameter of the chest in patients with emphysema. In these patients the ribs do not leave the spine at a 45 degree angle but traverse the chest almost horizontally so that the lower costal cartilage joins the sternum at a greater than 90 degree angle.

If the lower portion of the sternum is greatly depressed, and the ribs extend markedly farther forward than the sternum, the condition is referred to as "funnel chest" and is characterized by lateral displacement of the heart and other mediastinal structures. If the sternum protrudes farther forward than the ribs, the condition is referred to as "pigeon breast." Neither condition interferes with respiratory efficiency.

Physical examination of the thorax should be used to confirm and follow up data obtained in the medical history and review of systems. A detailed occupational history should have been taken on any patient with respiratory symptoms, since several chronic lung diseases result from occupational hazards (silicosis, anthracosis, asbestosis).

When the patient is prepared for examination of the thorax, his clothing should be removed to the waist and he should be seated facing the practitioner. The patient should first be observed for dyspnea and cyanosis. Dyspnea, or difficult breathing, is a subjective symptom but may be apparent from marked increase in the rate or depth of respiration, from tightening of the scalene and sternocleidomastoid muscles, or from flaring of the alae nasi. The degree of dyspnea or breathlessness can be roughly evaluated by noting the number of words which the patient can utter before having to take the next breath.

Cyanosis, or bluish discoloration of the skin and mucosa, occurs when the concentration of reduced hemoglobin in the blood exceeds 5 grams per 100 ml. Therefore, cyanosis does not occur in a severely anemic patient with respiratory difficulty (his hemoglobin level is so low that, even if most of the hemoglobin in the blood were to be in reduced form, the concentration would not reach 5 grams per 100 ml. of blood). On the other hand, a patient with polycythemia vera may develop cyanosis in conjunction with a normal arterial partial pressure of oxygen (his hemoglobin concentration is so much greater than normal that when only a small proportion of that hemoglobin is in reduced state, the quantity of reduced hemoglobin may exceed 5 grams per 100 ml.).

Next, the practitioner should observe the patient's breathing pattern; degree of chest wall expansion; use of accessory muscles of respiration; posture; symmetry of rib cage movement; presence or absence of cough; chest scars; and any orthopedic abnormalities that would interfere with normal ventilation. In inspiration the diaphragm normally moves downward, and contraction of intercostal muscles pulls the ribs upward and outward, thereby increasing intrathoracic volume, decreasing intrathoracic pressure, and pulling air into the lungs. Expiration occurs when relaxation of the diaphragm and intercostal muscles causes the diaphragm and ribs to fall back to their rest positions, compressing the lung and forcing air to the outside. In males respiratory movement is predominantly diaphragmatic: in females rib movements are more marked than diaphragmatic movements. On observation, the inspiratory phase seems slightly shorter than the expiratory phase. Normal respirations are of regular rate and rhythm, and the ratio of respirations to pulse rate is about 1:4.

The patient's breathing pattern, in regard to rate, depth, rhythm, and duration of inspiration as compared with duration of expiration, provides information of diagnostic significance. Rapid respiration is seen in febrile states, in acidosis, in anemia, in cardiac failure, in hyperthyroidism, and in anxiety. Slow respiration is seen in deep relaxation, in sleep, and in drug-induced depression of the respiratory center. In Cheyne-Stokes respirations repetitive cycles of hyperventilation and apnea occur in which breathing is first slow and shallow, then gradually increases in rapidity and depth to a quite rapid rate, at which point a 30- to 40-second period of apnea occurs, followed by reappearance of slow, shallow respirations. Cheyne-Stokes respirations, which are typically seen in central nervous system disease, severe cardiac disease, and certain toxic states, indicate disturbance in central nervous system control of respiration.

In obstructive pulmonary disease, such as bronchial asthma, the expiratory phase of respiration is prolonged and a gasping type of inspiration is accomplished through the use of accessory muscles of respiration (the internal intercostals, the sternocleidomastoids, the scalenes, and the trapezius). Patients with chronic obstructive lung disease, such as emphysema, often purse their lips during exhalation in an effort to increase intrapulmonary pressure so as to prevent alveolar collapse. Greater than normal inspiratory effort is called for when lung compliance is decreased and additional force is needed to impel air into terminal airways. In patients with decreased lung compliance, intercostal retractions of skin and muscle can be observed during inspiration.

Fever, insomnia, anxiety, hypoxia, hypercapnia, and acidosis may cause hyperventilation or increase in rate and/or depth of respiration. In order to identify the cause of hyperventilation it is necessary to determine whether both rate and depth of respiration are increased (hyperpnea) or only the respiratory rate (tachypnea). A patient without pulmonary disease who is acidotic will develop increase in both rate and depth of respiration, while patients with chronic fibrotic lung disease will often demonstrate rapid but shallow breathing.

During the physical examination the practitioner may observe that the patient can breathe comfortably only in an upright or sitting position (orthopnia). Further questioning may reveal that the patient elevates his head on several pillows in order to sleep and that, in spite of so doing, he frequently wakens during the night with extreme dyspnea and must sit upright on the edge of the bed to "catch" his breath (paroxysmal nocturnal dyspnea). Orthopnea and paroxysmal nocturnal dyspnea result from pulmonary congestion in left ventricular heart failure.

Dilation of superficial veins of the anterior chest wall is characteristic of superior vena caval obstruction.

Palpation

Normally, chest wall circumference increases about three inches with maximal inspiration. Pre-inspiratory and post-inspiratory measurement of chest circumference at both the level of the axillae and the level of the xiphoid process will demonstrate that chest expansion is greater at the level of the lung bases than at the level of the lung apex. The degree of chest wall expansion can be determined in part by observation. The short, panting respirations associated with congestive heart failure obviously result in less than normal chest expansion. The deep blowing Kussmaul respirations of diabetic acidosis clearly represent greater than normal chest expansion. In most instances, however, chest expansion can be best evaluated by palpation. With the patient in recumbent position, the practitioner should place her hands palm downward on the anterolateral chest, with thumbs along the costal margin and fingers pointing toward the axillae. The practitioner should then observe her hands rise and fall as the patient breathes both quietly and deeply. Differences in expansion between the two sides of the thorax will be obvious with this method. Limitation of motion of one hemithorax may occur in pneumonia, pleurisy, or rib fracture. Movement of the posterior thorax should be similarly tested, the practitioner placing her outstretched hands on the patient's back, with her thumbs lateral to the spinous processes of the vertebrae and the fingers extended laterally to the mid-axillary line on each side. As the patient inspires, the practitioner's thumbs will rise and move outward. Differential expansion of the two hemithoraxes will be evidenced by less movement of one hand than the other. In emphysema there is decreased expansion of the lower rib cage, due to flattening of the dome of the diaphragm and fixation of the thorax in the inspiratory position.

Decreased excursion of one part of the thorax may result from protective splinting in an effort to minimize pleuritic pain, or from focal failure of lung expansion due to consolidation, fibrosis, atelectasis, or pneumothorax. Exaggerated expansion of the lower rib cage may be seen in patients with hepatomegaly, which causes greater than usual elevation of the dome of the diaphragm.

Beginning with the posterior thorax and continuing to the anterior thorax, the practitioner should lightly palpate the ribs and intercostal spaces to determine whether there are any areas of pain, tenderness, or swelling. Pain, swelling, crepitation, or abnormal movement will indicate a rib fracture. Tenderness of intercostal tissues may be due to neuritis or myositis. The position of the trachea should be determined by placing the index finger in the supra-

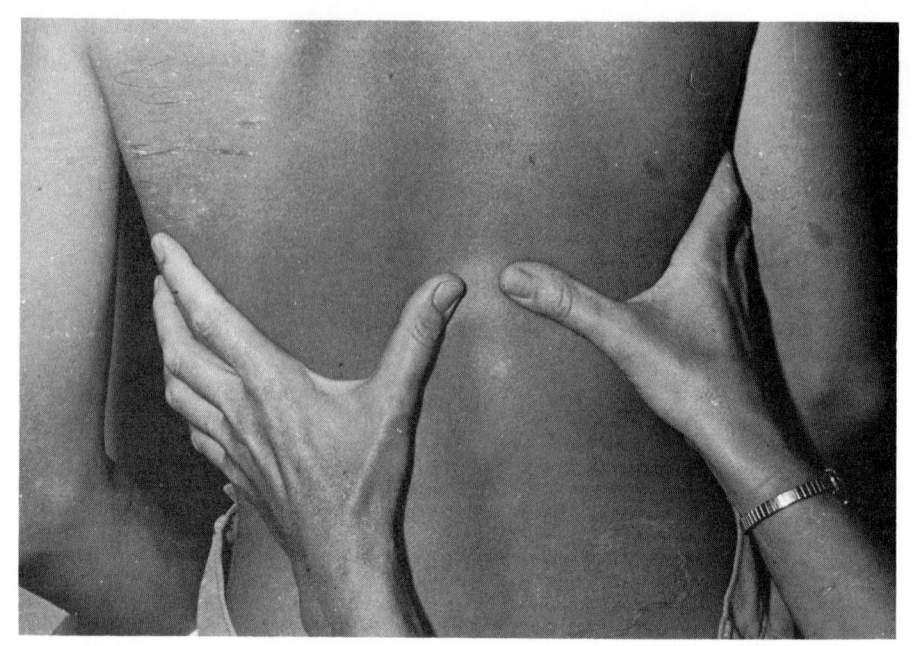

Figure 25. Determining chest wall expansion.

sternal notch, and comparing the distance between the right clavicle and the right side of the trachea with the distance between the left clavicle and the left side of the trachea. Tracheal palpation is facilitated by gently flexing the patient's head on his neck while keeping his chin centered over the suprasternal notch. Deviation of the trachea to one side or the other may be due either to displacement of neck structures by an enlarged thyroid gland or hypertrophied lymph nodes or to displacement of mediastinal structures by pleural effusion, pneumothorax, atelectasis, or tumor. Fremitus, or vibration of the chest wall, which arises from respiratory structures, can sometimes be palpated and is helpful in identifying pathological changes in underlying tissues. Fremitus may be classified into the following types: vocal, tussive, pleural friction, and rhonchal. Fremitus can best be perceived by applying the palmar surface of the fingers or the ulnar surface of the hand to the chest wall.

The practitioner should test for vocal fremitus by applying the palmar surface of the fingers of one hand first to one side of the patient's chest and then to the other, while the patient intones "one, two, three" and "ninety-nine" several times, using the same pitch and intensity with each utterance. By thus palpating symmetrical points at different levels of the thorax, the practitioner may identify areas where vocal fremitus is significantly increased or decreased. Since vocal fremitus arises from laryngeal vibrations and these are transmitted through the bronchial tree, vocal fremitus is most pronounced at those points where the large air passages are most superficial; that is, at the base of the neck anteriorly and posteriorly, between the scapulae, and on either side of the upper portion of the sternum. Increased vocal fremitus can be detected over areas of pneumonic consolidation that lie adjacent to a patent bronchus and extend to the lung periphery, since a solid medium of uniform density (coagulum filled alveoli) transmits sound vibrations more effectively than does a porous structure of varying density (normal lung tissue). Decreased or absent vocal fremitus is found in bronchial obstruction, pleural effusion, or pneumothorax, since all of these conditions interfere with transmission of sound vibrations from the larynx through the air passageways to the chest wall.

Palpable vibrations of the thoracic wall can also be produced by coughing (tussive fremitus), by the grating of inflamed pleural surfaces as they move against one another (pleural friction fremitus), and by the passage of air through secretions in the air passages (rhonchal fremitus). Tussive fremitus is, of course, coincident with coughing. Rhonchal fremitus can be differentiated from pleural friction fremitus by having the patient cough, since coughing, by removing secretions from the tracheobronchial tree, will eliminate rhonchal fremitus. Pleural friction fremitus will be unaffected by coughing.

Percussion

The density of underlying tissues can be estimated by systematically tapping the body surface with the fingers, causing the structures below the striking finger to emit tactile and audible vibrations. Tissue vibration and consequent sound intensity vary with the density of the structure being percussed. Direct percussion consists of tapping the body wall directly with the tip of the middle finger. More commonly used is mediate percussion, in which the distal two phalanges of the middle finger of the left hand (the pleximeter) are placed firmly against the chest wall parallel to the ribs in the intercostal space and the middle finger of the right hand (the plexor) is used to strike a quick blow to the proximal portion of the terminal phalanx of the pleximeter. The examiner then notes both the sound produced and the vibrations palpated by the pleximeter.

In performing chest percussion the practitioner should apply sufficient pressure to the pleximeter to keep the skin beneath it taut in order to prevent vibration of that tissue; he should keep all fingers but the pleximeter off the patient's skin so as to avoid damping the percussion note; he should hold the right forearm stationary and deliver each blow with equal force of the plexor. Too-heavy percussion should be avoided, as a heavy blow to the chest wall will produce vibration of all chest structures, making it difficult for the examiner to differentiate the density of tissues at specific points as the pleximeter is moved from one part of the chest to another.

Chest percussion should be performed in the following systematic fashion. Place the patient in sitting position and examine the anterior thorax by percussing the supraclavicular fossa, then the first interspace, then each succeeding interspace in a downward direction, comparing the two sides of the chest at each level. The cardiac outline should be identified by percussing the first few interspaces from the anterior axillary line medially toward the cardiac border on the left and toward the sternum on the right. On the right side at about the level of the fourth intercostal space the percussion note will change from resonant to dull owing to the presence of liver tissue behind the lower lobe of the lung. From about the level of the sixth interspace to the lower costal margin the percussion note will be flat because lung tissue no longer overlies the liver.

The lower border of the left lung cannot be similarly identified because as the left anterior hemithorax is percussed in a downward direction the note of pulmonary resonance gradually merges with the note of gastric tympany (due to the gastric air bubble).

After the anterior thorax has been thoroughly percussed, the patient should raise his arm and place his hand on his head while the lateral chest wall is percussed from the axilla to the costal margin.

To facilitate examination of the posterior chest the patient should lean forward slightly with his arms extended and crossed at waist level in order to move the scapulae as far apart as possible. The practitioner should percuss along the superior border of the trapezius, from the side of the neck toward the shoulder, until the flat percussion note changes to resonance, and then percuss from the shoulder toward the neck until resonance is detected. The two to three inch interval between these two points is occupied by the lung apex. The interspaces should then be percussed from above downward, comparing at each level one side with the other (Fig. 26). The range of motion of the diaphragm is determined by instructing the patient to take in a deep breath and hold it, then percussing downward in a vertical line from the tip of the scapula until resonance is replaced by dullness, at which point the skin should be marked with a non-irritating substance. The patient is then instructed to exhale completely, percussion is repeated and the new level of dullness is marked. The distance between the two marks is measured and recorded as the extent of diaphragmatic motion. The opposite side of the thorax is examined in like manner, and the diaphragmatic level and degree of movement on the two sides are compared. The extent of normal diaphragmatic movement between forced inspiration and forced expiration is between four and six centimeters and is equal on the two sides.

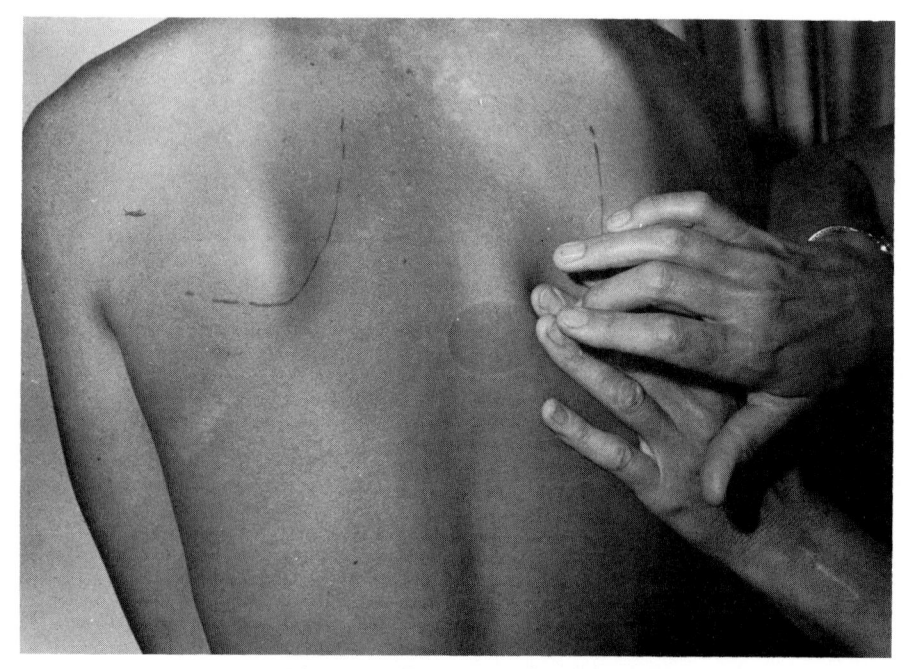

Figure 26. Percussion, chest (posterior).

Percussion receives its diagnostic value from the fact that air-filled tissue, such as normal lung tissue, is elastic and is easily set into motion by a blow to the chest wall, while fluids and dense tissues are not elastic, are not set into motion by the usual percussion stroke, and serve to decrease or alter the percussion note. The sound waves produced by vibration of different structures vary in frequency, amplitude, quality, and duration. The greater the frequency of vibrations of an object, the higher the pitch of the sound produced. The greater the amplitude of vibrations, the greater the intensity or loudness of the sound produced. The sounds elicited by percussion can be classified as resonance, hyperresonance, tympany, flatness, and dullness.

Resonance, the percussion sound produced by normal, air-containing lung, is vibrant, low pitched, and of long duration. Hyperresonance, the percussion sound emitted by emphysematous lungs, is lower in pitch, of longer duration, and louder than resonance. Tympany, the percussion sound elicited over a closed space containing predominantly air, such as the stomach and intestines, is a somewhat musical sound of higher pitch and greater intensity than resonance. Flatness, the percussion sound elicited over solid tissue like the liver, is the absence of resonance, in that it is nonvibrant, higher in pitch, of shorter duration, and of less intensity than resonance. Dullness or impaired resonance, the percussion note elicited over an area of predominantly solid tissue with some overlying air-containing lung, as in atelectatic or consolidated lung tissue, is less vibrant and less intense than resonance, and is of short duration.

All the percussion sounds except hyperresonance are found in percussing the normal chest. Resonance will be heard over most of the anterior chest, although there will be less over the apices than over the bases of the lungs, owing to the relatively greater muscle to lung ratio over the upper than the lower thorax. As mentioned earlier, dullness will be heard between the fourth and sixth interspaces of the right anterior chest owing to the fact that in that area the lower lobe of the lung overlies the right lobe of the liver. Flatness will be heard from about the sixth right interspace to the lower costal margin because liver tissue alone underlies that area.

Auscultation

There are two methods of listening to respiratory sounds—immediate auscultation, in which the examiner's ear is placed directly against the chest wall, and mediate auscultation, in which a stethoscope is used to convey sound from the chest wall to the examiner's ear. The stethoscope bell is best suited for transmitting low-pitched sounds, the diaphragm for transmitting high-pitched sounds. To increase the accuracy of information obtained by this method of examination, the practitioner should carry out chest auscultation in as quiet an environment as possible. She should avoid production of adventitious sounds herself by breathing heavily on the stethoscope tubing, by allowing one portion of the tubing to rub against another, by sliding her finger on the chest piece, by permitting the chest piece to rub against the chest skin or hair, or by positioning the bell so that one part of its rim is not in contact with the patient's skin.

The respiratory sounds that are evaluated through auscultation are breath sounds, adventitious sounds, and changes in vocal resonance. In order to obtain maximum information from lung auscultation, the practitioner should investigate breath sounds fully before attending to any adventitious sounds that may be present. Perception of breath sounds will be enhanced by instructing the patient to breathe normally or with just slightly increased depth and with his mouth open.

Breath Sounds

Breath sounds, which result from vibrations produced by the movement of air through the respiratory tree, should be analyzed as to pitch, intensity, quality, and duration. Normally, three different types of breath sounds can be heard over different portions of the lung. Vesicular breath sounds are soft, low pitched, low intensity, sighing sounds produced by movement of air in and out of the alveoli. In vesicular breath sounds, the inspiratory phase is of slightly higher pitch and is longer than the expiratory phase. Vesicular breath sounds are heard normally over most of the lung fields, but are decreased over emphysematous lung, diminished or absent over an area of pleural thickening or pleural effusion, and absent over an area of atelectasis.

Bronchial or tubular breath sounds, which are produced by the movement of air through the trachea and bronchi, are almost the opposite of vesicular breath sounds in that they are loud, harsh, blowing, rather high pitched sounds in which expiration is slightly louder and longer than inspiration. Normally tubular breath sounds are heard anteriorly only in the midline over the trachea and when heard over any portion of the lung parenchyma indicate consolidation of lung tissue, since tissue of uniform density (consolidated lung) transmits vibrations from deep-lying bronchi to the surface more readily than does tissue of varying density (normal air-filled alveoli).

Bronchovesicular breath sounds are a mixture of tubular and vesicular breath sounds and as such are higher, louder, and harsher than vesicular breathing, but lower and softer than tubular breathing. Bronchovesicular breath sounds are normally heard over those portions of the lung where both large bronchi and alveoli lie close to the chest wall, as over the right apex and first and second intercostal spaces anteriorly and between the scapulae posteriorly. Bronchovesicular breath sounds heard over an area of the lung in which vesicular sounds are expected suggest incomplete consolidation of lung tissue, as in beginning pneumonia.

Adventitious Sounds

Adventitious sounds, or those not usually heard over the lung parenchyma, include rhonchi, rales, wheezing, pleural friction rub, and stridor.

Rhonchi are coarse, rumbling, low pitched sounds of relatively long duration which result from passage of air through narrowed trachea, bronchi, and bronchioles. Rhonchi are usually present on both inspiration and expiration but may be heard only on inspiration. Since they usually result from partial obstruction of the bronchi by secretions, they may change in character from one minute to the next and are particularly likely to change in quality, to decrease or disappear immediately following a cough. Rhonchi are of different types, having a snoring, bubbling, or musical quality depending upon the consistency of secretions and the size of the passageways occluded. Higher-pitched rhonchi result from obstruction of small bronchi; lower-pitched rhonchi are heard with obstruction of the trachea or large bronchi. Rhonchi result from any condition in which secretions accumulate in the trachea and bronchi, and may therefore be heard in upper respiratory infection, bronchitis, asthma, or any condition in which the cough reflex is impaired.

Rales, which are produced by the movement of air into alveoli containing fluid, are short high-pitched sounds similar to those produced by crushing cellophane or by rubbing hairs together in front of the ear. Rales are usually heard near the end of inspiration, tend to be exaggerated on deep breathing, and are not cleared by coughing. When rales are detected the practitioner should carefully note their location, their timing in regard to the respiratory cycle, and whether they are of high, medium, or low pitch. If fluid is located in the alveoli only, the rales will tend to be high pitched and will occur late in the inspiratory phase. If fluid is located in the respiratory or terminal bronchioles the rales will be lower in pitch (due to the greater diameter of the tube occluded) and will appear earlier in the inspiratory cycle. Rales due to left heart failure or to bronchiectasis are typically seen in the dependent portions of the lung. In bronchial pneumonia, rales tend to be widespread throughout the lung due to the scattered distribution of pulmonary inflammation. In lobar pneumonia, rales are usually localized in one lobe of one lung.

Wheezing respirations are high pitched, musical or whistling sounds due to diffuse obstructions of bronchial air flow which may occur on either inspiration or expiration but are most pronounced on expiration. Bilateral wheezing is suggestive of asthma or emphysema. Unilateral wheezing may result from bronchial obstruction by tumor.

A pleural friction rub is a coarse, scratching, creaking, or grating sound which results from the rubbing of inflamed pleural surfaces against each other. The character of the sound is the same during inspiration and expiration. A pleural friction rub is most often heard over the lower anterolateral chest wall, since that is the region of greatest thoracic movement.

Stridor is a harsh, high-pitched crowing sound produced by the passage of air through a partially obstructed larynx or bronchial tree, as in laryngotracheal bronchitis of infancy. Stertorous breathing is characterized by snoring sounds, and results from vibration of the soft palate or of thickened secretions in the upper air passages.

Coughing

Coughing is a periodic paroxysm of forceful expirations against a partially closed glottis. Each forceful expiration is preceded by a preliminary inspiration of slightly greater than usual depth, and often results in the elevation of secretions from the lung, through the bronchial passages, and into the oral cavity. Cough may be moist and productive, as in pulmonary edema or bronchiectasis, or may be dry and unproductive, as in emphysema or non-cavitary tuberculosis. If the patient has a productive cough, the amount, color, odor, and viscosity of sputum raised should be noted and recorded. A brassy cough results from paralysis of the recurrent laryngeal nerve; a shrill cough occurs in acute laryngitis; and a short, convulsive cough followed by a whoop is typical of pertussis. A hiccup is a short, sharp inspiratory cough caused by spasmodic lowering of the diaphragm followed by spasmodic closure of the glottis. Hiccups may result from many causes, such as irritation of the diaphragm, irritation of the phrenic nerve, toxic stimulation of the respiratory center, or hysteria.

Changes in Vocal Resonance

Laryngeal vibrations produced by vocal effort are transmitted through the air passages to the lung periphery and the chest wall. Normally, the patient's spoken words cannot be distinguished by auscultation. Over an area of consolidated lung, however, vocal sounds can be clearly perceived through a stethoscope. To test for changes in vocal resonance the patient should be directed to repeat "One, two, three" or "Ninety-nine" several times while the practitioner compares voice transmission through one side of the chest with a comparable point on the other side. An even more sensitive test consists of auscultation after directing the patient to whisper certain words or phrases. Normally whispered vocal sounds are heard only indistinctly throughout the chest, but whispered words can be heard over consolidated lung tissue with such clarity that even individual letters can be distinguished.

Vocal resonance, the indistinguishable murmur normally heard through the chest wall when the patient speaks, is usually loudest over those areas where the trachea and main bronchi lie near the chest wall. Decreased vocal resonance will result from any condition that interferes with transmission of laryngeal vibrations through the air passages to the chest wall, such as bronchial occlusion, atelectasis, and pleural effusion.

CARDIAC EXAMINATION

Much information about cardiac functioning can be obtained from study of the pulse and blood pressure. Discussion of pulse is given in those sections of this chapter relating to physical examination of the neck and of the extremities. Discussion of blood pressure determination is included in Chapter 7.

Examination of the heart requires that the patient be disrobed from the chest up, although a drape towel should be used to prevent undue exposure. The cardiac examination should begin with the patient in supine position but should include palpation and auscultation in the left lateral and sitting position as well.

In order to correctly interpret findings obtained on cardiac examination the practitioner must be aware that the normal heart lies obliquely behind the sternum, with about two thirds of its diameter to the left of the midline, and with its left border extending from the second left rib to the fifth left intercostal space. Because of its oblique position in the chest the anterior surface of the heart is made up predominantly of the right ventricle and the right atrium, with the left ventricle comprising a narrow strip along the left cardiac border. In cardiac disease, enlargement of one or another of the cardiac chambers will modify these normal relationships.

Inspection

Observation of the point of maximum impulse (P.M.I.), or the faint heaving of the anterior chest wall caused by the forward thrust of the contracting ventricle, helps to locate the apex of the heart, which lies one-half centimeter to the left of this point. The apex beat can best be seen in a tangential view of the chest from the foot of the examining table. Normally, the P.M.I. is located in the fifth left intercostal space in the mid-clavicular line or eight to ten centimeters to the left of the midsternal line. In the patient with a dilated heart the point of maximum impulse, and therefore the apex, is often located in the sixth interspace and to the left of the mid-clavicular line (sometimes in the anterior or mid-axillary line). Elevation of the diaphragm caused by pregnancy, ascites, or abdominal tumor will cause the point of maximum impulse to be displaced laterally. The point of maximum impulse is usually visible in persons who are thin or of average weight. It may not be visible in obese patients, owing to the cushioning effect of fat, or in emphysematous patients, in whom inspiration brings a segment of overdistended lung over the cardiac apex so as to prevent its contacting the chest wall.

The rate and magnitude of chest wall movement at the point of maximum impulse tend to be increased in febrile, anemic, hyperthyroid, or nervous patients. In the latter, the precordial impulse usually becomes less noticeable as the examination proceeds and the patient becomes more comfortable with the examiner and the procedure.

Next, the practitioner should observe the entire chest wall for symmetry, venous pattern, and abnormal pulsations. Marked cardiac enlargement or massive pericardial effusion may produce bulging of the left anterior chest. Dilated superficial veins of the chest wall provide collateral circulation in hepatic cirrhosis. Aneurysm of the ascending aorta may produce visible pulsations in the second right intercostal space.

A rough estimate of venous pressure can be made by observation of the neck veins. Normally, when the body is supine the neck veins are distended, but when the head is elevated at a 45 degree angle the neck veins are collapsed. To measure neck vein distention the patient should first be placed in a comfortable sitting position and his neck veins inspected. Then the patient's head should be lowered to a 45 degree angle, with the bed and his neck observed from the side. Distention of the neck veins in this position is suggestive of increased venous pressure, which may be due either to right heart failure or to superior vena caval obstruction.

Palpation

Palpation of the heart should begin with the patient in supine position and should be initiated by placing the flat of the hand lightly over the point of maximum impulse in order to determine the character of the apical impulse (Fig. 27). In a woman patient the examiner's hand should be placed against the chest wall under the left breast, retracting the breast tissue with the opposite hand if necessary. If the apical impulse is not readily palpable, the patient should be asked to sit up, lean forward, and exhale; this maneuver will cause the heart to fall forward against the chest wall. Normally, the apical impulse is felt as a quick light tap against the examiner's hand but in obese or

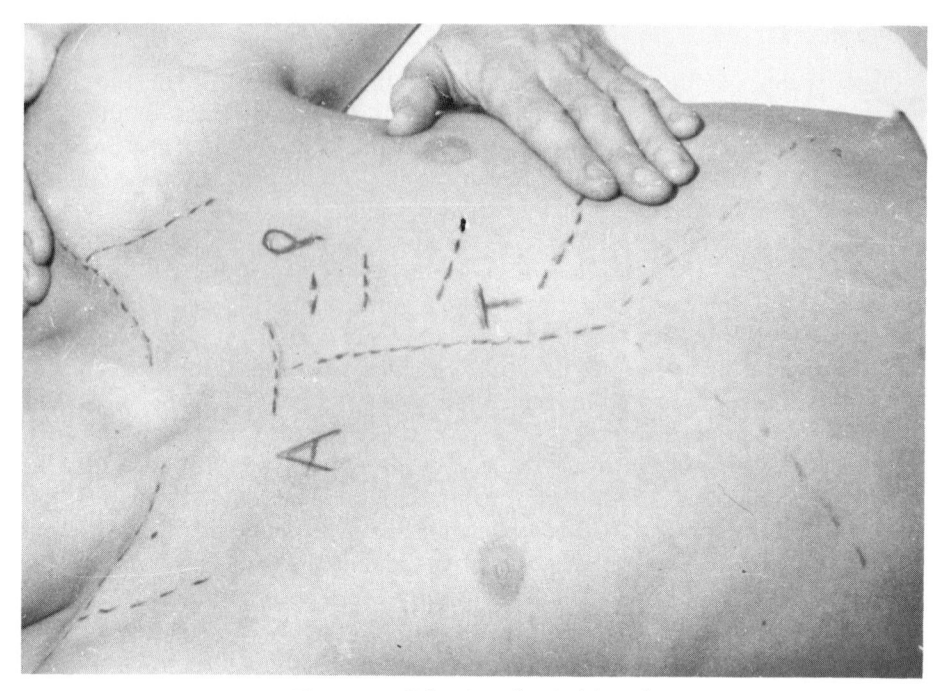

Figure 27. Palpation of apical impulse.

barrel-chested patients the apex impulse may not be palpable at all. In left ventricular hypertrophy a prolonged lifting or heaving force can often be felt over the apex. Through palpation the examiner can often identify disturbances in rate and rhythm that were first suspected on inspection. Aneurysm of the ascending aorta may produce pulsations that are palpable in the second interspace to the right of the sternum.

A thrill, or "palpable murmur," is a body surface vibration similar to that felt in touching a purring cat, and results from turbulent blood flow through a damaged heart valve or a septal defect. A thrill is best felt when the patient exhales forcefully and, depending upon the structural defect present, may be best perceived when the patient is either leaning forward or in the left lateral position. In palpating for thrills the examiner should apply the palmar aspects of the index, middle, and ring fingers to the apex, the left heart border, the second left interspace (the pulmonic area), the second right interspace (the aortic area), and the suprasternal notch. It is important to determine when in the cardiac cycle a thrill occurs. To determine whether a thrill coincides with systole or diastole, the thrill should be palpated simultaneously with the carotid pulse, which is precisely coordinated with the first heart sound.

Percussion

Percussion of the heart borders is useful in determining cardiac size. The same method of mediate percussion is used to investigate the heart as was used to investigate the lung: striking the proximal aspect of the terminal phalanx of the left middle finger with the right middle finger. A light percussion stroke is more effective than a forceful stroke in effecting the slight change in sound that occurs at the point at which lung tissue overlies cardiac tissue. To locate the heart borders, the pleximeter finger should be placed parallel to the heart border being investigated, and percussion should begin laterally and proceed toward the midline in the third, fourth, and fifth interspaces, since a change from resonance to dullness is more easily perceived than the reverse. Detection of cardiac dullness below the fifth left interspace, beyond the left mid-clavicular line, or to the right of the sternum is characteristic of marked cardiac hypertrophy and dilation. Mild to moderate degrees of cardiac hypertrophy are not usually detectable by thoracic percussion. Increased dullness over the base of the heart may be seen in aortic aneurysm. A decrease in the area of cardiac dullness may be seen in emphysema, owing to the fact that the segment of lung which overlies the heart is so over-distended that the change in percussion note normally heard over this area is not discernible.

In patients with pericardial effusion the area of cardiac dullness shifts as the patient changes position. The effect of gravity on accumulations of pericardial fluid is such that with the patient in sitting position the area of dullness at the apex is increased, and with the patient in supine position the area of dullness at the base of the heart is increased.

Auscultation

Many cardiac sounds are of such low amplitude as to be undecipherable against a high level of background noise. Therefore, auscultation of heart sounds, like auscultation of the lungs, should be carried out in as quiet an environment as possible. Noisy breath sounds may also obscure a low-pitched murmur. For this reason the practitioner should direct the patient to "breathe naturally" or "breathe quietly" during cardiac auscultation, and may even for brief periods of time direct the patient to "stop breathing" in order that she may listen for low-pitched sounds. When this is done the practitioner should hold her breath at the same time in order to know when to tell the patient to resume breathing. In order to derive maximum diagnostic information from heart sounds the practitioner should understand the several mechanical events comprising each cardiac cycle and should interpret cardiac sounds as manifestations of certain of those events. During auscultation the practitioner should first focus her attention on one such event throughout several cardiac cycles, then focus on another event through several cycles, and so on until all aspects of the cycle have been studied.

The four classic areas used for cardiac auscultation derive from the fact that the vibrations and therefore the sound produced by the closure of each cardiac valve is projected in the direction of blood flow. Thus the mitral area is in the region of the cardiac apex in the fifth interspace in the mid-clavicular line; the tricuspid area is near the lower end of the sternum; the pulmonic area is in the second interspace to the left of the sternum, and the aortic area is in the second interspace to the right of the sternum (Figs. 28 and 29). In order not to overlook significant findings, it is advisable to always follow a fixed sequence in listening to heart sounds in these areas. In addition, auscultation should be carried out at various points between the mitral, tricuspid, pulmonic, and aortic areas, as well as in the epigastric and supraclavicular

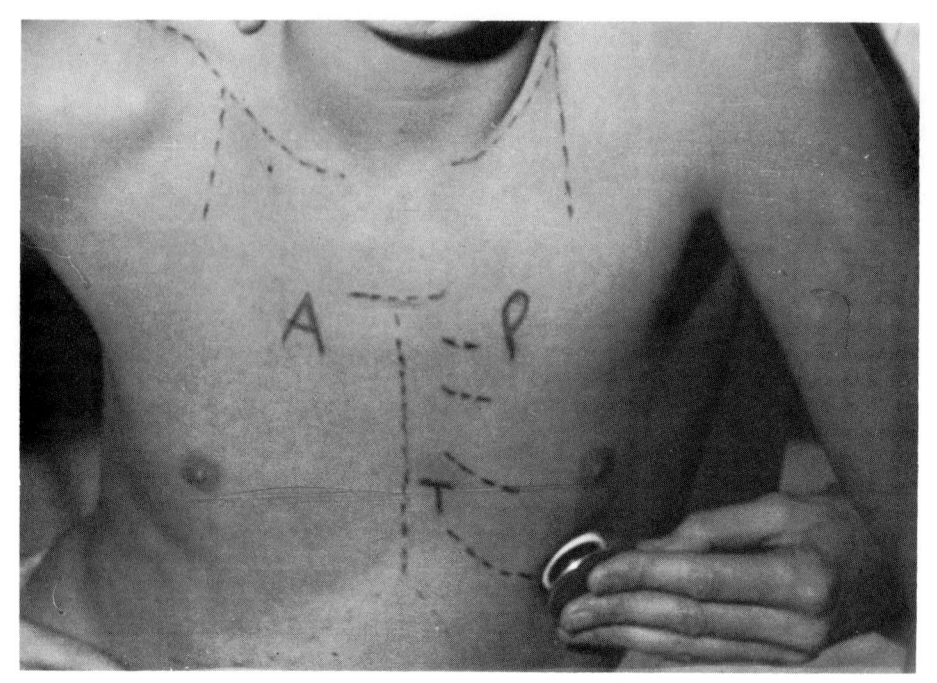

Figure 28. Four classic areas for cardiac auscultation: auscultating with the bell of the stethoscope.

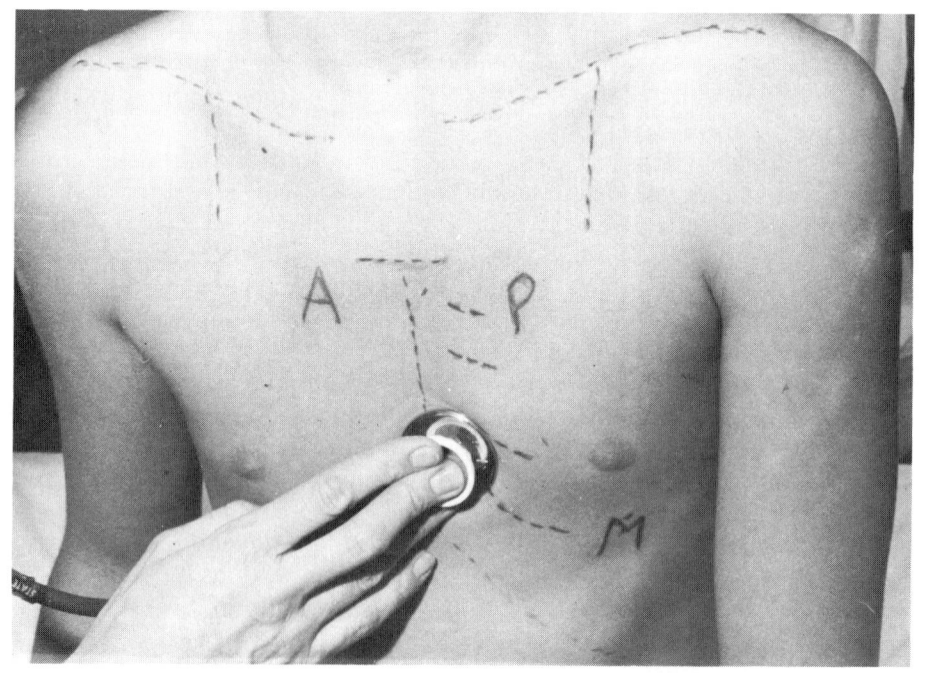

Figure 29. Four classic areas for cardiac auscultation: auscultating with the diaphragm of the stethoscope.

areas. At each point, auscultation should be carried out with both bell and diaphragm; the bell is most useful in detecting low-pitched sounds, and the diaphragm is more useful in detecting high-pitched sounds.

Auscultation may reveal an arrhythmia that was not detected on inspection and palpation or may corroborate irregularities noted earlier. Sinus arrhythmia, which results from vagal stimulation and which is frequently seen in healthy young persons, is characterized by a speeding of cardiac rate during inspiration and a slowing during expiration. A premature ventricular contraction is a small beat that follows shortly after a normal beat and is itself followed by a longer than normal, or compensatory, pause before the next regular beat occurs. In atrial fibrillation the rate of atrial contraction is so rapid that the ventricles can respond only to occasional impulses reaching the atrioventricular node, hence the cardiac rhythm is perceived as completely irregular.

Heart Sounds

There are four main heart sounds, only the first two of which are usually heard in the normal heart. The first heart sound (S_1), "lub", is produced by closure of the mitral and tricuspid valves. It is best heard over the apex but usually can be heard over the entire precordium and can be differentiated from the second sound by the fact that the first sound is synchronous with carotid pulsation. When heard at the apex the first sound is louder, lower in pitch, and longer in duration than the second sound. Since the mitral valve closes slightly in advance of the tricuspid, the first sound may be split so that two components are audible when the sound is heard over the tricuspid area (to the right of the sternum in the fourth interspace). However, since vibrations from the mitral valve are well transmitted to the apex and vibrations from the tricuspid are not, the first heart sound is usually not split when heard at the apex. The first heart sound tends to be faint in aged persons and in patients with emphysema, myocardial weakness, or mitral incompetence. The first heart sound tends to be accentuated in patients with hyperthyroidism, hypertension, and mitral stenosis.

The second heart sound (S_2), "dup", which is shorter and higher pitched than the first, occurs at the end of systole and is produced by closure of the aortic and pulmonic valves. When heard at the base of the heart the second sound tends to be louder than the first and is almost wholly the result of aortic closure. The pulmonic component of the second heart sound is normally heard only in the region over the pulmonary valve (the second left intercostal space). In the well person there may be slight splitting of the second sound at the pulmonic area at the end of inspiration due to the effect of increased venous return flow in prolonging right ventricular contraction (physiological splitting). In conditions of increased blood flow or increased pressure in the right ventricle (atrial septal defect or pulmonary artery stenosis) there may be fixed splitting of the second sound; that is, the two components of the sound may be audible throughout the entire respiratory cycle. Accentuation of the second sound may be due to arterial or pulmonary hypertension. Faintness of the second sound may be associated with either pulmonary or aortic stenosis.

The third heart sound (S_3) is a faint, low-pitched sound occurring in early diastole shortly following the second sound, and results from ventricular vibrations produced by rapid filling. The third sound, which is best heard at the apex, is found in some normal children and adults, and may be accentuated with respiration, but probably has no significance in young persons. When heard in an older adult the third sound is suggestive of either diastolic overloading of the ventricles (as in mitral or tricuspid regurgitation) or impaired myocardial tone.

The appearance of a third heart sound gives rise to a triple, or gallop, rhythm, which is usually heard best at the apex. Since the third heart sound results from decreased myocardial tone, a gallop rhythm is strongly suggestive of myocardial disease (infarction or myopathy).

The fourth heart sound (S_4), which is not heard in the normal adult, occurs in late diastole immediately prior to the first heart sound. The fourth sound, which is heard best at the apex, results from atrial and ventricular vibrations produced by forceful contraction of an enlarged atrium. It may be heard in systemic and pulmonary hypertension.

Events of the Cardiac Cycle

In order to interpret correctly the significance of cardiac sounds, they must be related to the electrical and mechanical events occurring throughout the heart cycle. Normally, the impulse which initiates each cardiac cycle originates in the sinoatrial node, is transmitted throughout the atrial musculature to the atrioventricular node and thence by way of the bundle of His and the Purkinje network to the ventricular musculature. During the delay (0.01 second) in impulse transmission through the atrioventricular node, atrial contraction is completed. Then, as the atria relax, the ventricles are stimulated and contract. Each cardiac cycle, then, consists of a period of contraction or systole, in which blood is forced from the heart into the pulmonary artery and aorta, and a period of relaxation or diastole, in which the heart receives blood from the venae cavae and pulmonary veins.

At the same time that these electrical impulses traverse the heart and trigger contraction of first the upper and then the lower heart chambers, certain volume and pressure changes occur within the heart and the great vessels of the thorax. As blood flows from the great vessels into the right and left atria, pressure increases in these chambers to the point that the tricuspid and mitral valves open, allowing much of the blood in the atria (70 per cent) to flow passively into the ventricles. Then the atria contract, forcing the remaining blood in the upper chambers (30 per cent) to flow into the lower chambers.

As the ventricles fill with blood, pressure in these chambers increases to the point that intraventricular pressure exceeds intra-atrial pressure, at which point the tricuspid and mitral valves close, producing the first heart sound (S_1). Shortly following closure of the tricuspid and mitral valves ventricular contraction begins, further increasing intraventricular pressure. When the pressure within the ventricles exceeds that in the pulmonary artery and the aorta, the pulmonary and aortic valves are forced open and blood is pushed into the two arteries leaving the heart.

The large volume of blood pumped into the pulmonary artery and aorta markedly raises the pressure in those vessels at the same time that ventricular relaxation causes intraventricular pressures to drop suddenly. This difference in pressure causes the pulmonary and aortic valves to close, producing the second heart sound (S_2). As the ventricle continues to relax and blood continues to pour into the atria, atrial pressures again increase to the point that they exceed ventricular pressures, and the tricuspid and mitral valves are again forced open.

A number of disease conditions can upset this series of electrical and mechanical events, resulting in a modification of cardiac functioning and a change in heart sounds. Rheumatic inflammatory damage to leaflets of the mitral, aortic, or tricuspid valve may produce either stenosis or insufficiency of the valve. A rigid, stenosed valve opens with difficulty and to a smaller than normal diameter, hence a "snap" may be heard as the inflexible leaflets pull apart on opening, and a murmur may be heard as the blood is forced through the narrowed valve opening past rigid and unyielding leaflets. On the other hand, in an insufficient or incompetent valve the leaflets are incapable of complete approximation. Therefore, even when the valve is in "closed" position, blood is allowed to leak backward through the valve into the preceding chamber, creating a systolic murmur in the case of the mitral or tricuspid valve and a diastolic murmur in the case of the aortic or pulmonary valve.

In hyperthyroidism and anemia the greatly increased rate of blood flow produces abnormal vibrations of valve leaflets and heart muscle, giving rise to a systolic murmur at the apex or the pulmonic area.

In myocardial infarction, rheumatic carditis, and alcoholic myocardiopathy there may be such a decrease in myocardial tone that blood flow through the heart produces increased vibrations of the heart wall, giving rise to a third or fourth heart sound. If at the same time heart rate is unusually rapid, a gallop rhythm may develop.

In systemic or pulmonary hypertension, the increased vascular pressure is referred backward to the ventricle. At the same time, the ventricular muscle undergoes compensatory hypertrophy as it is called upon to force blood into the vascular bed against an increasing head of pressure. The rise in intraventricular pressure, combined with an increased force of ventricular contraction, causes valve leaflets to close with greater than normal force, accentuating both the first and second heart sounds.

Murmurs

Murmurs are audible vibrations of the heart and great vessels produced by turbulent blood flow. Such turbulence may result from various causes: increased rate of blood flow (as in anemia), obstruction to blood flow (as in valvular stenosis), or counter-currents of blood flow (as in valvular insufficiency). Thus, the presence of a murmur does not necessarily signify heart disease. In general, a murmur is best heard over the area of the valve responsible for its production, and a murmur differs from a normal heart sound in that the murmur is longer and of a different quality. Most murmurs are either systolic or diastolic, though a few are heard throughout both phases of the cardiac cycle. A diastolic murmur usually signifies organic disease: a systolic may or may not indicate structural abnormality. In order to diagnose the structural or functional cause for a particular murmur, it must be analyzed as to its timing, location, pattern of radiation, intensity, pitch, quality, and constancy.

Systolic

A systolic murmur, or one which occurs between S_1 and S_2, may be present during all or part of systole. From a physiologic point of view systolic murmurs may be of two types: ejection or regurgitant. A systolic ejection murmur is heard in mid-systole and occurs when the rate of blood flow is disproportionate to the size of the orifice through which it must pass or when blood is pumped from a high pressure area to a low pressure area through abnormal valves. Systolic ejection murmurs are frequently associated with aortic or pulmonary valve stenosis, and are best heard at the base of the heart. Stenosis of the aortic valve may result from rheumatic fever or arteriosclerosis. Stenosis of the pulmonary valve is usually a congenital defect.

A systolic regurgitant murmur is usually pansystolic and results from backward flow of blood from the ventricle into the atrium through an incompetent valve. The most common systolic regurgitant murmur is that due to rheumatic mitral insufficiency, which is best heard at the apex and is usually characterized as harsh or blowing. Other possible causes for such a murmur are papillary muscle dysfunction following myocardial infarction, rupture of the chordae tendineae, or severe cardiac dilatation, since all these conditions would prevent normal approximation of the valve leaflets in the closed position.

Diastolic

Diastolic murmurs occur between S_2 and S_1, always indicate organic heart disease, and are of two types: filling and regurgitant. A diastolic filling murmur results from disproportion of blood flow rate to orifice size, such as the flow of blood from atrium to ventricle through a stenosed valve. The low-pitched, rumbling murmur of mitral stenosis, which is best heard at the apex with the patient in left lateral position, begins in mid-diastole and may intensify as the atria contract, just before the first heart sound. The diastolic filling murmur of tricuspid stenosis is best heard to the left of the lower sternal border.

A diastolic regurgitant murmur results from the backward flow of blood through an incompetent valve and begins at S_2, decreasing in intensity during most of diastole. Diastolic regurgitant murmurs due to aortic or pulmonary valve insufficiency are heard best at the base of the heart. The high pitched, blowing murmur of aortic regurgitation is loudest in the third left interspace near the sternum.

Section IV. Examination of the Abdomen

Although percussion and auscultation are the most valuable means of examining thoracic structures, palpation is the most valuable means of examining abdominal structures; however, it is not the method that should be employed first.

Before beginning the abdominal examination, the nurse practitioner should instruct the patient to remove his underwear, assist him to assume the supine position with a small pillow under his head and his hands crossed over his chest, and adjust the drape sheets so as to expose the abdomen completely from the xiphoid process of the sternum to the symphysis pubis. The nurse should then take her position at the patient's right side. Since the patient's abdominal musculature must be as relaxed as possible to permit adequate palpation of the abdominal viscera, the nurse should reassure him with a remark such as, "I will be as gentle as possible in examining your abdomen. You can assist by relaxing completely." Here again, as during the thoracic examination, both the room air and the nurse's hands should be warm enough that the patient is not chilled, since chilling causes an increase in skeletal muscle tone.

In order to systematize the abdominal examination and accurately indicate the location of any abnormal structures palpated, the anterior surface of the abdomen is divided into four quadrants by two intersecting imaginary lines, a vertical line extending from the xiphoid process to the symphysis pubis and a horizontal line transecting the abdomen at the level of the umbilicus. In order to identify abdominal structures through percussion or palpation, the nurse should recall that the normal contents of each of the abdominal quadrants is as follows:

Left upper quadrant
Left lobe of liver
Spleen
Stomach
Left kidney
Body and tail of pancreas
Splenic flexure of colon

Left lower quadrant
Sigmoid colon
Left uterine tube
Left ovary
Left ureter

Right upper quadrant
Right lobe of liver
Gallbladder
Pylorus
Duodenum
Head of the pancreas
Upper part of right kidney
Hepatic flexure of colon

Right lower quadrant
Lower portion of right kidney
Cecum
Appendix
Ascending colon
Right uterine tube
Right ovary
Right ureter

Midline
Uterus
Urinary bladder

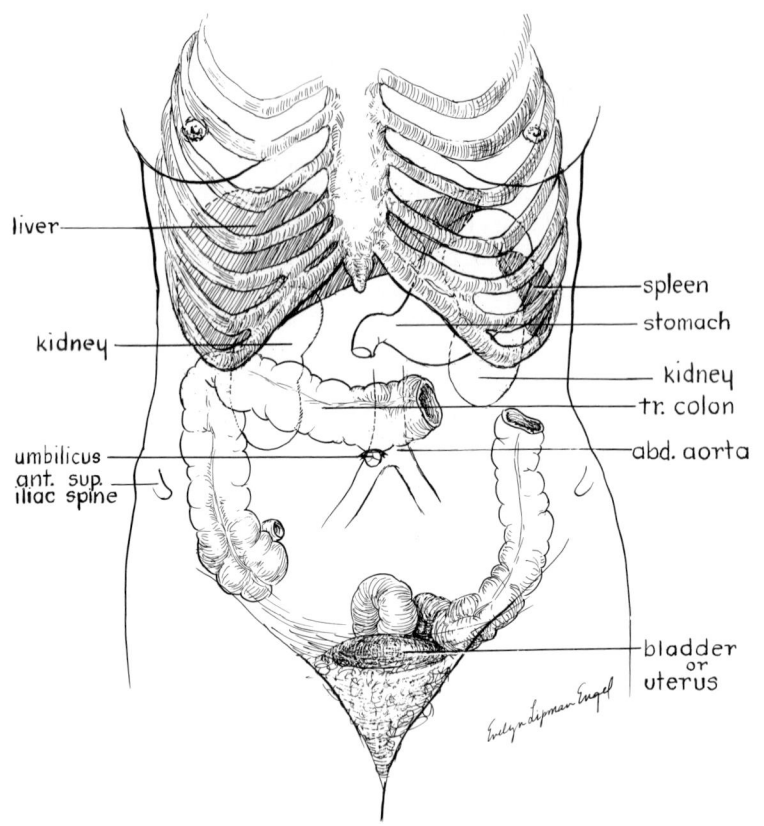

Figure 30. Position of the abdominal organs. (From Morgan, W. L., Jr., and Engel, G. L.: *The Clinical Approach to the Patient.* Philadelphia, W. B. Saunders Co., 1969.)

Inspection

Examination of the abdomen should begin with inspection, which requires both good overhead lighting and a source of oblique illumination to visualize certain subtle abnormalities in surface contour. The abdomen should be observed for symmetry, general contour, visible masses, and condition of the skin. Asymmetry of the abdomen may be more evident when the nurse stands at the foot of the examining table than when she sits at the bedside, hence the abdomen should be viewed from both viewpoints. Asymmetry may suggest the presence of such underlying masses as a greatly enlarged liver, spleen, kidney, or ovary, which should then be further investigated by percussion and palpation.

When the abdomen is viewed from the side, with the eyes on a level with the body surface, the abdominal contour can be described as flat, rounded, or scaphoid. If flat, the anterior abdominal wall extends in a straight line from the lower costal margins to the symphysis pubis. A flat abdomen is usually seen in healthy young persons of athletic build. In a rounded abdomen the anterior abdominal wall presents an outward convexity when viewed from the side. The rounded abdomen is abnormal except in young children. In older persons it is commonly due to deposition of excess subcutaneous fat or to lack of abdominal muscle tone. Generalized abdominal fullness may result from ascites or intestinal distention, which can later be differentiated by percussion and palpation. The scaphoid abdomen is one in which the anterior abdominal wall presents an outward concavity when viewed from the side. In mild degree the scaphoid abdomen may be seen in thin persons of all ages; in severe degree it is suggestive of malnutrition, dehydration, or marked weight loss.

The normally smooth contour of the anterior abdominal wall may reveal a local protrusion as a result or hernia, tumor, cyst, abscess, or distended hollow viscus. Sometimes in pyloric or intestinal obstruction, vigorous peristaltic contraction in the part proximal to the obstruction can be seen through the anterior abdominal wall. The location and shape of any protuberance, together with its character and consistency as determined by palpation, should be related to the patient's clinical history in order to diagnose the abnormality.

The skin of the abdomen may be better suited than the skin of the face, neck, and upper chest for observation of significant changes in color and character since abdominal skin is less subject to the effects of weather exposure. Therefore, the pallor of anemia, the yellowish tint of jaundice, or the bronze discoloration of Addison's disease may be more readily noted on the abdomen surface than in the facial skin. A line of increased pigmentation may appear in the midline of the abdomen from umbilicus to pubis (replacing the linea alba) during pregnancy. In addition, there are several skin lesions that are commonly found on the abdomen. Striae, white lacy stretch marks paralleling the long axis of the body, may be seen over the lower abdomen of the person who has borne children or who has experienced a rapid weight gain for some other reason. Lesions of tinea corporis and scabies are often found on the skin of the abdomen.

The normal pattern of pubic hair distribution in women is triangular, with the base of the triangle overlying the pubic bone; while in men, pubic hair distribution is roughly diamond shaped, so that hair extends over the lower abdomen coming to a point at the umbilicus. In a woman with virilizing tumor of the adrenal gland pubic hair may be distributed according to the male pattern. In a man with cirrhosis, pubic hair may be distributed according to the female pattern as a result of the liver's inability to detoxify estrogens.

Superficial veins in the abdominal wall may dilate, providing increased collateral circulation and facilitating venous return to the heart in obstruction of portal circulation (portal vein thrombosis or hepatic cirrhosis) or obstruction of the inferior or superior vena cava. The veins of the anterior abdominal wall radiate outward from the umbilicus, and the normal direction of flow is away from the umbilicus. In portal hypertension the normal direction of blood flow is maintained. In vena caval obstruction the direction of blood flow in the superficial abdominal vessels is reversed; that is, in obstruction of the superior vena cava blood flows *downward* through the venous collaterals in the upper abdomen to make its way via the umbilical veins to the inferior vena cava and thus to the heart. In obstruction of the inferior vena cava, blood flows *upward* through the venous collaterals in the lower abdomen, thence through the collaterals in the upper abdomen, to veins of the upper trunk to enter, finally, the superior vena cava.

In order to identify the pathophysiology underlying such venous abnormality, the nurse should determine the direction of blood flow in the dilated veins on both the upper and lower abdomen. This can be done by compressing the vein with both index fingers, then stripping the vein of blood for a short distance by moving one index finger away from the other for a few centimeters along the course of the vein. One of the two compressing fingers is removed, and it is observed how rapidly the emptied vein segment refills with blood. The same segment of vessel is again emptied of blood, the opposite compressing finger is released, and speed of filling is again noted. The rate of filling will be noticeably faster in the direction of blood flow.

In the patient with cirrhosis a radiating network of dilated veins may encircle the umbilicus, and small cutaneous angiomas or spider nevi may be seen on the abdomen and chest. A spider nevus consists of a central dilated arteriole from which a series of capillaries radiate. Nevi can be differentiated from petechiae by the fact that compression of the central arteriole will cause blanching of the capillaries that radiate from it.

Auscultation

Auscultation of the abdomen should be performed prior to palpation since, when the bowel wall is irritated, palpation may either decrease or increase peristalsis. In listening for evidence of peristalsis, the practitioner should apply the diaphragm of the stethoscope lightly over each of the four quadrants of the abdomen and over the epigastrium and evaluate the character, pitch, intensity, and frequency of the sounds detected. Most sounds relating to intestinal peristalsis arise from activity of the small bowel (the contents of which are fluid) and are relatively high pitched, soft, and gurgling in nature. Generally, the frequency of bowel sounds roughly matches the respiratory rate, though the number tends to increase following the ingestion of food. Because there is considerable variation from one person to another in regard to usual degree of viscerotonia, it is difficult to evaluate decreased bowel sounds. Before the nurse decides that bowel sounds are completely absent, which would indicate cessation of peristalsis such as that resulting from traumatic handling of the bowel during surgery, from peritonitis, or from decreased serum potassium levels, the nurse should listen carefully over all four abdominal quadrants for at least five minutes. Increased peristalsis is revealed by increased frequency and intensity of bowel sounds (borborygmi) and may occur in enteritis or small bowel obstruction. In bacterial or viral enteritis, bowel sounds may be loud and continuous. In bowel obstruction there will typically be rushes of peristalsis yielding a loud, high-pitched, metallic tinkling sound alternating with periods of silence in which the exhausted intestinal musculature recovers its contractility.

A peritoneal friction rub, or rough grating sound created by the rubbing of parietal peritoneum over an area of inflamed visceral peritoneum, may sometimes be heard over the lower left costal margin in infarction of the spleen or in the right or left upper quadrant over a pointing amebic liver abscess.

Occasionally auscultation of the abdomen will reveal a bruit, or purring, blowing, rasping, or humming sound, which occurs during cardiac systole and represents abnormal vibrations created by the flow of blood through narrowed or occluded arteries. A bruit heard over the epigastrium may be due to an aneurysm of the abdominal aorta. A bruit heard in the flank or in the costovertebral angle may be due to sclerotic narrowing of the renal artery. Since bruits are typically soft, high-pitched sounds they are easily missed when auscultation is carried out in a room with a high level of background noise. The nurse should be particularly alert for the existence of bruits in patients with known arteriosclerosis or hypertension.

Percussion

Abdominal percussion is used principally to determine whether the liver or spleen is enlarged and whether abdominal enlargement is due to gaseous distention of the bowel or to accumulation of free fluid in the peritoneal cavity.

It is advisable for the practitioner to follow a routine sequence in percussing the abdomen, examining structures in first one quadrant and then the next in clockwise progression in order not to overlook significant pathology. Beginning with the right upper quadrant the examiner should percuss down the lower right anterior thorax to locate the upper limit of hepatic dullness (usually at about the fifth to seventh interspace), then continue percussing downward until liver dullness is replaced by tympany (usually at the lower costal margin). If the upper border of the liver is percussed at the fifth, sixth, or seventh interspace and the lower border extends below the lower costal margin (that is, if the liver diameter is more than 10 cm.), the organ is enlarged. Normally, the liver descends from two to four centimeters on inspiration, so apparent liver size can be checked by percussing upper and lower liver borders during full inspiration and full expiration to determine whether and how much each border moves.

Similar percussion over the left anterior chest should reveal a change from normal lung resonance to tympany over the splenic flexure of the colon at about the ninth interspace. Dullness in this area might result from enlargement of the spleen, enlargement of the left kidney, or even marked enlargement of the left lobe of the liver.

Percussion in the epigastric region slightly to the left of the midline will reveal an area of tympany over the gastric air bubble. Enlargement of the spleen or of the left lobe of the liver will displace the area of gastric tympany downward.

Unless the bladder is distended with urine, the rest of the abdomen should be tympanitic to percussion, as a result of the presence of gas in the small and large intestine. Percussion over any visible mass will enable the practitioner to differentiate distended loops of bowel (tympanitic) from solid tumor masses (dull) and accumulations of peritoneal fluid (dull and shifting with changes in position).

Palpation

Abdominal palpation should be carried out with the patient in the supine position. Since abdominal muscle tension renders palpation of viscera difficult, the practitioner should encourage the patient to relax by diverting him conversationally or by placing a hand on his arm or shoulder in a reassuring gesture. If the patient seems unusually tense, he might be advised to flex his hips and knees slightly and to breathe deeply with his mouth open in order to achieve the desired muscle relaxation.

First, light palpation with the palmar aspects of the fingers should be used to make a general survey of the four quadrants of the abdomen. Here, the practitioner's primary purpose is to determine whether tenderness or increased muscle tone is present, but it may also be possible to detect severe organomegaly or large tumor masses by light palpation. Additionally, the soft, gentle pressure of light palpation tends to relax abdominal muscles, thereby facilitating later deep palpation. In investigating the character of the abdominal wall the practitioner should palpate comparable areas on either side of the body in order to identify any focal areas of tenderness or increased tension. Light stroking or scratching of the abdominal skin in one area may result in sharp pain over a circumscribed area of inflamed peritoneum elsewhere in the abdomen.

In deep palpation of the abdomen the nurse should explore last any area of tenderness identified by history or light palpation, but should otherwise move from one quadrant to another in clockwise rotation. By starting in a pain-free area the practitioner demonstrates her concern for the patient's comfort and maintains as long as possible the muscle relaxation engendered by light palpation. Although the degree of pressure required for deep palpation tends to decrease the tactile sensitivity of the examiner's fingertips, this disadvantage can be offset somewhat by placing the extended fingers of one hand against the abdominal wall in relaxed fashion and covering them with the extended fingers of the other hand, which are then used to press the passive examining fingers into contact with the structures to be explored (Fig. 31).

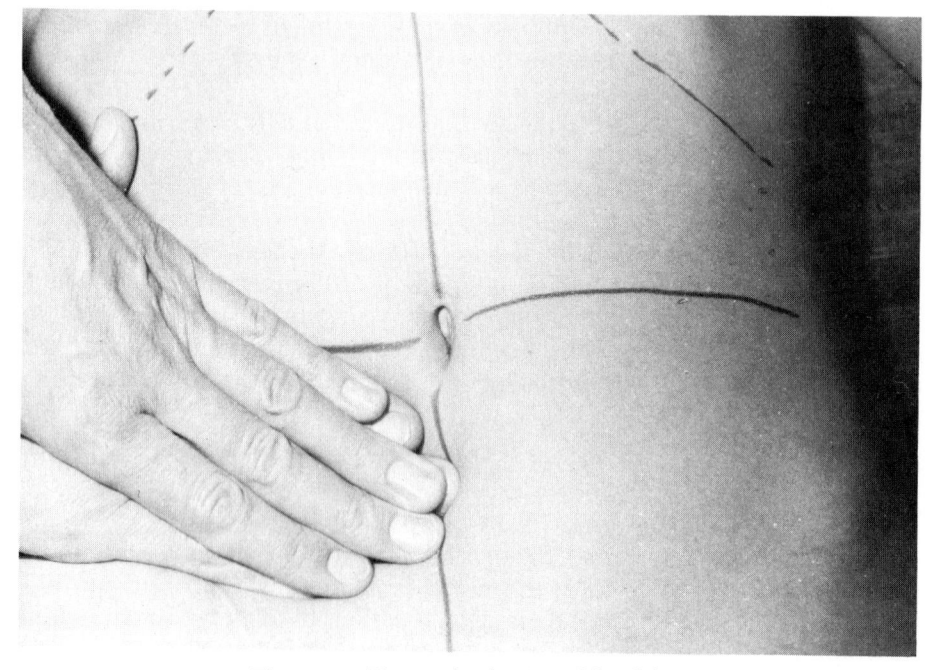

Figure 31. Bimanual palpation of the abdomen.

Throughout deep palpation the practitioner should check for tenderness and abdominal rigidity. The evocation of dull pain is suggestive of visceral pathology, while sharp pain is more likely to derive from involvement of such somatic structures as the parietal peritoneum, abdominal muscles, or skin.

A specific type of discomfort termed "rebound tenderness" indicates inflammation of an area of peritoneum overlying an inflamed viscus, such as an infected appendix. The phenomenon can be tested for by applying firm pressure to a part of the abdominal wall considerably removed from the area of discomfort, then suddenly releasing the pressure. If rebound tenderness is present, sharp pain is felt in the diseased area of the abdomen when the pressure on the distant point is *released*.

If the examination is impeded by abdominal muscle rigidity, palpation may be facilitated by instructing the patient to breathe deeply in and out, then maintaining pressure on the examining hand throughout both cycles of respiration. Since the abdominal muscles tend to relax somewhat during expiration, the examiner's fingers will be allowed to advance slightly with each expiration. Then, if pressure is not released during subsequent inspiration, still further penetration of the muscular barrier can be achieved in each successive expiration.

When palpating any abdominal mass the practitioner should note its position, size, shape, consistency, surface characteristics, sensitivity, and mobility. Several abdominal organs are normally palpable in the subject of average weight with a relaxed abdominal wall. The liver, right kidney, abdominal aorta, descending colon, and sigmoid are usually palpable in the healthy individual. The cecum, urinary bladder, and lumbar spine may sometimes be palpated in the normal subject. Generally, the stomach, spleen, gall bladder, small intestine, and transverse colon cannot be palpated unless they are diseased.

Liver

To palpate the liver the practitioner should stand at the patient's right side, place her left hand under the patient's right flank with the extended fingers parallel to the ribs and lateral to the paraspinous muscles, and lift upward or push the liver toward the anterior abdominal wall, then place her right hand flat on the anterior abdominal wall with the fingers parallel to the long axis of the body in the midclavicular line and below the percussed level of liver dullness (Fig. 32A). While exerting firm pressure on the abdominal wall with her right hand the practitioner should instruct the patient to take a deep breath. On descent of the diaphragm with inspiration the liver edge will be forced downward and, if palpable, will be felt as a firm structure which slips under the examining fingertips, deflecting them upward. The ability to palpate the liver below the costal margin on inspiration does not necessarily indicate hepatic enlargement, since the organ is typically low lying in thin, visceroptotic subjects and the liver tends to be deflected downward in patients with emphysema or with massive pleural effusion.

When the liver edge is palpated the practitioner should note whether it is moderately firm and sharp, as is characteristic of the normal liver, or blunt, as in passive congestion of the liver, or nodular, as in portal cirrhosis. The liver may be tender to palpation as a result of acute inflammatory disorders.

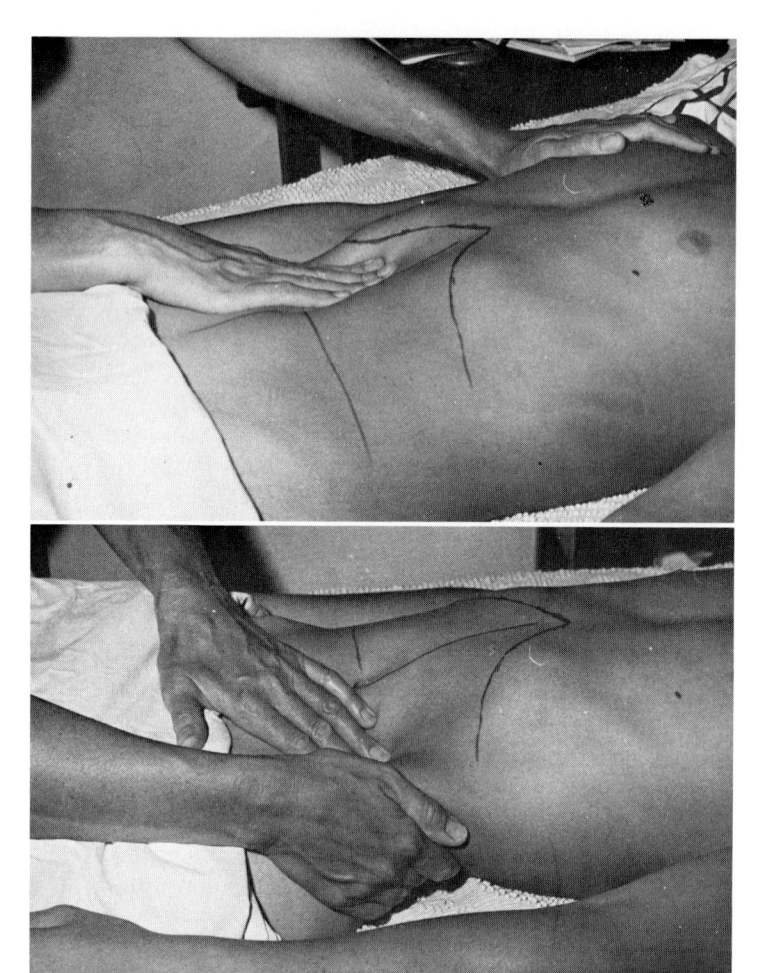

Figure 32A. Position of the examiner's hands in palpation of the liver.

Figure 32B. Position of the examiner's hands in palpation of the left kidney.

Gall Bladder

The normal gall bladder is not palpable, but the gall bladder that is distended because of cystic duct or common duct obstruction may be felt as a pear-shaped, fluctuant mass underneath the liver edge in the midclavicular line. In acute cholecystitis the gall bladder, if enlarged, will be tender to palpation.

Kidneys

Because the upper poles of both kidneys touch the diaphragm, the kidneys descend on inspiration. To palpate the right kidney, which is more easily felt than the left since it is more low lying, the practitioner should place her left hand in the patient's right flank and her right hand on the anterior abdominal wall in the midclavicular line at the level of the umbilicus. As the patient inhales deeply the practitioner applies moderate pressure to the anterior abdominal wall. By slightly increasing pressure with the examining hand as the patient begins to exhale, the practitioner may feel the kidney slip upward between her two hands as the diaphragm ascends. To examine the left kidney the practitioner should employ the same procedure, reaching across the abdomen to place her right hand under the patient's left flank, and using her left hand to palpate the left kidney through the anterior abdominal wall as the patient takes a deep breath (Fig. 32B).

Normally, the lower pole of the right kidney is palpable, but the left kidney is palpable only in very thin persons with poorly developed abdominal musculature. Occasionally the kidney will be tender to palpation as a result of acute inflammatory change. Since, however, it may be difficult or impossible to palpate the kidneys in obese subjects or those with abdominal muscle rigidity, renal tenderness can be looked for by applying a light blow with the closed fist over the costovertebral area.

Spleen

In palpating for the spleen the practitioner should, while standing at the patient's right side, place the fingers of her right hand under the eleventh and twelfth ribs posteriorly and gently insert the fingers of her left hand under the left anterior costal margin lateral to the midclavicular line (Fig. 33). While the patient inhales deeply the practitioner gently lifts forward the patient's lower rib cage with her right hand and applies gentle pressure with her left hand. The spleen, if palpable, will be felt as a firm mass, which taps against the examiner's finger at the height of inspiration. In the adult the spleen is not palpable unless enlarged. If the spleen is massively enlarged, it may extend into the left lower quadrant or into the right side of the abdomen. Therefore, if a large, firm mass is encountered in examining the left upper quadrant, the

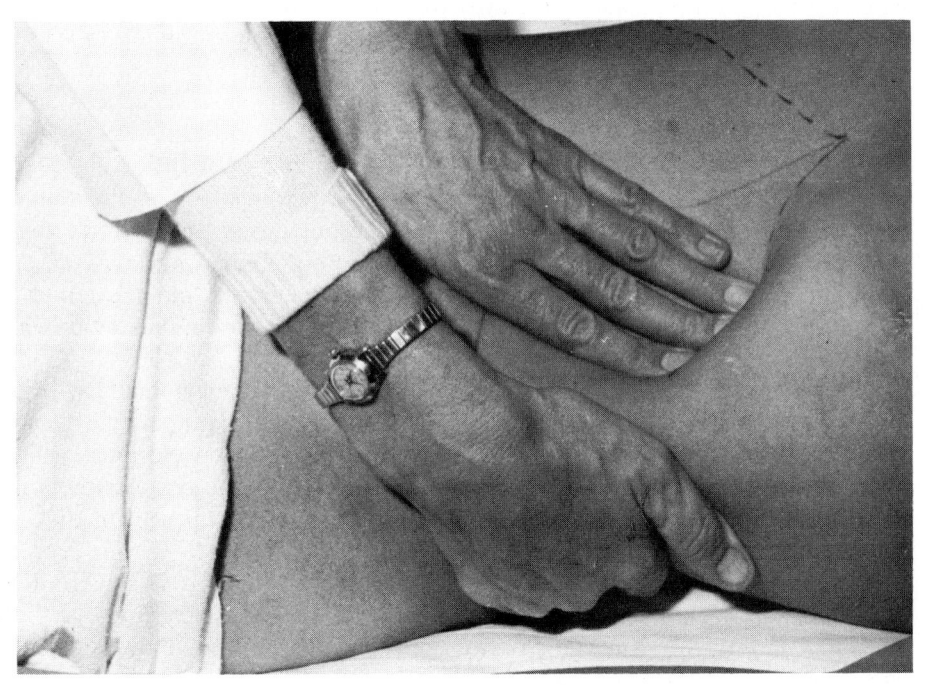

Figure 33. Palpation of the spleen.

practitioner's left hand should be moved lower and lower and farther toward the right side of the abdomen in an attempt to locate the splenic border.

If the spleen is not felt with the patient in the supine position, he should be turned to his right side with his upper leg flexed, and the practitioner should again use bimanual palpation to search for the organ. In this position gravity may cause the spleen to drop forward to a point where deep inspiration will make it accessible to the examiner's fingers. When the spleen is palpated the practitioner should record its location, size in centimeters, shape, consistency, surface characteristics, and sensitivity to pressure. The spleen that is enlarged due to infection or infarction is tender to palpation.

If the spleen cannot be palpated, it may be possible to approximate its size and shape by percussion. The spleen is best percussed with the patient lying on his right side, in which position the spleen will fall forward of the stomach and colon. In attempting to outline the spleen the practitioner should percuss the patient's left lower thorax, left upper abdominal quadrant, epigastrium, and right upper quadrant in an oblique direction. The normal spleen is identified as an area of dullness of about seven centimeters in length under the left lower ribs.

Stomach

Percussion over the stomach air bubble in the upper part of the stomach will produce a fairly loud tympanic sound that is lower in pitch than that heard over gas-filled intestine. Following a meal, percussion over the mixture of liquid and solid food components in the body of the stomach will yield a dull sound similar to that heard over any fluid-filled sac. If it has been some time since the patient has eaten, the area of gastric tympany will be roughly half-moon or crescent shaped, following the normal contour of the empty stomach. Either a large left pleural effusion, enlargement of the left lobe of the liver, or splenomegaly may displace the area of gastric tympany downward and medially. Because the gastric musculature adjusts gastric capacity to the volume of food stored, and since there is considerable individual variation in gastric muscle tone, the size of the gastric air bubble is of little significance unless the stomach is massively distended. In gastric obstruction the stomach may be grossly distended to the point that the outline of the organ is visible through the anterior abdominal wall. In addition, vigorous waves of peristalsis can often be seen to sweep across the upper left quadrant and the epigastrium, proceeding from the left or fundic side to the right or pyloric side of the stomach.

Inflammatory changes in the peritoneum overlying the stomach will give rise to tenderness on gastric palpation. In both the infant and adult with pyloric obstruction peristaltic activity may be audible even without a stethoscope and rocking the patient from side to side will elicit a succussion splash as the accumulation of excessive gastric content strikes the wall of that distended organ.

Because the pancreas is retroperitoneal and most of it lies behind the stomach, it is rarely palpable on physical examination. Occasionally, however, in a very thin individual a tumor or cyst of the pancreas may be palpated as a mass in the right epigastrium.

Abdominal Aorta

Except in the obese individual, pulsations of the abdominal aorta, which overlies the bony spine, can be felt in the midline of the upper abdomen down to the level of the umbilicus, at which point the aorta bifurcates into right and left iliac arteries. To palpate the aorta the thumb and fingers of the examining hand should be held slightly apart and parallel to the midline in the epigastric region. There, as the patient breathes deeply in and out, the examining fingers are advanced further and further through the anterior abdominal tissues as the patient's abdominal muscles relax increasingly with each successive expiration. When the practitioner's thumb and fingers finally span the aorta, the width of the vessel and the character of its wall should be evaluated. Severe arteriosclerosis may produce a rigid aortic wall with nodular plaques scattered along its course. Occasionally, severe arteriosclerosis may so weaken the vessel wall as to produce an aortic aneurysm, giving rise to a pulsatile abdominal mass that is palpable in the upper abdomen, slightly to the left of the midline. Any pulsating mass should be carefully explored to determine whether the pulsations spread equally in all directions, which would be characteristic of an aortic aneurysm, or are transmitted only in an anterior direction, which would suggest a tumor mass overlying the aorta and thrust forward with each aortic pulsation.

Small Intestine

Normally, the small intestine is not palpable. Rarely, an inflammatory or tumor mass may be palpated in the ileocecal region. Obstruction of the small bowel causes the portion of the bowel proximal to the obstruction to become distended with gas and fluid. Such distention is usually first seen in the lower abdomen since the majority of the small bowel lies in the pelvis. A distended portion of the intestine is usually tender to palpation.

Large Intestine

Of the large intestine only the cecum and the sigmoid flexure are normally palpable. Other portions of the colon are palpable only if diseased, distended, or filled with fecal material. To palpate the colon the palmar surface of the fingers should be placed on the anterior abdominal wall over the normal course of the bowel and at right angles to its length. Firm pressure should then be exerted against the bowel so as to roll it against the lateral abdominal wall (or liver in the case of the transverse colon). When this is done, the cecum can often be felt as a soft, compressible, gas- and fluid-filled, slightly movable tube in the right lower quadrant and the sigmoid is felt as a more firm, feces-filled, slightly movable tube in the left lower quadrant. Palpation of a firm mass in the right lower quadrant would be suggestive of a neoplasm of the cecum or ascending colon. Tenderness to palpation in the region of the cecum may be suggestive of terminal ileitis or appendicitis. A hard, irregular tumor in the region of the sigmoid may be due either to impacted feces, in which case the mass is moveable, or to malignant tumor, in which case the mass may be fixed to surrounding tissue.

The appendix is the most frequent site of intra-abdominal inflammation. The symptoms of appendicitis vary with the position of the appendix. If the appendix lies in the normal position, palpation will usually reveal muscle guarding in the right lower quadrant, tenderness at McBurney's point (a little over halfway between the umbilicus and the anterior superior iliac spine), rebound tenderness, and a mass in the right iliac fossa. If the appendix lies in the pelvis, pain may be predominantly suprapubic.

In diverticulitis there may be tenderness to palpation over that portion of the bowel in which the inflamed diverticuli are found (most commonly the sigmoid and descending colon). Abscess formation in an acutely inflamed section of bowel may give rise to a palpable, warm tumor mass.

Urinary Bladder

The normal bladder, when empty, cannot be palpated through the anterior abdominal wall. When distended with urine, however, the bladder can be percussed and palpated as a smooth, firm mass in the midline over the symphysis pubis. When markedly distended, as in the patient with urinary obstruction due to prostatic hypertrophy, the bladder may be visible as a convex swelling in the lower abdomen. Manual pressure over an acutely distended bladder will usually stimulate a desire to urinate. The patient with urinary retention (as in prostatism) may experience no such sense of urinary urgency but his suprapubic swelling will be relieved by catheterization.

Hernia

Palpation, as well as inspection, is used in diagnosing different types of hernias. The musculofascial defect underlying the hernia may be due either to a congenital weakness or to the strain of increased intra-abdominal pressure. If the abdominal wall defect is of sufficient size, abdominal fat, peritoneum, or a loop of bowel may enter the hernia sac. At first, these structures may move into the sac on coughing or straining and disappear back into the abdomen when the patient relaxes in reclining position—and the hernia is said to be reducible. An incarcerated or strangulated hernia is one which cannot be reduced; that is, the contents of the hernia sac cannot be made to disappear within the abdomen on gentle pressure. If in the strangulated hernia there is compression of the bowel lumen and impairment of circulation to the tissue, gangrene of the bowel will result and symptoms of bowel obstruction will develop rapidly.

An umbilical hernia, when seen in a newborn infant, is usually the result of a congenital muscle weakness and may disappear spontaneously within the first year of life. Typically, the umbilical hernia is a small, soft swelling just above the umbilicus that appears during crying, coughing, or straining and is easily reduced with simple pressure. In the adult, umbilical hernias are most common in patients with numerous pregnancies, marked obesity, or ascites.

Diastasis recti, or separation of the abdominal rectus muscle in the midline, is often seen in multiparous women and may be associated with an umbilical hernia. The separation can best be observed by directing the patient to rise from the recumbent position without using her arms; this action will cause contraction of the two halves of the muscle with bulging of abdominal tissues through the muscular defect.

Incisional hernias, which are a more frequent complication of vertical than of horizontal muscle splitting incisions, are caused by infection or impaired healing of a surgical wound. Palpation of an incisional hernia may reveal several defects in the surgical scar with septa of intact tissue dividing the apertures. When an abdominal scar is present and palpation reveals no underlying muscular defect, the patient should be asked to cough. If a hernia is present, an increase in intra-abdominal pressure may cause a bulge to appear in the incisional line.

Inguinal hernias, much the most common type in males, are classified as indirect or direct. An indirect inguinal hernia, most often seen in male infants and young adults, is one in which a peritoneal sac (which may or may not contain a loop of bowel) penetrates the internal or abdominal inguinal ring, traverses the inguinal canal, emerges through the subcutaneous or external inguinal ring, and may descend into the scrotum. A direct inguinal hernia is one in which the peritoneal sac (which may contain a loop of bowel) penetrates the abdominal wall directly at the location of the external inguinal ring. Direct hernias are most common in males over 40 years of age and are due to an abrupt increase in intra-abdominal pressure in a thin, visceroptotic individual.

Occasionally, an inguinal hernia will be visible when the patient is in the recumbent position. More frequently, it can be observed when the patient is standing. In order to palpate for hernia, the nurse should direct the patient to stand with his ipsilateral leg slightly flexed and his weight borne on the opposite leg. The practitioner should, by inserting her index finger low into the scrotum, invaginate the scrotal skin so as to advance the examining finger through the external inguinal ring and, if possible, 4 to 5 centimeters through the inguinal canal to the internal inguinal ring (Fig. 34). The patient is then asked to bear down. If pressure is felt against the finger tip an indirect hernia is present. If pressure is exerted against the side of the finger, a direct hernia exists.

A femoral hernia, or protrusion of a peritoneal sac through the opening in the abdominal wall through which the femoral artery passes in entering the thigh, is most common in middle-aged women. The femoral hernia is iden-

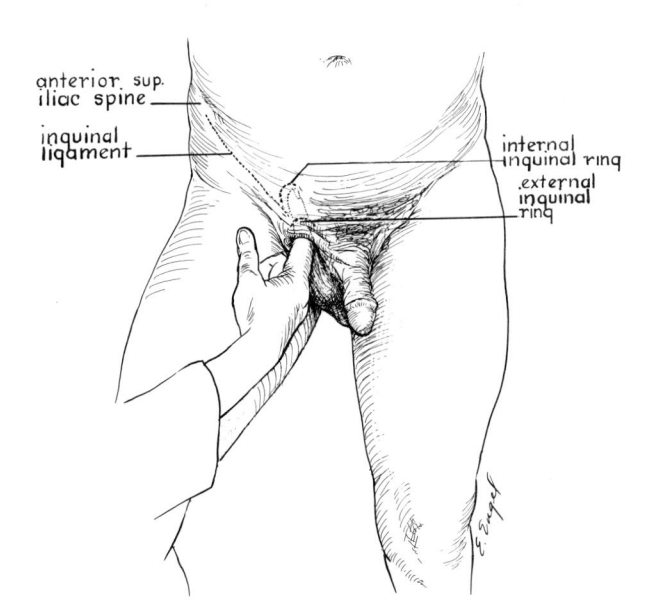

Figure 34. Palpation for an inguinal hernia. (From Morgan, W. L., Jr., and Engel, G. L.: *The Clinical Approach to the Patient.* Philadelphia, W. B. Saunders Co., 1969.)

tified as a palpable swelling in the groin just medial to the femoral artery. Although a femoral hernia may resemble a direct inguinal hernia if it curves upward over the inguinal ligament, on careful palpation the neck of the femoral hernia will be felt below the inguinal ligament.

Section V. Examination of the Pelvis

RECTAL EXAMINATION

Although most patients find the rectal examination embarrassing and uncomfortable, it should routinely be included as part of the physical examination since 75 per cent of rectosigmoid carcinomas can be diagnosed by digital examination of the rectum. If the male patient is bed bound, he may be placed in the left Sims position or the knee-chest position for the rectal examination. If he can stand, he should bend forward over a waist-high examining table. In the female patient, the rectal examination is usually carried out in the lithotomy position, immediately following the pelvic examination.

In preparing for the rectal examination, the practitioner should assist the patient to assume the desired position, drape him so as to minimize exposure and prevent chilling, provide an additional light source if needed, and don a rectal glove. The examination should begin by spreading the buttocks to inspect the perianal region for discolorations, inflammations, skin lesions, scars, fissures, fistulas, or hemorrhoids. The location, size, color, consistency, and sensitivity of any lesion should be noted and later recorded.

Lesions that may be encountered include skin excoriations resulting from scratching in pruritus ani, flat hypertrophic papules in secondary syphilis, moist, wartlike condylomata acuminata, radiating anal cracks or fissures, small perianal abscesses, and thrombosed external hemorrhoids.

After the anal orifice has been inspected for skin tags, hemorrhoids, and rectal prolapse, the patient should be asked to bear down and the anus again examined for prolapse. Next, surgical lubricant jelly is applied to the gloved index finger, which is then used to apply gentle pressure against the anus. When after a few seconds the anal sphincter relaxes, the examining finger should be slowly and gently inserted through the anal sphincter (Fig. 35). After noting the tone of the anal sphincter, the practitioner should slightly flex her examining finger and then rotate it so as to palpate the anterior, posterior, and lateral walls of the rectum for internal hemorrhoids, polyps, or tumors. After the lower portion of the rectum has been palpated, the patient is asked to bear down, by which maneuver a higher, previously inaccessible rectal mass may be brought within reach of the examining finger.

Finally, in the male patient, the examining finger should be directed anteriorly to palpate the prostate. The prostate can be felt by the palmar aspect of the distal phalanx of the fully extended index finger. Normally, the gland is firm, small, and rubbery in consistency, and presents as two symmetrical lateral lobes separated by a median furrow. If the gland is hard and irregular, a malignancy may be present. In prostatitis, the gland is soft and tender. With prostatic abscess there is unilocular pain and swelling.

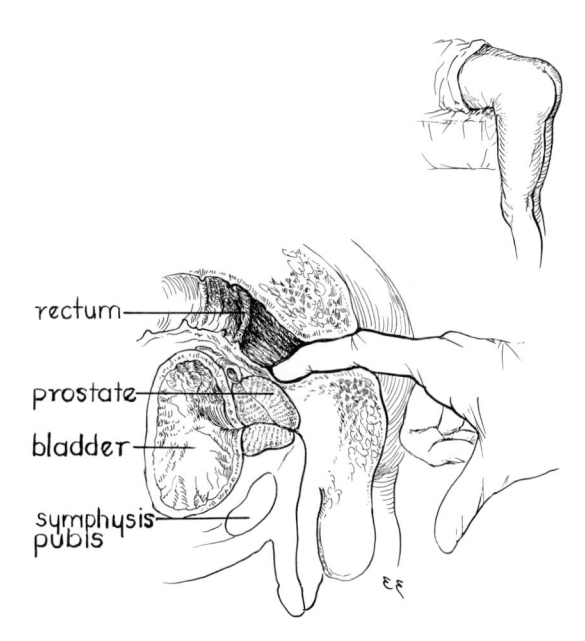

Figure 35. Digital examination of the rectum in the male patient. (From Morgan, W. L., Jr., and Engel, G. L.: *The Clinical Approach to the Patient.* Philadelphia, W. B. Saunders Co., 1969.)

In the female, the cervix can be felt as a small, round mass adjacent to the anterior wall of the rectum.

EXAMINATION OF THE MALE GENITALIA

Examination of the male genitalia should begin with observation of the amount and distribution of pubic hair, which in the male should extend upward from the pubis as a triangle with its apex at the umbilicus. Next, the practitioner should inspect and palpate the inguinal lymph nodes, which are often enlarged in infections and malignancies of the perineal area.

Observation may reveal that the genitals are abnormal in size. An unusually small penis and scrotum may result from hypopituitarism, mumps orchitis, or undescended testis. An unusually large penis and scrotum may result from an adrenal tumor, edema of cardiac failure, or obstruction of local lymph channels.

In examining the penis, it should be noted whether the foreskin is absent or present. If present, the foreskin should be easily retracted. On retracting the foreskin, smegma, a cheese-like secretion of sebaceous glands, may be noted in the coronal sulcus of the unclean patient. Phimosis, or narrowing of the preputial opening so that the foreskin cannot be pushed back over the glans, may result from a congenital defect but is more often due to infection.

Inflammation of the glans penis may be due to either venereal or nonspecific infection but commonly occurs in a person with poor personal hygiene in whom filth is allowed to collect under the foreskin. If inflammation is severe the mucosa of the glans is swollen, erythematous, and excoriated, and purulent material collects around the corona.

While the prepuce is retracted, the urethral orifice should be inspected. In hypospadias the external meatus is located on the lower or ventral surface of the penis. In epispadias, a condition which is often associated with exstrophy of the bladder, the urethra opens on the dorsum of the penis. Both deformities require surgical correction.

The presence of purulent discharge at the urethral opening may suggest gonorrhea. A syphilitic chancre, a shallow, painless indurated ulcer with clearly defined border, is usually found just behind the glans or on the prepuce and may be associated with an enlarged inguinal lymph node. Condylomata acuminata or venereal warts are friable, moist, erythematous papillomas of viral etiology that may appear on both the glans and the shaft of the penis as well as on the scrotum and perianal skin. Condylomata acuminata are most likely to occur in persons with excessive preputial secretion and poor personal hygiene.

The scrotal sac is normally pear shaped, with a median furrow traversing the structure vertically and with the skin arranged in transverse folds which permit elongation and shortening of the scrotum with increases and decreases in environmental temperature. Normally, the left side of the scrotum is larger than the right. Each testis should be palpated separately between the thumb and first two fingers. The normal testis is firm, smooth, and freely moveable within the scrotal sac. The epididymis is a crescent-shaped structure that is normally palpable on the posterolateral surface of the testis, and the spermatic cord can be palpated as it extends upward from the epididymis to the external inguinal ring. The testes, which are located intra-abdominally during fetal life, normally descend into the scrotum shortly before birth. In cryptorchidism, or failure of the testis to descend into the scrotum, it may be possible to palpate the small undescended testis within the inguinal canal.

Normally, the two testes are of the same size and rubbery consistency. Atrophy of one testis may result from trauma or from mumps orchitis. A hard irregular testis or nontender testicular lump may suggest a malignancy. Occasionally the scrotum may be considerably enlarged by the presence of a varicocele, or mass of dilated and engorged veins. The varicocele feels like a bag of worms above and behind the testis and may cause the patient to complain of a dull aching sensation in the scrotal area. A varicocele is best observed with the patient in the standing position, since the dilated vessels tend to empty when the patient is supine.

Scrotal enlargement may sometimes be caused by hydrocele, or marked accumulation of serous fluid in the tunica vaginalis of the testis. A rapidly developing hydrocele is usually a result of inflammation of the testis or epididymis. A slowly developing hydrocele may occur without apparent cause. In hydrocele, scrotal enlargement is painless, the mass is fluctuant, and scrotal skin appears tight and shiny.

Acute epididymitis is a common disorder and results from direct or hematogenous spread of bacteria from urinary tract infections or from prostatitis. The scrotal skin overlying the epididymis may be red and warm to touch, the epididymis may be enlarged, and there may be marked tenderness to palpation in the posterolateral aspect of the testis.

A rectal examination should be performed to investigate the size, consistency, and surface contour of the prostate gland.

EXAMINATION OF THE FEMALE GENITALIA

Before beginning the pelvic examination, the practitioner should ascertain the patient's previous experience with and attitude toward the procedure with some such question as, "Have you ever had an internal or pelvic examination—an examination of your female parts?" If the patient's answer indicates any fear or reluctance toward the procedure the practitioner should explain that, while the examination will cause some discomfort, it will provide much needed information, and then she should describe briefly what the examination consists of. Under these circumstances, most patients will allow the practitioner to proceed.

In order that vaginal discharge can be properly evaluated and that cytological studies and bacteriological smears and cultures not be interfered with, the patient should not douche during the 24 hours preceding a pelvic examination. So that the rectal approach can be used to investigate the cul-de-sac, the rectum should be emptied shortly before the examination is begun. In preparation for the examination, the practitioner should assemble the needed instruments and supplies, have the patient empty her bladder, place her in dorsolithotomy position with her feet in stirrups and her buttocks at the edge of the examining table, cover her abdomen and legs with a drape sheet, adjust the light source, and don sterile gloves.

The perineal area should be inspected for amount and distribution of pubic hair, skin lesions, swelling or discoloration of the labia, and evidence of abnormal vaginal discharge. The normal female pattern of pubic hair distribution is that of an inverted triangle, the base of which overlies the symphysis pubis. Such lesions as excoriations, condylomata, chancres, and ulcerations may occasionally be seen on the labia minora, labia majora, or the surrounding skin. In aged females, atrophy and fibrosis of vulvar structures may cause dryness and itching, which are revealed by skin excoriations resulting from repeated scratching.

In the virgin, the labia majora are usually full and rounded and meet in the midline. In the multipara, the labia majora are thinner and are separated so that the labia minora are visible. Palpation of a tender and fluctuant tumor mass in the posterior portion of the labia majora would suggest a Bartholin's gland abscess, which is often gonococcal in origin. By spreading the labia majora, the practitioner can inspect the clitoris, labia minora, and fourchette. An unusual enlargement of the clitoris may indicate the masculinizing effect of an ovarian or adrenal tumor. In the person with poor personal hygiene, an accumulation of smegma may be noted in the furrow between the labia majora and the labia minora. Redness of the urethral meatus indicates urethritis. Reddening and excoriation of the entire vestibule is characteristic of pruritis vulvae due to monilial or trichomonas vaginitis. Purulent secretion may sometimes be seen at the external urethral meatus in the patient with gonorrhea.

Rarely, there may be no opening in the hymen, or membranous fold which partially covers the vaginal orifice in the virgin. Obstruction of the vaginal orifice would, of course, produce complications with the onset of menstruation. Scars in the fourchette probably represent the healing of lacerations associated with childbirth. Second degree lacerations, with injury to

104 CHAPTER 3 – SECTION V

perineal fascia and levator ani muscle, may weaken the perineum so as to cause gaping of the introitus.

In the patient with a rectocele or a cystocele the posterior or anterior rectal wall may bulge into the introitus. In uterine prolapse the cervix may be visible at the vaginal orifice or may even protrude below it.

In the patient with a marital introitus, a speculum examination should be performed. A bivalve speculum is lubricated with water (any other lubricant will interfere with the Papanicolaou smear), the perineum is depressed, and the speculum is inserted into the vagina at an oblique angle and with the blades closed, so as not to exert pressure on the urethral meatus or urethra. When the speculum is completely inserted, the handle should be rotated downward and the blades separated in order to visualize the cervix and the vaginal vault (Figs. 36, 37, 38). At this point in the examination, materials should be obtained for the Papanicolaou cytological study for cancer detection and microbiological smears or cultures of vaginal secretions. (See Chapter 5 for details of this technique.)

Normally, the uterus is anteflexed and the cervix is directed posteriorly. In patients with uterine retroversion, the cervix will be directed anteriorly. The cervix is normally 2 to 3 centimeters in diameter and protrudes into the upper vagina approximately the same distance. The external cervical os is seen as a small round dimple in the middle of the cervix in the nulliparous woman and as a longitudinal slit or a stellate opening in the multipara. In premenopausal women it is normal for the cervix to be covered with clear mucus which is greatest in amount at the time of ovulation. The normal cer-

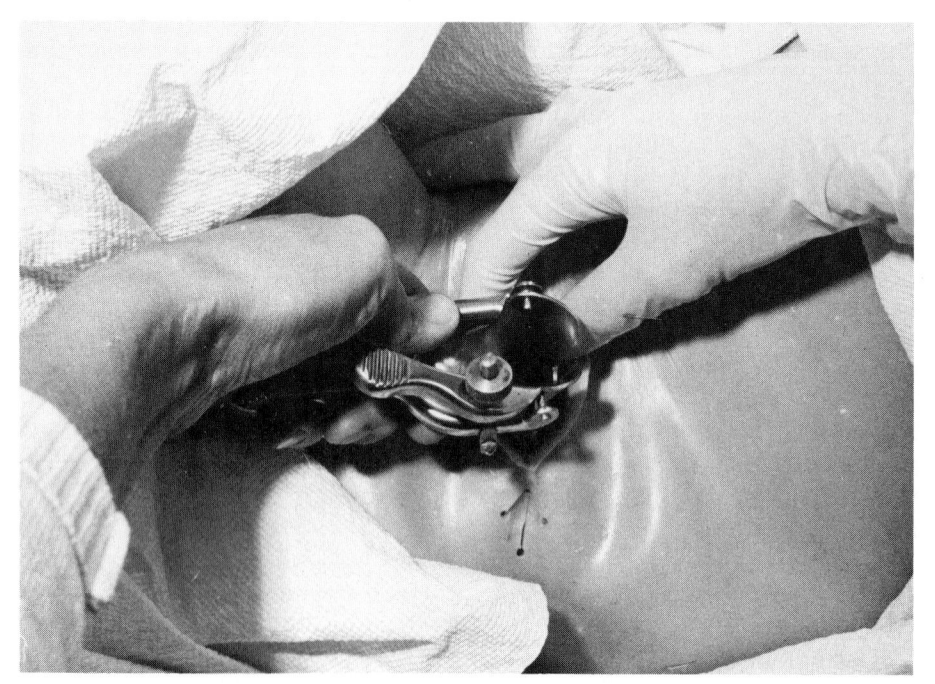

Figure 36. Insertion of the vaginal speculum.

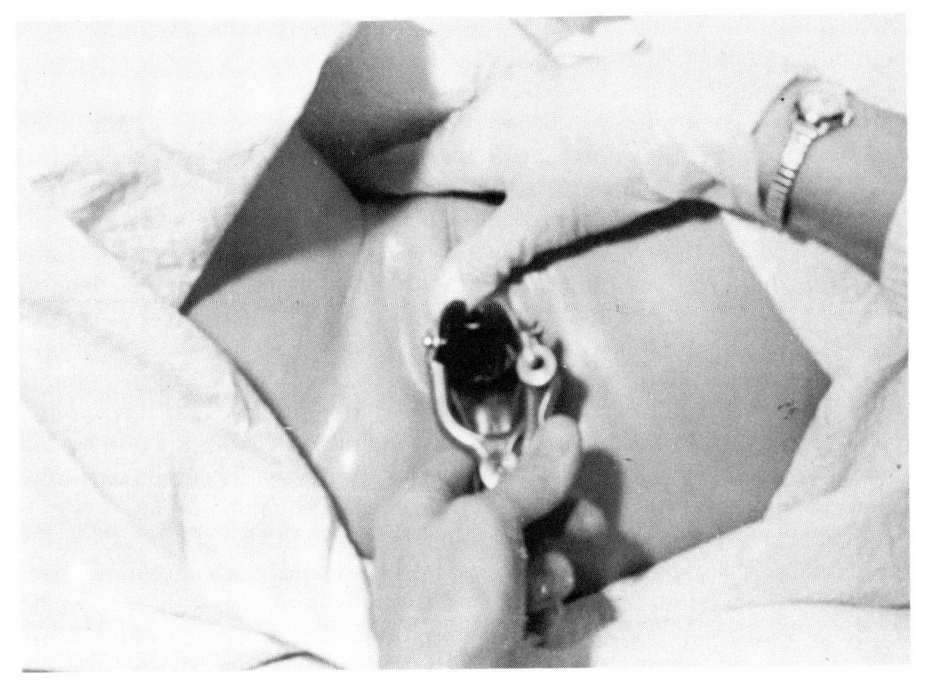

Figure 37. Insertion of the vaginal speculum.

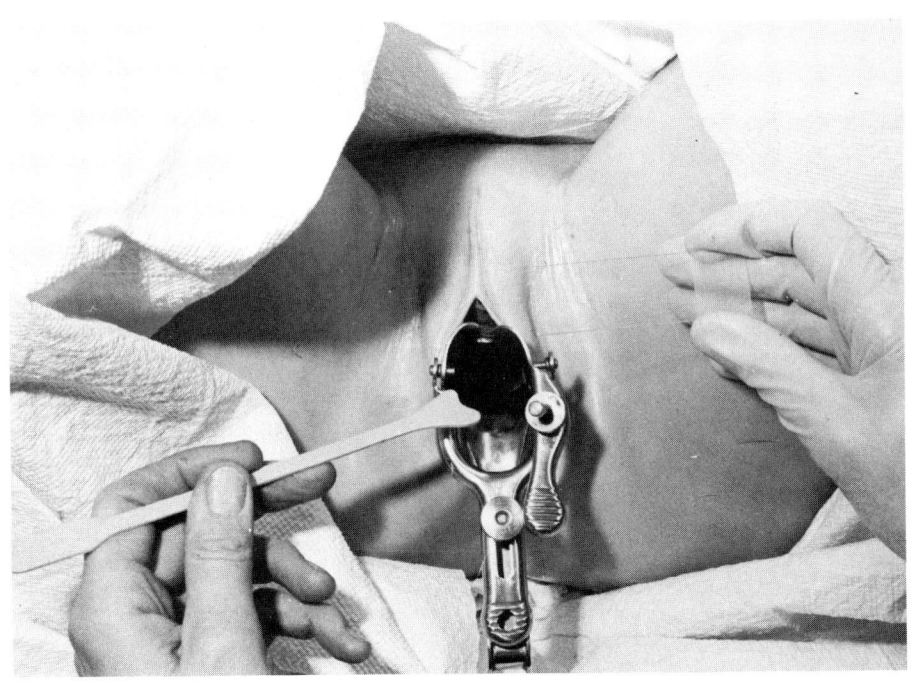

Figure 38. Equipment for obtaining a cervical smear for cytological study.

vical mucosa is pale pink. In pregnancy the cervix becomes dusky blue. A reddening of the mucosa is seen in cervicitis. There may be exudation of purulent material from the external os in endocervical or intrauterine infections. Cervical polyps are bright-red, globular structures which protrude through the cervical os and tend to bleed easily when traumatized. Early cervical carcinoma may appear as a bright-red erodent lesion with an irregular margin. Advanced cervical carcinoma usually appears as a fungating or cauliflower-like mass, which is friable and bleeds easily.

The lateral walls of the vagina should be examined while the speculum is in place. The normal vaginal mucosa is pink, smooth, and glistening but may display a bluish cast just before onset of menstruation. The appearance of cheesy or curdlike white exudate on the vaginal mucosa is suggestive of Candida albicans infection. Extreme reddening of the mucosa and the presence of copious thick, yellow, frothy discharge are characteristic of infection by Trichomonas vaginalis. The anterior and posterior vaginal walls can be examined by rotating the speculum 90 degrees. In the normal premenopausal adult the vaginal mucosa lies in transverse folds or rugae. In the postmenopausal patient these rugae are less obvious. The rugae and the general tone of the vaginal wall should be noted as the speculum is removed. If there is weakness of the anterior or posterior vaginal wall, the cystocele or rectocele will bulge into the vaginal lumen as support by the speculum is removed.

After the speculum has been removed a bimanual pelvic examination should be performed. The gloved and lubricated second and third fingers of one hand are inserted as far as possible into the vagina and the other hand is used to apply pressure on the lower anterior abdominal wall to bring the pelvic structures within reach of the examining fingers in the vagina (Fig. 39). To find the uterus the practitioner should place her hand in the patient's midline, slightly below the umbilicus, and exert pressure with the palmar as-

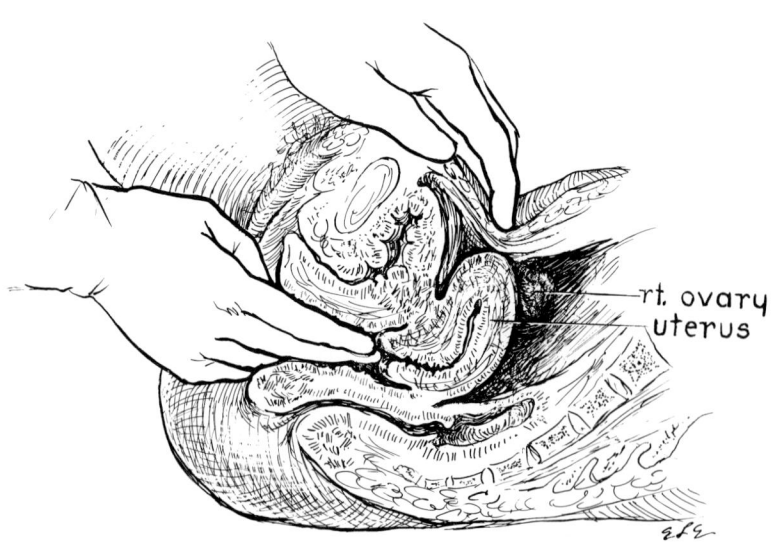

Figure 39. Bimanual palpation of the uterus. (From Morgan, W. L., Jr., and Engel, G. L.: *The Clinical Approach to the Patient.* Philadelphia, W. B. Saunders Co., 1969.)

pect of the fingers toward the sacrum. If the uterus is not felt the practitioner should move her hand gradually toward the symphysis pubis, exerting pressure at each point until the uterine mass is felt between the two hands.

In early pregnancy the cervix softens and the uterus softens and enlarges. Motion of the cervix should not be painful. In infection of the uterine tubes (usually gonococcal or tuberculous) or in ectopic pregnancy movement of the cervix will produce severe pain.

As the uterus is held between the examiner's two hands the size, shape, position, mobility, and surface contour of the uterus should be evaluated. In the normal adult the uterus is a firm, pear-shaped organ, which is roughly 5 cm. long, 4 cm. broad, and 2.5 cm. thick. Irregular or nodular enlargement of the uterine body is characteristic of leiomyomata. Irregular enlargement of a uterus in association with decreased mobility of the organ is suggestive of uterine malignancy.

Although in the obese patient the normal uterine tube is not palpable and the ovary (normally 3×4 cm.) may be difficult to palpate, tubal infections and ovarian cysts and tumors may often be identified through bimanual pelvic examination. To investigate the tube and ovary the practitioner's vaginal examining fingers should be directed somewhat lateral and anterior to the uterus, and her abdominal examining fingers, positioned slightly above and to the side of the uterine body, should exert deep pressure toward the midline. Through this maneuver the ovary may be palpated against the palmar surfaces of the fingers of the two hands. An ovarian cyst is usually smooth, tense, and somewhat compressible. A firm, irregular, or nodular ovarian tumor suggests malignancy. Acute tenderness on palpation of adnexal structures is typical of tubal infection or ectopic pregnancy.

Section VI. Examination of the Back

With the patient in the sitting position the nurse should examine his back, posterior thorax, and lungs. The practitioner should assist the patient to sit on the edge of the bed or examining table with his feet supported on a straight chair by the bedside. If the patient is too ill to sit upright by himself, a second nurse may stand in front of him and support him by placing her hands on his shoulders. The nurse practitioner should then demonstrate how he is to extend his arms and cross one over the other in order to separate the scapulae during percussion of the posterior lung fields, and should show him how to breathe normally with his mouth open during auscultation of breath sounds. The practitioner should then stand behind the patient and undrape him, to fully expose the back.

First, the skin of the back should be observed for color, turgor, moistness, edema, and presence of discolorations or lesions. If the patient has been bedridden for some time, areas of skin irritation or breakdown may be noted over the scapular spines, the vertebral spines, the sacrum, or the coccyx. In herpes zoster, or shingles, a viral inflammation of the posterior root ganglia, a unilateral vesicular eruption may be noted that begins at the side of the spinal column and extends transversely around the trunk, following the distribution of the spinal nerve. Ecchymoses, abrasions, or lacerations may indicate recent physical trauma. Focal brawny discoloration may suggest prolonged use of a heating pad or hot water bottle.

The scaling dull-red plaques of psoriasis are often found on the skin of the back. So also are the fawn-colored oval patches of pityriasis rosea, the ring-shaped vesicles or vesicopustules of tinea corporis, the nonpruritic pink macules of secondary syphilis, the small, erythematous vesicles of miliaria (prickly heat), and the inflamed cysts and pustules of acne. The skin of the back is also a common location for lipomas, or fatty tumors, a smooth soft mass which is non-adherent to underlying tissue.

Next, the patient's posture should be observed, with attention directed specifically to the relative positions of the scapulae, spine, ribs, and iliac crests, and to the contour, symmetry, and mobility of the thorax. The cervical concavity, dorsal convexity, and lumbar concavity seen in the normal spine are moderate in degree. Accentuation of the dorsal curve (kyphosis) may be seen in Marie Strumpell arthritis (a variant of rheumatoid arthritis which is usually seen in men), in Potts' disease (tuberculosis of the bony spine with collapse of vertebral bodies), in Paget's disease (osteitis deformans), and in senile osteoporosis. Lordosis, or exaggeration of the lumbar curve, is seen in pregnancy, marked obesity, ascites, bilateral hip dislocation, and spondylolisthesis. Scoliosis, or lateral curvature of the spine, may be congenital or may be caused by poliomyelitis or thoracoplasty. Most deformities of the bony spine result in structural changes in the thorax. In kyphosis there is an increase in the anteroposterior diameter of the chest. In scoliosis there may be marked shortening and narrowing of the hemithorax toward which the thoracic concavity is directed, causing crowding and displacement of the lungs and heart.

In examining the spine the practitioner should, while standing or sitting behind the patient, locate the spinous process of the seventh cervical vertebra (the visible prominence at the base of the neck posteriorly) and then run her fingers down along the spinous processes to the gluteal cleft. By so doing the practitioner can determine, more accurately than by simply viewing the back, whether the spine is straight and whether any of the normal spinal curves is exaggerated. The spinous processes should be lightly percussed to determine whether or not there is undue bone sensitivity, such as that seen in tuberculosis of the spine, multiple myeloma, and osteoporosis. A soft, fluctuant tumor protruding from the lumbar or sacral spine may be a meningocele, or herniation of the meninges, through a spina bifida. If the sac that has herniated through the defect in the spinal canal contains portions of the cord as well as meninges (meningomyelocele) the patient probably will have paralysis and loss of sensation in the lower extremities. A dimple, small lump, or small tuft of hair over the lumbosacral spine may indicate a spina bifida occulta, a simple defect in closure of the vertebral arch without associated neural pathology.

Mobility of the cervical spine should be tested by having the patient tip his head forward and backward, roll his head toward first one shoulder and then the other, and turn his head to the right and to the left. Mobility of the dorsal spine can be tested by having the patient elevate and depress each shoulder, rotate both shoulders forward and then pull them back, and rotate each shoulder in an arc. Movement of the lumbar spine can be tested by grasping the patient's iliac crests to immobilize his hips, then directing him to bend forward and back at the waist; and then having him twist at the waist to face first to one side then to the other.

The scapulae should be examined for position and symmetry. In Sprengel's deformity, a congenital disorder, the scapula is elevated and attached to the lower cervical vertebrae by a band of fibrous tissue. In "winging" of the scapula the bone is displaced posteriorly as a result of paralysis of the serratus magnus muscle.

Using the palmar aspects of the fingers, the practitioner should palpate the paravertebral and the trapezius muscles for tenderness or spasm, which may indicate either disease of the spine or neuromuscular disorder. For instance, spasm of paraspinous muscles commonly occurs following rupture of an intervertebral disc; tenderness of paraspinous muscles is found in rheumatoid arthritis of the spine. In fibromyositis the paraspinous muscles become painful following minor trauma or exposure to cold and dampness.

If the patient's chief complaint or history of past illness suggests the possibility of renal disease, the practitioner should test for renal tenderness by light fist percussion over the costovertebral angle. Percussion is best applied by placing the open hand palm-down over the costovertebral angle and applying a light blow to the dorsum of the outstretched hand with the closed fist of the other. Resulting pain suggests pyelonephritis or stag-horn calculus.

Section VII.   Examination of the Extremities

Fractures, tumors, and deformities of bones often can be diagnosed simply by palpating the bone throughout its length. Abnormal angulation, abnormal movement, crepitation, pain and soft tissue swelling are commonly associated with a fracture. Bone swelling and pain may be indicative of bone tumor. Unusual angulation of long weight-bearing bones may be seen in rickets and in osteitis deformans.

UPPER EXTREMITY

As part of the examination of the upper extremity the axillary and epitrochlear lymph nodes should be palpated. As indicated earlier, the axillary nodes should be palpated while the arm is rotated through full range of motion so that an enlarged node is not hidden by overlying fat or muscle tissue. The epitrochlear lymph nodes should be sought by flexing the forearm, then palpating the indentation immediately above and behind the medial condyle of the humerus. The location, size, consistency, tenderness, and mobility of any enlarged nodes should be noted and recorded for comparison with findings on later re-examination of the same area. Enlargement of axillary nodes may be found in leukemia, lymphoma, or breast malignancy. Enlargement of epitrochlear nodes often occurs in infection of the hand and lower arm.

The size, shape, position, and color of each upper extremity should be noted. Swelling of one arm may be the result of carcinomatous involvement or surgical removal of axillary lymph nodes. Swelling of both arms is seen in superior vena caval obstruction. In generalized edema due to congestive heart failure or nephrotic syndrome there may be swelling of all four extremities. Atrophy of one arm may be a congenital defect, may be due to such neurological disease as anterior poliomyelitis or may result from primary muscle atrophy.

Absence of the radial pulse may result from obstruction of blood flow through the subclavian artery by pressure from an aortic aneurysm. Following trauma, a palpable thrill or a bruit over an arm vessel may indicate an arteriovenous fistula. Palpation of hard plaques along the course of the radial artery indicates a severe degree of arteriosclerosis. The fingers may be cold, pale, and numb, due to prolonged vasospasm. In lymphangitis, following infection of the hand or arm, the path of the inflamed lymphatic may be visible as a red streak running up the inner aspect of the arm toward the axilla.

Examination of the hands may occasionally reveal such congenital deformities as webbing of the fingers or the presence of supernumerary digits. The condition of the hands and the nails often yields information about the patient's occupation, personal hygiene, and temperament. The manual laborer typically has callused, stained, or scarred hands. The professional or business worker will more often have soft, well-manicured hands. The slovenly person may have dirty nails. Bitten fingernails or nicotine-stained fingers help to identify the tense or nervous individual.

In acromegaly the hands are disproportionately large, with broad palm and thick fingers. In myxedema the hands and arms appear to be enlarged because the soft tissues are thickened and doughy. In certain chronic lung diseases the distal phalanx of the fingers may be clubbed or bulbous (pulmonary osteoarthropathy).

In osteoarthritis or hypertrophic arthritis small nodules tend to develop on the dorsal surface of the distal interphalangeal joint. In rheumatoid arthritis it is common to see fusiform swelling and muscle atrophy of the proximal interphalangeal joint. As rheumatoid arthritis progresses there may be sufficient joint destruction to produce severe ankylosis of involved joints, shortening of the digits, and ulnar deviation of the hand. In acute rheumatic fever many joints may be swollen, inflamed, and painful, and subcutaneous nodules may be found along the extensor tendons of the involved joints. In hypocalcemic tetany carpopedal spasm may develop in which there are extension of the interphalangeal joints, flexion of the metacarpophalangeal joint, and adduction of the thumb into the palm. Inability to extend the wrist (wrist drop) may be seen following cerebrovascular accident or peripheral neuritis.

The palms of the hands should be examined as well as the dorsum. In severe anemia there is marked pallor of the palmar lines as well as the palmar surface. In portal cirrhosis there is marked reddening of the thenar and hypothenar eminences. In polycythemia the palms tend to be bluish red in color. Certain types of hypochromic anemia may cause spoonlike deformation, or concave curvature of the nails. There is often longitudinal ridging of the nails in long-term chronic infection. In hypothyroidism the nails are brittle and break easily. In bacterial endocarditis small "splinter" hemorrhages may appear in the nail bed, signifying embolization to the end arterioles.

A tremor of the hand may be seen in the patient with chronic alcoholism, general paresis, or hyperthyroidism as he extends his arms and spreads his fingers. In Parkinsonism there is typically a "pill-rolling" movement (rolling of the thumb against the palmar aspects of the second and third finger) and a tremor of the hand at rest, which disappears with voluntary activity. In multiple sclerosis, on the other hand, there is typically intention tremor, or a tremor which is initiated by voluntary movement. In moribund patients there often may be involuntary purposeless picking at the bedcovers.

The degree of mobility of the shoulder, elbow, wrist, and hand joints should be evaluated. To test range of motion the patient should be directed first to flex his elbow 90 degrees, then to flex, extend, abduct, adduct, internally rotate, and externally rotate the shoulder. The position of the scapula should be observed as the patient performs each of these motions, since movement of the scapula with every movement of the humerus would indicate some limitation of shoulder joint motion. Limited or painful shoulder motion may result from arthritis, fracture of the humerus, or primary nerve or muscle disease. Evaluation of the elbow should include observation of the carrying angle, or angle at which the forearm deviates from the upper arm when the arms are extended at the sides with palms forward. Inequality of the carrying angle of the two arms may indicate an imperfectly aligned healed fracture of one arm. The patient should then be directed to flex and extend the elbow, and pronate and supinate the forearm. Limitation of elbow flexion and extension may be due to arthritis. Limitation of pronation and supination may be due to radial or ulnar fracture as well as to joint disease.

Flexion, extension, radial deviation, and ulnar deviation of the wrist should be tested. Limitation of wrist motion, together with joint tenderness and swelling, may occur in arthritis. Limitation of wrist motion may also occur in fracture of the lower portion of the radius or ulna. Flexion and extension of metacarpophalangeal and interphalangeal joints may reveal pain or limitation of motion caused by arthritis, sprain, dislocation, or fracture. In general, children and young adults demonstrate much greater joint mobility than do the elderly. In order to identify small decreases in joint mobility it may be necessary to compare the degree of motion in the joint in question with the degree of motion in the corresponding joint in the opposite extremity.

LOWER EXTREMITY

Since gravity has a marked effect on circulation in the legs and feet, it is advisable to examine the lower extremity with the patient in both the recumbent and erect positions whenever possible. First, the general size, shape, and position of the limb should be evaluated. In achondroplastic dwarfism the legs are disproportionately shorter than the trunk. In acromegaly the feet are disproportionately large. In Cushing's syndrome the thighs and legs are normal but the trunk is obese. Atrophy of one leg may be the result of peripheral nerve damage or of poliomyelitis. Atrophy of both legs may be a result of primary muscle disease.

The most common cause for swelling of the lower extremities is the edema of congestive heart failure. This swelling pits on pressure and shifts with changes in position to the most dependent portions of the body. Thus, the edema of heart failure is seen in the feet when the patient ambulates or sits up in a chair but shifts to the sacral area when the patient is recumbent. Edema of the lower extremities can also be seen in the nephrotic syndrome and in the severe hyproproteinemia associated with malnutrition or chronic liver disease.

Unilateral swelling of the leg and foot may result from venous or lymphatic obstruction. For example, in late pregnancy, the enlarged uterus compresses the pelvic veins. In femoral or saphenous phlebothrombosis, clots and intimal swelling occlude the inflamed vein. The edema secondary to pregnancy or to thrombophlebitis usually disappears following termination of pregnancy or resolution of the venous inflammation; however, the edema caused by enlargement of inguinal nodes in lymphoma or metastatic tumor is usually not reversible.

Varicose veins, or dilated, tortuous veins, commonly occur in the legs and are most easily seen when the patient is in standing position and the veins are maximally distended. Varicosities are most common on the medial and posterior aspect of the lower leg and the inner aspect of the thigh. Bilateral varicosities suggest a familial weakness of the venous walls. Unilateral varicosities may follow trauma or thrombophlebitis. Mechanical trauma to the thin atrophic skin overlying a varicosity may cause the vessel and overlying skin to rupture, giving rise to an ulcer which heals slowly due to impaired circulation. The skin surrounding a chronic varicose ulcer is often thickened and discolored (stasis dermatitis). In the patient whose superficial veins are severely varicosed, it is helpful to know whether the valves of the communicating veins are competent and whether there is obstruction to blood flow through the deep veins. To test valvular competence in the communicating veins the patient should be placed in supine position, a tourniquet should be tightly applied around the upper thigh, the patient should be directed to stand, and the speed of vein filling should be noted. If the superficial vessels fill rapidly from below, the valves in the communicating veins are not competent. If there is little or no filling for 30 seconds or more, the communicating veins are competent.

In phlebothrombosis the involved area is often swollen, tender, and inflamed. Even when swelling is not evident on inspection, measuring the circumference of both calves or thighs will often reveal that one is larger than the other.

In examining the lower extremities the inguinal and popliteal lymph nodes should be palpated and the femoral, popliteal, posterior tibial and dorsalis pedis pulses should be palpated. The dorsalis pedis pulse is usually found between the first and second metatarsal bones, though in a few persons it may be located in an anomalous position (Fig. 40). If the dorsalis pedis pulse is not felt, the posterior tibial artery should be palpated posterior to the internal malleolus (Fig. 41). If the posterior tibial pulse is not felt, the practitioner should search for the popliteal pulse by turning the patient onto his abdomen, flexing his lower leg at a 30 degree angle, and palpating the popliteal space. If the popliteal pulse cannot be felt, the femoral pulse should be palpated just below the inguinal ligament and halfway between the anterior superior iliac spine and the symphysis pubis.

In severe arteriosclerosis of the lower extremities the dorsalis pedis and

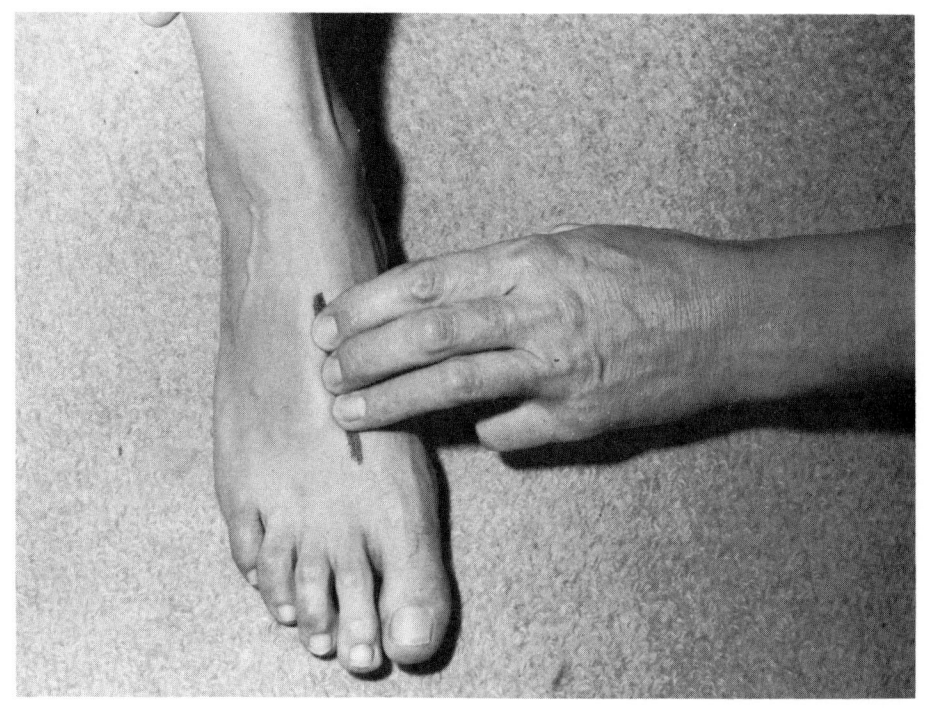

Figure 40. Palpation of dorsalis pedis pulse.

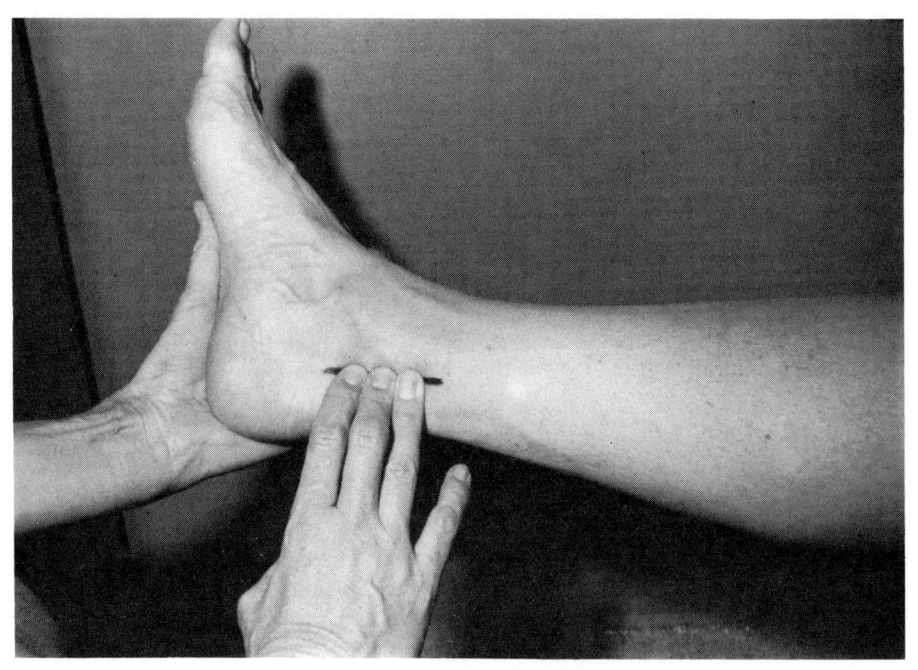

Figure 41. Palpation of posterior tibial pulse.

posterior tibial pulses may be decreased or absent, the foot is cold to touch, and there is absence of hair on the dorsum of the foot. Patients with arterial insufficiency of the lower extremity typically complain of intermittent claudication, or cramping of the calf muscles, precipitated by walking and relieved by rest. In the diabetic patient with severe arteriosclerosis, trauma or infection of the feet may sufficiently embarrass the already impaired circulation to produce gangrene of a toe, foot, or leg.

Restriction of arterial blood supply causes trophic changes of nails and skin, and even minor trauma may produce chronic ulceration and gangrene. In patients with sickle cell anemia it is common to find circulatory ulcers over the anterior surface of the tibia or over the internal malleolus. These ulcerations result from trauma of tissues inadequately perfused as a result of vascular thrombosis.

A number of orthopedic deformities may be seen in the lower extremities. In congenital dislocation of the hip there are shortening of one leg, asymmetry of the gluteal folds, and limitation of abduction. Genu varus (bowleg) may result from rickets or osteitis deformans. In congenital syphilis the tibia may be bowed anteriorly as a result of periosteal inflammation. Genu valgum (knock-knee) may result from birth injury or from rickets. In tabes dorsalis, or tertiary neurosyphilis, as a result of loss of pain sensation there may be repeated trauma to the knee and destruction of joint tissue resulting in an enlarged, hyperextensible joint.

Talipes, or clubfoot, a congenital deformity, may be of the equinus variety, in which the patient walks only on the anterior portion of the foot, or of the calcaneus variety, in which the patient walks only on the heel. In either variety the foot may be everted, so that weight is borne on the inner aspect of the foot (valgus position); or the foot may be inverted in such manner that weight is borne on the outer edge of the foot (varus position). In pes planus, or flatfoot, weakness of foot muscles and ligaments is responsible for loss of the longitudinal arch of the foot. In hallux valgus the great toe is deviated laterally in such a way that the toes override each other. In hammer toe the proximal phalanx of the second toe is dorsiflexed and the distal phalanges are plantar flexed. These two latter deformities may be congenital or acquired. A bunion, or inflammation and thickening of the bursa of the metatarsophalangeal joint of the great toe, usually results from ill-fitting shoes. In gout this same first metatarsophalangeal joint may become swollen, inflamed, and exquisitely painful.

Dermatophytosis, or "athlete's foot," is a fungus infection characterized by maceration and fissuring of the skin between the toes and around the nails.

Section VIII. Neurologic Examination

To perform the neurologic screening examination the practitioner should have available an ophthalmoscope, a small flashlight, tongue blades, cotton, safety pins, a drawing compass, a reflex hammer, and a 128 cycle per second tuning fork.

Although the neurological examination is usually performed at the end of the physical examination, the practitioner should have noted the patient's gait and stance when he first walked into the examining room and evaluated the patient's intellectual functioning and spoken language ability during history taking. The neurological screening examination involves minimal investigation of the functioning of the cerebrum, cerebellum, cranial nerves, spinal cord, and peripheral nerves.

In evaluating cerebral functioning the practitioner should consider the patient's state of consciousness, orientation, mood, memory, and ability to think critically and abstractly.

LEVEL OF CONSCIOUSNESS

As the practitioner questions the patient about his present and past illnesses, she should note his general level of consciousness. In conditions of heightened neuromuscular excitability, as seen in hyperthyroidism, anxiety, or amphetamine intoxication, the patient will jump at loud noises in the environment, will display an increase in the amount and speed of muscle movement, and may exhibit tremor of the extremities. Hyperactivity may also be seen in patients with febrile delirium, or manic excitement. Decreased levels of neuromuscular activity may result from emotional depression, administration of sedative medications, and various debilitating diseases. Still further depression of activity is seen in stupor and coma. In stupor the patient is unconscious but can be roused by loud commands. In coma the patient is unconscious, cannot be aroused, and usually demonstrates abnormal reflexes. If a comatose patient does not respond to verbal commands the practitioner should apply painful stimuli (such as firm supraorbital or testicular pressure) to determine whether he is likewise unresponsive to pain, which finding would indicate a very severe degree of cerebral depression. Stupor or coma may be seen in drug intoxication, acute febrile diseases, diabetic acidosis, hypoglycemia, cerebrovascular hemorrhage, and severely increased intracranial pressure.

In the patient with progressive deterioration of cerebral functioning, it is typical to note, first, disorientation to time; next disorientation to place; and last, disorientation to person. In order not to offend the patient when questioning in this area the practitioner might say, "Now I need to ask you some questions to determine whether you're having any trouble with memory. For instance, can you tell me what day of the week this is and what today's date is?" In determining orientation to place, it is customary to ask, "Can you tell me what kind of place this is?" If the patient answers, "A hospital," the practitioner should then ask, "Which hospital?" Finally, in testing the patient's orientation to person, the practitioner should ask, "What kind of person am I?" and, "What is your name?" Disorientation may be found in such toxic, inflammatory, traumatic, and degenerative disorders as uremia, meningitis, subdural hematoma, and cerebral arteriosclerosis.

MOOD

The patient's mood may have diagnostic significance. Occasionally the schizophrenic patient may seem silly or giddy. Manic-depressive patients may be euphoric or despairing, depending on the phase of their illness. Following cerebrovascular accident patients may demonstrate abrupt mood swings.

MEMORY

The quality of the patient's memory may be revealed by the volume of detail he can provide in relating his health history. Patients with disease of the frontal cortex often attempt to conceal their memory defects by circumlocution (talking around an issue without really answering the question) and confabulation (relating imaginary experiences rather than admitting inability to remember past events).

COMPLEX FUNCTIONS

The patient's ability to reason abstractly is usually tested by asking the patient to explain the meaning of a proverb such as "A stitch in time saves nine." A person with ability to reason abstractly would respond by saying that, frequently, a precautionary or reparative effort undertaken when a problem first becomes apparent will avert more serious later difficulty. A patient without abstract reasoning ability would talk about the number of stitches required to mend a torn garment. Another means of testing the patient's abstract reasoning ability is to ask him to identify what several objects, as an automobile, a train, a plane, and a ship, have in common. The expected answer is, "All are vehicles used to transport people from place to place." An abnormal response would be, "They cost a lot of money" or, "They don't have anything in common." A special form of abstract reasoning is the ability to perform mathematical calculations. The patient with cerebral deterioration will be unable to subtract serial sevens from one hundred or to execute simple problems in addition, subtraction, multiplication, and division.

Speech, reading, and writing are three more of the higher functions that should be evaluated in ascertaining the level of the patient's cerebral functioning. While the patient relates his health history, the practitioner should note his quality of articulation, his manner of syllabication, the aptness of his word choice, the completeness of his sentence structure, the amount of his vocal inflection, the strength of his voice, and his comprehension of the practitioner's questions. Impaired articulation may occur as a result of infarction of the dominant cerebral hemisphere, cerebellar dysfunction, lesions of the brain stem, or dysfunction of the fifth, seventh, ninth, tenth, or twelfth cranial nerves.

Cerebral dysfunction may result in aphasia, apraxia, or agnosia. Aphasia, or loss of language ability, can be either expressive (inability to send messages) or receptive (inability to comprehend messages received from others) and can relate either to spoken or written language. Global aphasia, or loss of all speech function, results from destruction of both motor and sensory speech areas in the dominant hemisphere (the left hemisphere is dominant in approximately 95 per cent of the population) and is most often seen following occlusion of the left internal carotid or middle cerebral artery, massive cerebral hemorrhage, or massive brain tumor. Motor or expressive aphasia is due to damage to Broca's area, the motor speech area in the anterior portion of the dominant cerebral hemisphere. Motor aphasia may be complete, in which case the patient will be unable to formulate any spoken language. If motor aphasia is not complete and the patient can utter a few words or phrases, these are apt to be words which are highly charged emotionally, as terms of profanity and vulgarity. If motor aphasia is still less severe the patient may demonstrate slow, poorly articulated speech and a tendency to omit pronouns, verbs, prepositions, and conjunctions.

Sensory or receptive aphasia is usually due to a lesion in the posterior temporal portion of the dominant hemisphere and is characterized by no reduction in the volume or tonal expressiveness of speech but by inability to comprehend the spoken language of others, inability to repeat test phrases, and frequent use of incorrect words or incorrect sentence structure. If the condition is severe the patient may utter a jumble of syllables having a similar sound to the intended word or phrase but having no real meaning.

Agnosia, or inability to recognize objects, may be visual, due to an occipital lobe lesion, or tactile, due to a parietal lobe lesion. In the former instance the patient is unable to identify and understand the function of a familiar object he can see. In the latter the patient is unable to identify and comprehend the use of an object he can touch and manipulate. The test for agnosia consists of pointing to or placing in the patient's hands such objects as a coin, a button, a key, a safety pin, and a safety clip and asking him to name the item and explain what it is used for.

Apraxia is the loss of the previously acquired ability to perform such simple skilled acts as tying one's shoes, buttoning a coat, opening and closing a safety pin, and fastening a belt buckle. Tests for apraxia might include asking the patient to tie his shoes, fasten a watchband, or imitate simple mouth and tongue movements demonstrated by the examiner, such as pursing the lips, extruding the tongue, licking the lips, and the like.

CRANIAL NERVE FUNCTION

Information about the functioning of some cranial nerves will have been gathered during earlier portions of the examination. It is desirable, however, to review here the function of each of the cranial nerves and to indicate means of testing their integrity.

Generally, the function of the first, or olfactory, nerve is not tested unless the patient complains of some disturbance in the sense of smell. To test olfaction the practitioner should occlude one of the patient's nostrils at a time, have him close his eyes, then give him such substances to sniff and identify as coffee, tobacco, and oil of peppermint. Obviously, the test will be of no value unless the patient's air passages are patent.

As indicated earlier, the head of the optic or second cranial nerve can be directly examined with an ophthalmoscope. In optic atrophy, or death of the nerve head, the optic disc will appear stark white, owing to disappearance of the tiny disc blood vessels. In papilledema, or venous congestion of the nerve head due to increased intracranial pressure, the disc margins are elevated and blurred. In glaucomatous injury to the optic nerve there is marked cupping or excavation of the optic disc. As described earlier, visual acuity should be measured by covering one of the patient's eyes at a time and directing him to read the smallest possible print on the Snellen chart at a distance of 20 feet. If vision is markedly impaired, it may be necessary to test the patient's sight by holding a hand a short distance in front of his face and asking how many fingers he can see.

To test the size of the patient's visual fields, the nurse should stand at arm's length in front of the patient, direct him to cover his right eye with his hand and fix his gaze on her nose. The examiner should then close her left eye, extend both arms at full length, and bring her waggling fingers in from the periphery of each visual quadrant toward the central field of her own and the patient's vision. The patient should be directed to inform the practitioner when her moving finger first becomes visible to him on each excursion from the periphery. Meanwhile, the practitioner notes when she herself can first see the same moving finger. The entire procedure is then repeated for the patient's other eye, and the practitioner then can judge the patient's field of vision by comparing it with her own. Visual field defects may be found in lesions of the optic nerve, optic chiasm, or the temporal, parietal, or occipital cortex, and the exact pattern of the visual defect can be very helpful in locating the underlying pathology.

The functions of the third (oculomotor), fourth (trochlear), and sixth (abducens) cranial nerves are tested together because of their coordinated effect on extraocular movements. The oculomotor nerve innervates several of the extrinsic eye muscles (not the superior oblique or the external rectus), the levator palpebrae superioris, the pupillary sphincter, and the ciliary muscle. Damage to the third nerve or its nucleus produces inability to turn the eye medially, lid ptosis, and pupillary dilation. Normally, the pupils are equal in size and constrict when exposed to light and when the gaze is fixed on a nearby object. Pupillary constriction is caused by stimulation of parasympathetic fibers; pupillary dilation is caused by stimulation of sympathetic fibers. Bilateral pupillary dilation may be seen in brain injury, following high dosages of sympathetic stimulants, and in the fourth stage of anesthesia. A unilaterally dilated pupil may result from multiple sclerosis or from increased intracranial pressure. In tertiary neurosyphilis the pupils may be small, unequal in size, irregular in outline, and poorly reactive to light.

The trochlear nerve innervates the superior oblique muscle. Damage to the trochlear nerve or its nucleus interferes with the directing of the eye downward and outward. The abducens nerve innervates the lateral rectus muscle, and injury to the sixth nerve or its nucleus will cause the eye to be deviated medially because of the unopposed pull of the internal rectus muscle. Eye movements can be tested by holding the patient's head steady with one hand and directing him to follow with his eyes the fingers of the examiner's other hand as she moves them to the left and right lateral, left and right temporal, and left and right nasal positions. A lesion of either the third, fourth, or sixth cranial nerves will, by interfering with conjugate movement of the two eyes, cause the visual image to fall on different points of the two retinas, producing diplopia or double vision. Diplopia may, of course, result from muscle weakness or disease as well as from neurological disorders.

The fifth, or trigeminal, nerve has a large sensory and a small motor component. The three sensory divisions of the fifth are the ophthalmic, which provides sensation to the skin of the anterior scalp and forehead and to the cornea; the maxillary, which provides sensation to the upper teeth and jaw, the cheeks, and the oral, pharyngeal, and nasal mucosa; and the mandibular, which provides sensation to the tongue, lower teeth and buccal surface. The motor fibers of the trigeminal nerve supply the masseter, temporalis, and pterygoid muscles, which are involved in mastication. To test the sensory divisions of the nerve, the patient should be asked to close his eyes, and the skin in all three regions tested for light touch (using a wisp of cotton), temperature (using vials of hot and cold water), and pain (using a pin-prick). The corneal reflex should then be tested by touching the corneal surface with a wisp of absorbent cotton that has been twisted to a point and directed toward the eye from the side. The normal response to corneal stimulation is a quick blink. To test the motor portion of the trigeminal nerve the practitioner should direct the patient to open his mouth and move his chin first to one side and then the other while she opposes the action with manual pressure against the ramus of the jaw.

In trigeminal sensory dysfunction there may be decreased or absent touch, temperature, and pain sensation in one or all of the areas supplied by the three sensory divisions of the nerve, and there may be failure of the blink reflex following corneal stimulation. In trigeminal motor dysfunction there may be facial asymmetry with deviation of the jaw toward the paralyzed side and decrease in the strength of the bite.

The seventh, or facial, nerve has a large motor and a small sensory component. The sensory portion of the nerve carries taste sensation from the anterior two thirds of the tongue, transmits sensation from the external auditory canal, and mediates secretion of the salivary glands. Facial nerve motor function is evaluated by noting the facial expression and by observing facial symmetry as the patient is directed to frown, close his eyes, and smile. Sensory function of the facial nerve can be evaluated by testing the accuracy of taste sensation. For this test the patient should moisten his tongue, protrude it, and hold it steady by grasping it with a square of gauze. The practitioner should then carefully place a small portion of each of the four test substances (sugar, vinegar, salt, and quinine) on the lateral portion of the anterior half of the tongue, asking the patient to identify, in writing, the flavor of each of the applied substances. The procedure should then be repeated for the opposite side of the tongue, and the taste perception of the two sides should be compared.

Following a cerebrovascular accident it is common to find weakness or paralysis of the lower facial muscles on the side opposite the cerebral lesion, causing widening of the palpebral fissure, erasure of the nasolabial fold, and drooping of the angle of the mouth. Lesions of the peripheral portion of the facial nerve cause paralysis of all facial muscles, producing inability to wrinkle the forehead or close the eye, as well as flattening of the nasolabial fold and sagging of the mouth.

The acoustic, or eighth cranial nerve has a cochlear branch, which mediates hearing, and a vestibular branch, which assists in maintaining equilibrium. As indicated earlier, a crude test of hearing ability consists of directing the patient to cover one of his ears with his hand and then asking him either to indicate when he can hear the tick of a watch that is moved toward him from a distance or to repeat words whispered by the practitioner as she stands outside his line of vision. A vibrating tuning fork held in front of the ear, placed against the mastoid process, and held against the midline of the forehead can be used to measure the relative effectiveness of air and bone conduction of sound. In damage to the cochlear portion of the eighth nerve, both air and bone conduction of sound are impaired on the affected side.

The function of the vestibular portion of the eighth nerve can be tested by means of the Romberg test, in which the patient is asked to stand with eyes closed and feet close together. In this position the patient with damage to the vestibular portion of the nerve will be unable to stand erect, and will sway and fall if not supported.

The functions of the ninth (glossopharyngeal) and tenth (vagus) nerves are tested together. Motor fibers of the glossopharyngeal nerve supply the muscles of the pharynx; sensory fibers of the same nerve transmit taste sensation from the posterior tongue and touch and temperature from the pharynx. Secretory fibers of the ninth nerve supply the parotid gland. Motor function of the glossopharyngeal nerve is tested by touching both sides of the posterior pharyngeal wall in an effort to elicit the gag reflex. Sensory function of the nerve can be evaluated by testing taste sensations on the posterior third of the tongue, using small quantities of sugar, vinegar, salt, and quinine. The most common sign of ninth nerve damage is dysphagia, or difficulty in swallowing.

Motor fibers of the vagus nerve supply the soft palate, pharynx, and larynx; sensory fibers carry impulses from a number of the thoracic and abdominal viscera. Unilateral vagal injury may produce deviation of the uvula to one side and hoarseness. Bilateral vagal dysfunction can produce dysphagia, accumulation of mucus in the mouth, and respiratory difficulty. To test the vagus nerve, the patient is directed to say "ah," and the practitioner observes the palate for asymmetry or immobility.

The completely motor eleventh, or spinal accessory, nerve supplies the sternocleidomastoid muscle and the upper portion of the trapezius. The function of the eleventh nerve can be tested by directing the patient to turn his head to the side while the practitioner opposes the motion by finger pressure against his jaw, and at the same time palpates the sternocleidomastoid on the opposite side. To test innervation of the trapezius the practitioner should place her hands on the patient's shoulders, press down, and direct the patient to shrug his shoulders. Lesions of the accessory nerve result in inability to execute these maneuvers against counterpressure.

The twelfth, or hypoglossal, nerve innervates the muscles of the tongue. Dysfunction of the nerve results in impaired articulation, impaired swallowing, fibrillation of tongue muscles, and paralysis of the tongue.

CEREBELLAR FUNCTION

The centers for balance and coordination are located in the cerebellum. Cerebellar disease may result in disturbance of posture or of voluntary movement. A lesion in one cerebellar hemisphere produces motor abnormalities on the ipsilateral side. Common signs of cerebellar disorder are staggering or lurching gait, inability to stabilize the trunk in an upright position, inability to adjust the strength of muscle contraction so as to execute voluntary actions smoothly, and inability to perform rapidly alternating movements. To test cerebellar function the practitioner should first observe the patient's posture and gait. The patient with cerebellar disease typically walks with a reeling gait, throwing first one foot and then the other forward in jerky fashion, and placing his feet far apart so as to maintain a broad base of support as a protection against falling. Because lack of skeletal muscle tone renders it difficult for the patient to hold his trunk upright, he tends to rock or jerk his trunk back and forth slightly when standing still. Posture and balance should be tested by asking the patient to stand erect, with his feet close together and his arms at his sides, first with his eyes open and then with his eyes closed. Although the normal person may sway slightly under these circumstances, he will be able to adjust his posture so as to remain upright. The patient with cerebellar disease will fall toward the side of his cerebellar lesion unless he is supported.

Muscle coordination of the upper extremities can be tested by directing the patient to extend and abduct his arms, then to touch his nose with first one index finger and then the other in rapid succession. The normal person can bring his arms from the outstretched position to touch his nose with first one index finger and then the other with his eyes either open or closed. The patient with cerebellar disease typically overshoots or undershoots the mark, even with his eyes open, because he is unable to grade muscle effort to achieve an exact degree of movement. Another means of testing muscle coordination in the upper extremities is to direct the patient to extend his arms in front of his body, then alternately pronate and supinate his arms in rapid succession. The normal patient can perform such motions quickly and smoothly, moving the two arms at the same time and to the same degree. The patient with cerebellar disease performs such motions slowly and awkwardly, and the two extremities do not move in phase with each other.

Muscle coordination in the lower extremities can be tested by directing the patient to place his right heel on his left shin just below the knee and run his heel down the entire length of the shin, then to reverse the procedure, using left heel and right shin. The normal person can perform this maneuver in such manner that the heel travels in a straight line down the entire length of the lower leg. When the patient with cerebellar disease attempts this test his foot moves jerkily down the opposite leg, slipping first to one side and then the other of the shinbone.

The patient with cerebellar disease may exhibit an intention tremor. That is, there is no tremor of the hand at rest, but a coarse tremor develops near the end of each purposeful movement, such as placing an object on a table, carrying a glass of water to the lips, or cutting a slice of meat.

MOTOR FUNCTION

Evaluation of muscle function should include observation of muscle structure and movement, evaluation of muscle tone, and testing of muscle strength. Throughout the entire physical examination the practitioner should note skeletal muscle mass and shape in each body part, comparing muscles in the two sides of the body for symmetry. Muscle atrophy may be indicative of neurological disease. Fasciculations, or involuntary, irregular twitching of groups of muscle fibers, in the patient with a lower motor neuron lesion may occur spontaneously when the part is at rest or can be precipitated by tapping the muscle lightly with a reflex hammer. Failure to move a body part in concert with other parts in the performance of complex activities suggests paralysis. Thus, failure to swing the arm at the side while walking and failure to elevate one corner of the mouth when smiling are two manifestations of hemiplegia resulting from cerebrovascular hemorrhage. Abnormal position of a part at rest may be indicative of neurological damage. Persistent severe plantar flexion of the foot (foot drop) may result from peroneal nerve injury. Persistent adduction of the arm together with elbow flexion, wrist flexion, and ulnar deviation of the hand are characteristic of the paresis or paralysis resulting from cerebrovascular hemorrhage.

Involuntary movements of the head or extremities accompany certain neurological diseases. A terminal intention tremor due to cerebellar dysfunction is seen in multiple sclerosis. A "pill-rolling" tremor at rest results from involvement of the basal ganglia in Parkinson's disease. In aged persons a fine tremor of the head, precipitated by movement, may result from cerebral ischemia (senile tremor.) Fine tremors of the hands, lips, and tongue are often seen in the alcoholic patient during periods of relative or absolute withdrawal from alcohol.

Some persons demonstrate rapid, repetitive, stereotyped muscle movements, such as facial twitching, jerking the head to one side, thrusting the chin forward, or blinking, when experiencing tension. Typically, such tics or habit spasms can be inhibited for brief periods by an act of will, but will recur when the patient's attention is diverted or his anxiety is suddenly increased.

The neurological examination should include evaluation of muscle tone, which is the slight resistance offered by normal muscle to passive motion. In an upper motor neuron disease, such as cerebrovascular accident, increased muscle tone or spasticity of the involved extremities is to be expected. Muscle spasticity may be constant throughout the full range of joint motion, or it may be phasic in that resistance is strongest when motion is initiated, but gives way suddenly as passive motion is continued. Disorders of lower motor neurons, such as spinal cord or peripheral nerve injuries, typically produce decreased muscle tone or flaccidity. Flaccid muscles are unusually soft to the touch, yield unduly to passive stretching, and may cause hypermobility of a part, such as hyperextension of the knee or plantar flexion of the foot.

Various methods should be used to test muscle strength, and in each test an effort should be made to compare the relative strength of muscle groups on the two sides of the body. To evaluate muscle strength in the upper extremities the practitioner should direct the patient to squeeze her hand; then with his arms outstretched at his sides to resist her attempts to depress his arm, flex his elbow, flex his wrist, and flex his fingers. Marked muscular weakness will be detectable through these maneuvers; minimal decrease in strength may be more difficult to detect, but by testing comparable muscles on the two sides at the same time unilateral muscle weakness may be detected.

Muscular strength in the lower extremity can be tested by having the patient perform the following motions against resistance: flex the hip, adduct the thigh, flex the knee, dorsiflex the foot, and evert the foot. The patient should then be directed to walk on his toes, walk on his heels, stand on one foot, and hop in place. In severe muscle weakness the patient will be unable to perform any of these latter activities.

REFLEXES

Several reflex arcs are tested as part of the neurological examination. When testing stretch reflex a normal reaction requires proper functioning of the sensory end organ, sensory nerve, spinal cord, efferent nerve, motor end plate, and the muscle itself. Injury to any of these structures will weaken or destroy the reflex. Disease of the upper motor neuron anywhere from the cerebral cortex to the anterior horn cell will result in hyperreflexia by releasing the reflex from the inhibitory control of higher centers.

The superficial reflexes that are tested as part of the neurological examination are the corneal, pharyngeal, abdominal, cremasteric, and plantar. Because many of the superficial reflexes are facilitated by the cerebral cortex, disease of either the upper or lower motor neuron will interrupt these reflexes. As indicated earlier the corneal reflex, which is mediated by the fifth cranial nerve, is tested by gently stroking the corneal surface with a piece of cotton wool that has been twisted to a point and introduced from the side of the eye. The normal response to such a stimulus is a quick blink. The pharyngeal reflex, which is mediated by the ninth cranial nerve, is tested by stroking the wall of the pharynx with a cotton-tipped applicator. The normal response to such stroking is to gag. To test the abdominal reflexes the patient should be placed in supine position with his abdomen bared, and a pin or applicator stick drawn across the skin of each quadrant. The expected response is a brief contraction of underlying muscle. Abdominal reflexes are typically absent on the paralyzed side following cerebrovascular accident and may be absent bilaterally in multiple sclerosis. The cremasteric reflex is tested by lightly stroking the inner aspect of the upper thigh; this action normally results in quick elevation of the ipsilateral testis. The plantar reflex is tested by running the thumbnail, a key, or the reflex hammer handle along the lateral border of the foot from the heel to the ball of the foot and thence medially. The normal response is flexion of the toes. In patients with an upper motor neuron lesion stimulation of the sole is followed by extension of the great toe and fanning of the other toes (Babinski reflex.)

Certain deep reflexes (stretch) are tested by tapping a tendon lying close to the body surface, thereby stimulating a stretch receptor and evoking a reflex contraction of the attached muscle. The biceps, triceps, radial, patellar, and Achilles reflexes are usually included in the neurological screening examination.

To test the biceps reflex with the patient in sitting position, the practitioner should support the patient's elbow in her hand while placing her thumb over his biceps tendon. When the examiner's thumbnail is struck with the reflex hammer the expected response is quick flexion of the forearm (Fig. 42). If the patient is in recumbent position, the elbow is flexed at a 90 degree angle, the forearm laid across the trunk, and the reflex tested in the foregoing manner. This reflex is mediated at the level of the fifth and sixth cervical vertebrae.

To test the triceps reflex the elbow should be slightly flexed, and supported in the practitioner's hand while the triceps tendon is given a blow with the reflex hammer (Fig. 43). The expected response is quick extension of the forearm. This reflex is mediated at the level of the seventh and eighth cervical vertebrae.

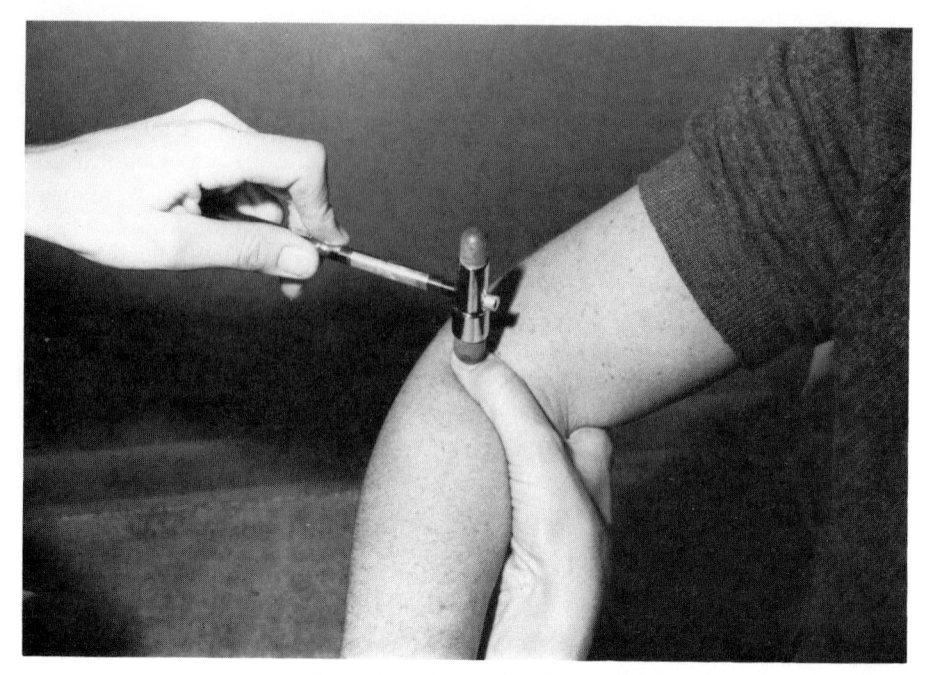

Figure 42. Testing the biceps reflex.

The radial reflex is tested by pronating the forearm, then tapping the lower third of the radius. The expected response is flexion of the forearm and the fingers. The radial reflex is, like the brachial, mediated at the level of the fifth and sixth cervical vertebrae.

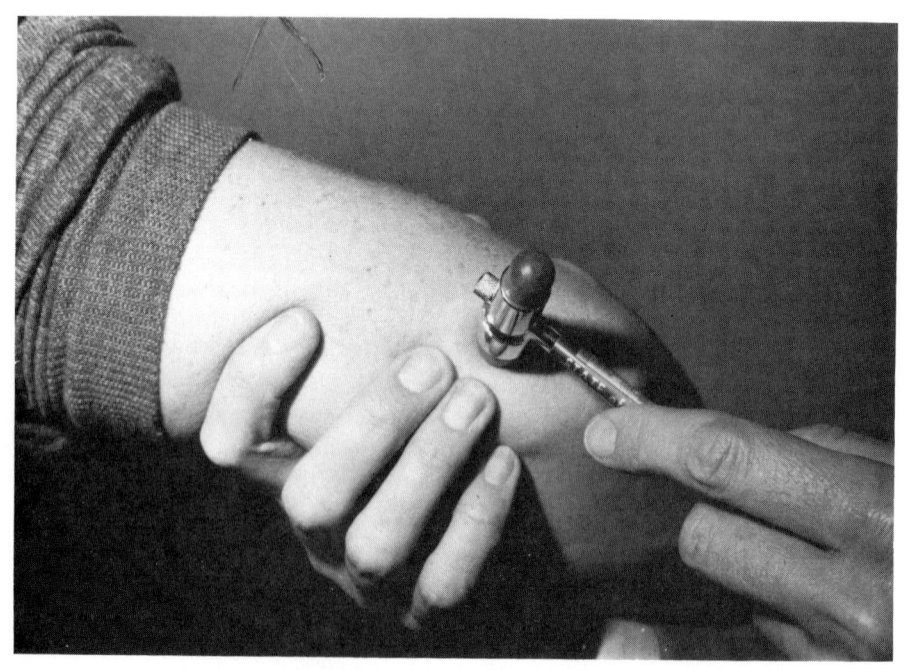

Figure 43. Testing the triceps reflex.

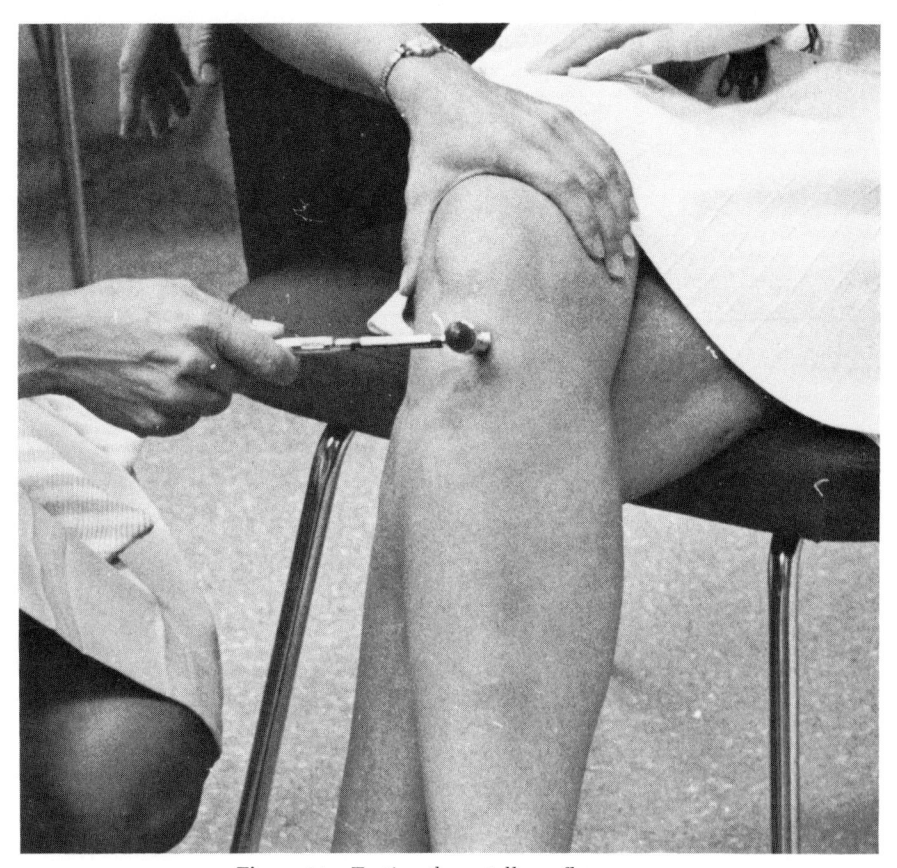

Figure 44. Testing the patellar reflex.

The patellar reflex is tested by having the patient hang his legs over the edge of the bed or, if sitting in a chair, cross one knee over the other (Fig. 44). If the patient is recumbent the practitioner should raise and support his knee in slight flexion. A light blow of the reflex hammer to the patellar tendon should cause quick extension of the knee. The patellar reflex is mediated at the level of the second, third, and fourth lumbar vertebrae.

The Achilles reflex is tested by directing the patient to kneel on a bed or chair with his feet extending over the edge. When the Achilles tendon just above the os calcis is tapped lightly with a reflex hammer the expected result is quick plantar flexion of the foot (Fig. 45). The Achilles reflex is mediated at the level of the first and second sacral vertebrae.

When reflexes are severely hyperactive, stretching the tendon may produce clonus, an involuntary, repetitive series of contractions. Clonus is most easily demonstrated by rapid and forceful dorsiflexion of the foot, which in the patient with extreme hyperreflexia will be followed by sustained back and forth movements of the foot against the examiner's hand.

Each reflex should be graded from 0 (no movement), through 1 plus (weak response), 2 plus (normal response), 3 plus (exaggerated response), to 4 plus (sustained clonus).

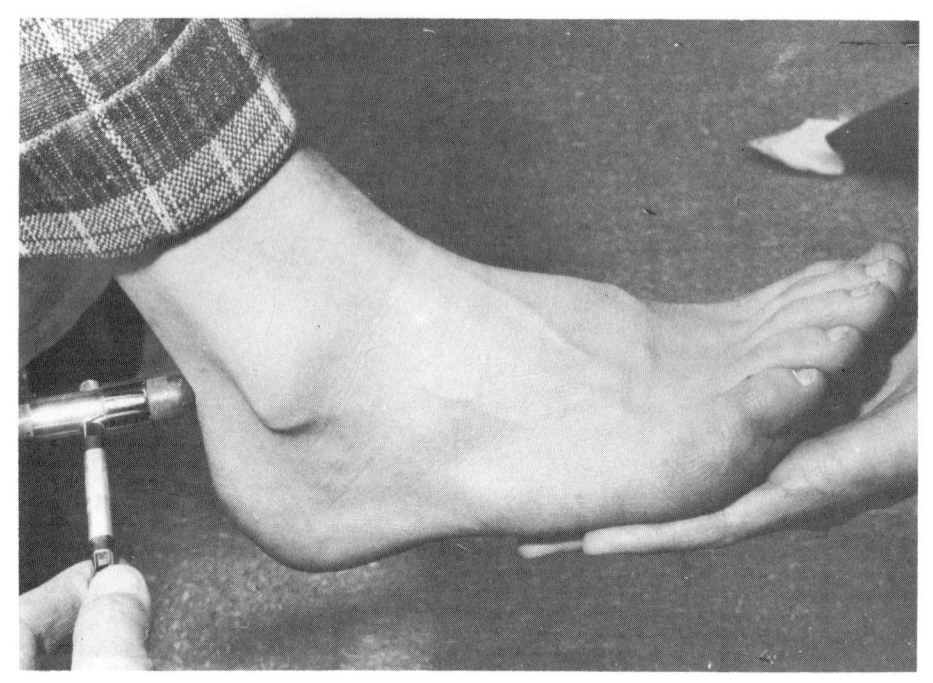

Figure 45. Testing the Achilles reflex.

SENSORY PERCEPTION

If the patient is alert and able to cooperate, the neurological screening examination should include testing his perception of light touch, superficial and deep pain, temperature, position, and vibration. In general, the face, trunk, arms and legs should be tested for light touch and pain. Additionally, the extremities should be tested for temperature, position and vibratory sense. In each type of test the two sides of the body should be compared. Light touch is tested by directing the patient to close his eyes, then touching the skin with a wisp of cotton at irregular intervals at several points in each body area. The patient is instructed to say "Now" whenever he perceives the stimulus. In areas where the skin is thickened or callused, such as the palms and soles, increased pressure may be required for the impulse to be perceived. Superficial pain sense is tested by directing the patient to close his eyes and then pricking the skin lightly with the sharp point of a pin. The patient is instructed to say "Sharp" whenever he perceives pain. For the test to be valid, the practitioner must be careful to exert the same amount of pressure on the pin with each skin prick.

Deep pain may be tested by exerting pressure on certain bones, muscles, tendons, and nerves. A commonly used test for deep pain sensation consists of squeezing the Achilles tendon. The normal patient will complain of pain or display avoidance behavior in response to such manipulation.

Temperature sense can be tested by having the patient close his eyes, then applying test tubes filled with hot and cold water to various body parts. The patient is instructed to say "Hot" or "Cold" each time a test tube is brought into contact with his skin.

To test position sense in each extremity the practitioner should direct the patient to close his eyes, then grasp the terminal phalanx of a digit by its sides and move it either upward or downward. The patient is asked to identify the direction of the motion. The sequence of position changes should be varied so as not to cue the patient to the proper response.

Vibratory sense can be tested by directing the patient to close his eyes, then applying a vibrating 128 cycles per second tuning fork to the top of the great toe, the medial malleolus, the patella, the tip of the middle finger, the distal radius, the styloid process of the ulna, and the olecranon process of the ulna (Fig. 46). The patient is asked to indicate whether the fork is vibrating and, if he says that it is, to indicate when he can no longer feel the vibrations. At that point the patient's threshold for vibration perception can be compared with the examiner's perception.

Two point touch discrimination can be tested by applying the two points of a compass to the skin at various points to determine whether the patient can differentiate between single point and double point stimulation. On the fingertips, two pinpricks separated by only 3 millimeters can be recognized as two point stimulation; on the palm the stimuli must be 1 centimeter apart to be distinguished from each other, and on the leg stimuli must be 3 centimeters apart to be recognized as being separate.

Loss of sensation is more often relative than absolute; therefore, if on initial testing there appears to be absence of sensation in some part, the part should be retested, using increasingly stronger stimuli until perception is

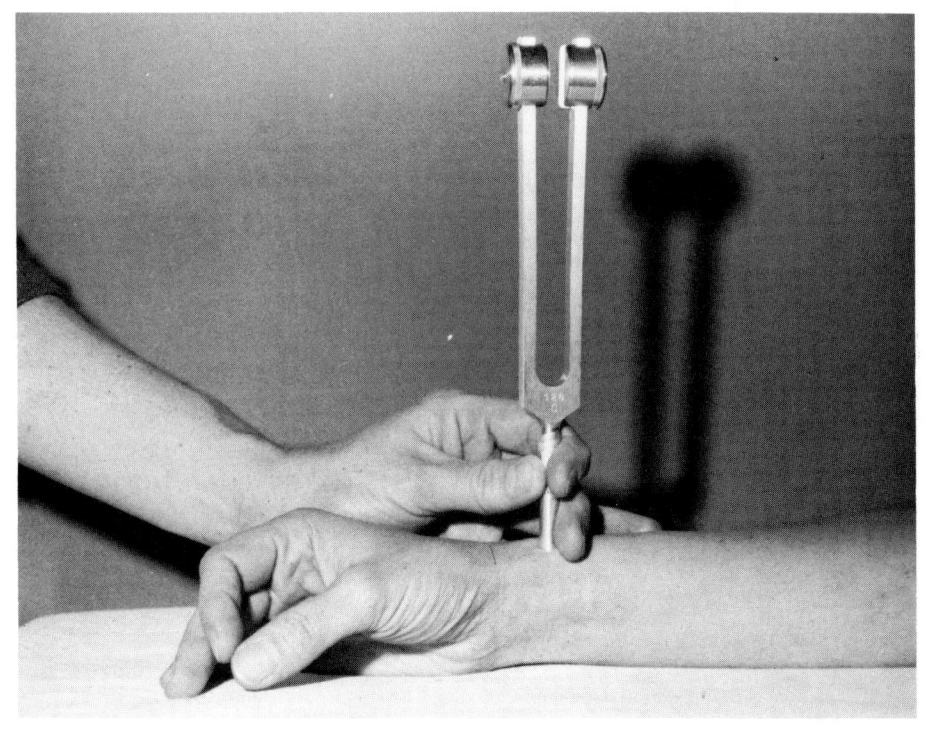

Figure 46. Testing vibratory sense.

finally achieved. The exact pattern of sensory loss should be carefully mapped out in order to determine whether the area of impaired sensation is one supplied by a particular peripheral nerve, which would suggest injury to that nerve; a dermatomal distribution, which would imply a lesion of the dorsal root; or an area so extensive as to suggest a spinal cord or brain disease. The hysterical patient may sometimes complain of numbness or paresthesias in an extremity. Such psychoneurotic sensory disturbances usually have a glove or stocking distribution; that is, disordered sensation is reported for the entire hand or foot, the entire lower arm or lower leg, or the entire extremity, rather than for an area supplied by a particular peripheral or spinal nerve. Although the specific location of a neurological lesion is the physician's responsibility, the practitioner can often unearth evidence in the neurological screening examination that points to the need for a more specific neurological workup.

BIBLIOGRAPHY: THE PHYSICAL EXAMINATION

Bates, Barbara: *A Guide to Physical Examination*, Philadelphia, J. B. Lippincott, 1974.
Beeson, Paul, and McDermott, Walsh, Eds.: *Textbook of Medicine*. 14th ed. Philadelphia, W. B. Saunders, 1975.
Buckingham, William, Sparberg, Marshall, and Brandfonbrener, Martin: *A Primer of Clinical Diagnosis*. New York, Harper and Row, 1971.
Conn, Howard, and Conn, Rex, Eds.: *Current Diagnosis 4*. Philadelphia, W. B. Saunders, 1974.
Cowdry, E. V., and Steinberg, Franz, Eds.: *The Care of the Geriatric Patient*. St. Louis, C. V. Mosby, 1971.
DeGowin, Elmer and DeGowin, Richard: *Bedside Diagnostic Examination*. 2nd ed. New York, Macmillan, 1969.
Delp, Mahlon, and Manning, Robert: *Major's Physical Diagnosis*. 8th ed. Philadelphia, W. B. Saunders Co., 1975.
Feinstein, Alsan: *Clinical Judgment*. Baltimore, Williams and Wilkins, 1967.
Fowler, Noble: *Examination of the Heart, Part II*. New York, American Heart Association, 1972.
Goss, Charles, Ed.: *Gray's Anatomy of the Human Body*. 28th ed. Philadelphia, Lea and Febiger, 1966.
Guyton, Arthur: *Textbook of Medical Physiology*. 5th ed. Philadelphia, W. B. Saunders, 1961.
Hochstein, Elliot, and Rubin, Albert: *Physical Diagnosis*. New York, McGraw-Hill, 1964.
Hopkins, Henry: *Leopold's Principles and Methods of Physical Diagnosis*. 3rd ed. Philadelphia, W. B. Saunders Co., 1965.
Hurst, J. Willis, and Schlant, Robert: *Examination of the Heart, Part III*. New York, American Heart Association, 1972.
Judge, Richard, and Zuidema, George: *Physical Diagnosis: A Physiologic Approach to the Clinical Examination*. 2nd ed. Boston, Little, Brown and Co., 1968.
Kampmeier, Rudolph, and Blake, Thomas: *Physical Examination in Health and Disease*. 4th ed. Philadelphia, F. A. Davis, 1970.
Kneeland, Yale, and Loeb, Robert: *Martin's Principles and Practice of Physical Diagnosis*. 3rd ed. Philadelphia, J. B. Lippincott, 1962.
Leonard, J., and Kroetz, F.: *Examination of the Heart, Part IV*. New York, American Heart Association, 1967.
Leopold, S.: *Principles and Methods of Physical Diagnosis*. 3rd ed., Philadelphia, W. B. Saunders Co., 1965.
Luckmann, J., and Sorensen, K.: *Medical-Surgical Nursing*. Philadelphia, W. B. Saunders, 1974.
Lynaugh, J., and Bates, B.: Physical diagnosis, a skill for all nurses? Amer. J. Nurs., 74:58–59, January, 1974.
Martini, P.: *Principles and Practice of Physical Diagnosis*. 3rd ed., Philadelphia, Lippincott Co., 1962.
Morgan, W., and Engel, G.: *The Clinical Approach to the Patient*. Philadelphia, W. B. Saunders Co., 1969.
Prior, J., and Silberstein, J.: *Physical Diagnosis*. 4th ed., St. Louis, C. V. Mosby Co., 1973.
Sodeman, W., and Sodeman, W. Jr.: *Pathologic Physiology*. 5th ed., Philadelphia, W. B. Saunders, 1974.
Stern, T.: *Clinical Examination*. Chicago, Year Book Medical Publishers, 1964.
Wintrobe, M., Thom, G., Adams, R., Bennett, I., Braunwald, E., Isselbacher, K., and Petersdorf, R. (Eds.): *Harrison's Principles of Internal Medicine*. 6th ed., New York, McGraw-Hill Book Co., 1970.
Wechsler, I.: *Clinical Neurology*, 9th ed. Philadelphia, W. B. Saunders Co., 1963.

4
LABORATORY TESTS AND SPECIAL EXAMINATIONS

In general, laboratory tests and diagnostic procedures can be thought of as serving the following functions: screening, qualitative determinations, quantitative determinations, and patient management. A particular test can at one time serve one of these functions and at some other time, another function.

Screening tests are relatively inexpensive, constitute little or no risk to the patient, and provide such basic information that they are of great value in identifying disease processes when applied broad scale to large numbers of sick and well individuals. Such tests are frequently referred to as "routine tests" and are usually a part of the general health work-up of any individual who presents himself for health care in either an inpatient or outpatient facility. Examples of such screening tests are the blood examination, including cell count, hematocrit, and hemoglobin determination; urinalysis for specific gravity, pH, sugar, acetone, albumin, and microscopic formed elements; tuberculin skin sensitivity test; serological test for syphilis; serum glucose determination; serum cholesterol determination on all adults; stool test for occult blood; Papanicolaou test on all women past menarche; chest x-ray; electrocardiogram on all persons over 40 years of age; and a proctoscopic examination on all persons over 40 years of age.

Qualitative tests are tests that enable the practitioner to confirm a diagnosis she suspects from information obtained through the medical history and/or physical examination. For instance, the practitioner may deduce, from the patient's history of polydipsia, polyuria, polyphagia, and weight loss, that diabetes mellitus is a likely diagnosis. In order to confirm the diagnosis she might order a two hour postprandial blood glucose determination or an oral glucose tolerance test. (See also Chapter 8.)

Qualitative tests may also be used, once a diagnosis of a chronic or multisystem disease has been made, to determine how widespread the structural and functional derangements are that result from the disease process; that is, to identify which organs or organ systems have undergone pathological change. For instance, for the patient who has been diagnosed as being hypertensive the practitioner may order electrocardiographic studies, renal function tests, or angiograms to determine whether the elevated pressure has caused secondary changes in the heart, kidney, or peripheral arteries. (See also Chapter 7.)

Quantitative tests are those the practitioner may use, once a diagnosis is made, to assess the severity or intensity of the disease process. For instance, in a patient with known chronic glomerulonephritis, phenylsulfonphthalein or para-aminohippuric acid clearance studies may be done to determine the degree of tubular damage present.

Certain tests that serve to monitor the effectiveness of certain drugs or treatments are used in therapeutic management of patients. For instance, after a patient has been started on a diabetic diet and insulin or an oral hypoglycemic drug, urine testing for sugar and acetone should be done on a regular basis to determine whether the patient's diet-drug-activity regimen is sufficiently balanced to prevent spillage of glucose in his urine (see Chapter 8). Or, after a patient in congestive heart failure has received digitalis for some time, an electrocardiogram may be taken to identify any subtle rhythm irregularities which may have developed as toxic effects of the drug (see Chapter 10).

Laboratory tests and diagnostic procedures are costly, and certain of these tests constitute some health risk to the patient; therefore, the practitioner should order no unnecessary tests. She should order only those tests that are essential to making or confirming a diagnosis, identifying the organs involved in a disease process, assessing the severity of a disease, or measuring the effectiveness of treatment.

Following are brief descriptions of the laboratory tests and diagnostic procedures the practitioner may employ in the health work-up and management of patients with diabetes mellitus, hypertension, chronic arteriosclerotic heart disease, degenerative arthritis, obesity, and alcoholism, together with a brief discussion of the possible interpretations and applications of the findings on each test. (For tables of Normal Laboratory Values see pp. 221–227.)

The practitioner herself can learn to perform many of the simpler, so-called "screening" examinations described in the following section (for instance, the hemogram, urinalysis, stool test for occult blood, and the tuberculin skin test) by following a standard laboratory manual. On occasion the practitioner may prefer to perform these tests herself rather than wait several days for the laboratory to report the data she needs to make a diagnosis or to follow up treatment results.

HEMOGRAM (HEMATOLOGIC STUDIES)

In most institutions and agencies the hemogram includes a red cell count, a white cell count, a differential count of the several types of white cells, hematocrit measurement, hemoglobin concentration, and, sometimes, the red cell sedimentation rate.

Red Cell Studies

The normal range of red cells (erythrocytes) in the male is 4.6 to 6.2 million per cubic mm. of blood; in the female it is 4.2 to 5.4 million per cubic mm. Red cells are increased above normal in polycythemia vera, a disease of unknown cause, in which there is marrow hyperplasia, with increased production of red cells, platelets, and often myeloid leukocytes. In polycythemia the red cells may number 7 to 10 million cells per cubic mm., and the patient typically appears plethoric or cyanotic and complains of headache, dizziness, tinnitus, dyspnea, and weakness.

Red cells may be *reduced* below normal numbers (anemia) as a result of deficient production, increased destruction, or blood loss. Deficiencies of either protein, iron, vitamin B_{12}, or folic acid will result in inadequate production of red cells. Iron deficiency produces a hypochromic (hemoglobin poor), microcytic (small cell) anemia. Vitamin B_{12} deficiency, folic acid deficiency, and chronic liver disease cause a macrocytic (large cell) anemia. Inadequate production of red cells may also result from depression of the marrow by toxic metabolites, such as the elevated urea and creatinine in uremia; by drugs, such as chloramphenicol; or by ionizing radiation.

The normal life span of an erythrocyte is about 120 days. As a result of either structural weakness of the erythrocytes (sickle-cell anemia, spherocytosis) or increased sequestration and hemolysis of erythrocytes by the spleen and other reticuloendothelial tissues, there may be an increased rate of red cell destruction.

Either acute or chronic blood loss will lead to a reduction in the number of red blood cells. Acute blood loss results in a normocytic (normal sized cell), normochromic (normal amount of hemoglobin) anemia since, following hemorrhage, interstitial fluid is drawn into the blood vessels to re-establish blood volume (thereby diluting the remaining normal red cells). Chronic blood loss gives rise to a microcytic (small cell), hypochromic (hemoglobin poor) anemia since the loss of a small amount of blood continuously over an extended period of time produces an iron deficiency.

Possible sources of error in counting the red cells include drawing up too much or too little blood or diluent into the pipette, coagulation of a portion of the blood sample, overloading the counting chamber, and faulty application of the cover glass. Excessive massaging of the finger from which the sample is taken or removal of the sample from a cold, pale, or cyanotic finger leads to inaccurate red cell counts because in rapid moving or stagnant blood the cell to plasma ratio is not representative of the blood volume as a whole.

In some institutions the red cell count has been abandoned in favor of the measurement of *hematocrit*, or the percentage of a sample of whole blood which is made up of erythrocytes. The normal hematocrit for males is 40 to 54 per cent and for females is 37 to 47 per cent. The hematocrit is increased in dehydration and in polycythemia and decreased in anemia. A possible source of error in hematocrit measurement is inadequate centrifugation of the blood sample.

Hemoglobin, or that component of the red blood cell to which oxygen and carbon dioxide are affixed for transport, can be measured by several means. In the commonly employed Sahli method the hemoglobin is converted to acid hematin by addition of dilute hydrochloric acid, and the yellow-brown color of this solution is then matched against one of a series of standards in a colorimeter. The normal concentration of hemoglobin ranges from 12 to 18 grams per 100 milliliters of blood, and the hemoglobin concentration of a sample should be reported in grams per cent, or grams per 100 milliliters of blood rather than as some percentage of normal, since authorities disagree as to what hemoglobin concentration is "normal." Frequent sources of error in hemoglobin measurement are the use of improperly calibrated pipettes and the presence of excessive fat in the blood sample, since the color of the fat will skew the comparison with the standard.

In addition to counting the number of red cells in a measured quantity of blood, a drop of blood is often smeared on a slide, colored with Wright's stain, and examined under a microscope in order to study the size, shape, and surface characteristics of the red cells. Erythrocytes are crescent shaped in sickle-cell anemia, spherical (rather than biconcave) in spherocytosis, abnormally shaped (poikilocytosis) and varied in size (anisocytosis) in hemolytic anemia; they are unevenly pigmented (target cells) in thalassemia and stippled (spotted) in lead poisoning. An increase in the number of reticulocytes indicates increased red cell production. The presence of nucleated red cells indicates marrow hyperactivity, as in erythremia.

The *red cell sedimentation rate* is the speed with which red cells settle out of a column of blood on standing. This rate of red cell settling is prolonged in pregnancy and in a number of inflammatory conditions, such as acute rheumatic fever, perhaps as a result of an increase in serum globulin and fibrinogen. The red blood cell sedimentation rate can be roughly evaluated by observing the rate at which cells settle out after being transferred from the syringe used for venipuncture to the hematocrit tube. If 10 per cent or more of the total column of blood in the tube is cleared of red cells on standing for 10 minutes, the sedimentation rate may be assumed to be increased and should be measured by a more sensitive test. Since there are a number of different methods for determining the sedimentation rate and since, for each test, there is a different "normal" rate, care must be taken to evaluate each test result against the standards for the specific test used. In the Wintrobe method the normal average red cell sedimentation rate in one hour is 0 to 5 mm. for men and 0 to 15 mm. for women. In the Westergren method the normal range for men is 0 to 15 mm. per hour and for women is 0 to 20 mm. per hour.

White Cell Studies

The normal leukocyte (white blood cell) count in the adult ranges from 5000 to 10,000 per cubic mm. The leukocyte count tends to be increased in bacterial infections, in leukemia, and sometimes in polycythemia (as a result of the marrow hyperactivity). The white cell count is decreased in some viral diseases (influenza), in agranulocytosis, in marrow depression by ionizing radiation or certain drugs (chloramphenicol), and in the aleukemic phase of certain acute leukemias.

There are three general types of leukocytes: granulocytes, which are formed in bone marrow; monocytes, which are formed in lymphatic tissue, and lymphocytes, which are formed in lymphoid tissue. The granulocytes are further divided into the following three types on the basis of whether their cytoplasmic granules stain with acidic, basic, or neutral dyes: neutrophils (also called polymorphonuclear leukocytes), basophils, and eosinophils.

The normal differential white blood cell count in adults is as follows:

Neutrophils (polymorphonuclear leukocytes)—57 to 67 per cent of total W.B.C.

Lymphocytes—25 to 33 per cent of total W.B.C.
Monocytes—3 to 7 per cent of total W.B.C.
Eosinophils—1 to 3 per cent of total W.B.C.
Basophils—up to 1 per cent of total W.B.C.

In leukemia there is usually an increase in only one type of leukocyte: of the granulocytes in myeloid leukemia, of lymphocytes in lymphatic leukemia, of monocytes in monocytic leukemia. In acute bacterial infections there is usually an increase in granular leukocytes. In certain viral infections, as infectious mononucleosis, there is an increase in lymphocytes. In certain chronic infections, as tuberculosis, there is an increase in monocytes. In allergic disorders there is often an increase in eosinophils.

URINALYSIS

In the normal person, an average of 1200 to 1500 milliliters of urine is produced in 24 hours. Typically this urine is amber in color, clear, faintly acidic in reaction, has a specific gravity of 1.003 to 1.030, contains no protein, glucose, acetone, bile, or casts, and no more than three red or white blood cells per high power field.

Methods of Specimen Collection

A voided urine specimen which is collected at random is usually suitable for routine qualitative testing. For quantitative tests urine should be collected for 24 hours, pooled, and a sample of that collection used in determining the total amount of a particular substance eliminated per unit of time.

Care must be taken in obtaining, labeling, storing, and transporting the urine specimen to ensure accurate findings on examination. For instance, if urinary infection is suspected and a urine specimen is needed for culture, steps must be taken to prevent introducing into the specimen contaminants from the external genitalia, the patient's or attendant's hands, the bed linen, or the specimen container. In the male, the glans penis should be cleansed with an antiseptic, the patient should void a small quantity (30 to 60 ml.) which is then discarded, and then the patient should void into a sterile specimen bottle, which is capped immediately. In the female, a urine specimen for culture may be obtained by catheterization or by the "clean catch" method, in which the labia are retracted and cleansed with soap and a mild antiseptic; then while the attendant holds the labia apart the patient first voids a small quantity, which is discarded, then voids directly into a sterile container, which is capped immediately. Since bacteria multiply rapidly in urine and cause decomposition of certain urinary constituents, each urine specimen should, ideally, be examined immediately after collection. When this is not possible the specimen should be refrigerated until the examination is performed.

In the male with a urinary infection, it may be desirable to collect a "three-glass specimen" in order to determine whether the infection is located in the upper or lower urinary tract. In this method, after the glans penis has been cleansed, the first 8 to 12 ml. that the patient voids is collected in the first sterile container; then the patient is allowed to void into the second container; finally, when the bladder is almost empty, the patient is directed to "squeeze out" the last few drops of urine into a third container. The first specimen of urine is considered to represent urethral contents, the second to represent urine from the bladder and renal pelvis, and the third to represent urine containing secretions that have been milked from the prostate gland. By centrifuging each specimen and examining the urinary sediment microscopically it may be determined that epithelial cells, pus cells, red blood cells, protein strands, or inflammatory debris are more plentiful in one specimen than in the others, which findings would suggest that the inflammatory process was localized in the area designated. A Papanicolaou smear preparation of the urinary sediment from the three containers may reveal malignant cells of the bladder, ureter, or kidney epithelium.

Specific Gravity

The specific gravity of the urine, or the relative weight of the urine as compared with that of an equal volume of water, is dependent upon the concentration of solutes in the urine. As the concentration of electrolytes and other particles in the urine increases, the specific gravity increases; as the concentration of such particles decreases, the specific gravity decreases. Therefore, when fluid intake is low, when there has been profuse perspiration, or when the urine contains sugar, acetone, bile, protein, casts, or blood cells, the urine specific gravity is high. If on the other hand fluid intake has been very high, there has been no fluid loss through excessive diaphoresis, bleeding, vomiting, or diarrhea, there has been no excessive intake of salt, and the urine contains no abnormal constituents, the urine specific gravity will be low.

The specific gravity of the urine is determined by floating a urinometer in a specimen of urine and then measuring the degree to which the fluid is displaced by the urinometer (a function of the density of the liquid). When the normal kidney concentrates urine to maximum density, the specific gravity of that urine is 1.040. When the kidney tubules are damaged, as in chronic glomerulonephritis, there is impaired ability to dilute and concentrate urine in response to changes in fluid intake, salt intake, or extrarenal fluid losses. Hence, the specific gravity tends to remain constant or "fixed" at a fairly low level (1.010 to 1.015) regardless of the state of body hydration.

pH

The pH of a fluid is an expression of its hydrogen ion concentration, that is, its acidity or alkalinity. The pH at which the number of hydrogen ions exactly equals the number of hydroxyl ions (chemical neutrality) is 7.0. Since the level of pH is a function of the *reciprocal* of the hydrogen ion concentration, the pH decreases as the hydrogen ion concentration increases and the pH increases as the hydrogen ion concentration decreases. Thus, a pH below 7.0 indicates acidity; a pH above 7.0 indicates alkalinity. Normally, the urine is slightly acid and a piece of litmus indicator paper will turn red when submerged in the urine. The urine may be alkaline for a few hours following a meal or during urinary tract infection by a urea splitting (therefore alkalinizing) organism such as Proteus vulgaris.

Glucose

In the normal person the renal threshold for glucose, or the serum concentration above which glucose is filtered from the blood in the glomerulus but not resorbed in the tubule, is about 170 to 180 mg. per 100 ml. of blood. Normally, the serum glucose concentration does not rise above this level, except after a very high carbohydrate meal. In the pregnant female, however, this renal threshold for glucose may be temporarily depressed, allowing glucose to spill over into the urine at a lower serum concentration. In the diabetic a lack of insulin interferes both with conversion of glucose to glycogen and with oxidation of glucose by tissue cells. Therefore, the blood glucose level gradually rises above normal levels until it exceeds the renal threshold for glucose and appears in the urine.

There are several ways to test urine for sugar. The most commonly used method is that of dipping small slips of chemically impregnated test paper into the urine specimen. The resulting color change is compared to a standard chart, which indicates the relative amount of glucose present for each shade of color reaction (none, trace amounts, 1 plus, 2 plus, 3 plus, and 4 plus reactions).

Acetone

At one stage in the process of fat digestion, acetone and ketone bodies are produced. In the normal person these intermediate products of fat digestion are further oxidized to carbon dioxide and water. Trace amounts of acetone may appear in the urine of a fasting individual as a consequence of the breakdown of fatty tissue as an energy source. In the diabetic patient the disturbance of carbohydrate metabolism results in impaired fat metabolism as well, with the result that acetone and ketone bodies are poorly oxidized and acetone accumulates in blood to the point that eventually it spills over into the urine. The accumulation of acetone in the blood serum is responsible for the metabolic acidosis that develops in the uncontrolled diabetic. Each time the diabetic patient's urine is found to contain glucose it should also be tested for acetone, the most common test for which consists of dipping a chemically impregnated test paper strip into the urine. The resulting color change, if any, is read against a standard color scale to determine the relative amount of acetone present in the sample (0, 1 plus, 2 plus, 3 plus, 4 plus).

Albumin

Although any of the blood proteins may be found in the urine, albumin is the one most commonly discovered, since the albumin molecule is smaller than the molecule of either globulin or fibrinogen and can therefore easily "leak" through a damaged glomerular membrane. Albumin may also exude from the capillaries of the lining of the bladder and/or urethra in inflammatory disorders of those structures. In a simple screening test for protein in the urine, a chemically impregnated test paper dipped into the urine turns from yellow to green-blue in the presence of protein. The intensity of color change can be matched against a standard to grade the reaction as trace, 1 plus, 2 plus, 3 plus, or 4 plus. Other tests for protein in the urine involve the use of heat, acetic acid, nitric acid, or sulfosalicylic acid to precipitate the protein in the sample. Protein is frequently found in the urine of the pregnant female and of patients with chronic glomerulonephritis, nephrosis, malignant nephrosclerosis, cystitis, prostatitis, and urethritis.

Microscopic Examination

As part of the urine examination 10 to 15 ml. of urine should be centrifuged for five minutes, the supernatant fluid discarded, and the urinary sediment placed on a slide, covered with a coverslip and studied under both low and high power microscopic lenses. Normal urine may contain some mucus shreds; a few crystals of various salts; a few epithelial cells shed from the lining of the kidney, ureter, bladder, or urethra; and an occasional red or white blood cell (no more than two of each per high power field). Excessive numbers of red blood cells may be found in the urine in renal trauma, acute glomerulonephritis, calculus, infection, benign or malignant malaria, tumor, and subacute bacterial endocarditis. Excessive numbers of white blood cells in the urine suggest infection.

Crystals normally seen in the urine include uric acid, urate, and calcium oxalate crystals, which tend to form in acid urine; and calcium carbonate and calcium phosphate crystals, which tend to form in alkaline urine. Calcium oxalate crystals may be numerous in the urine of a patient with urinary calculi. Certain of the less soluble sulfanilamide derivatives may precipitate in acid urine, occasionally accumulating in such quantities as to obstruct the renal tubules. Leucine and tyrosine crystals, resulting from the breakdown of protein molecules, are seen in the urine of patients with hepatic decompensation and necrotizing carcinomas.

Urinary casts are cylindrical molds of the renal collecting tubules which are composed of gelled protein. Hyaline casts, which contain no cells but may contain a few granules, are sometimes seen in small numbers in the urine of normal persons, especially following active exercise. Excessive numbers of hyaline casts indicate tubular exudation such as that which occurs in glomerulonephritis and certain febrile illnesses. Casts composed of clumped tubular epithelial cells, leukocytes, or erythrocytes are always abnormal and may be found in glomerulonephritis or nephrosis.

TUBERCULIN SKIN SENSITIVITY TEST

As a consequence of harboring a tuberculous infection, an individual's body tissue become sensitized to the protein of the tubercle bacillus in such a way that the introduction of even a small amount of tuberculin into the skin causes an allergic reaction. For testing purposes a purified preparation of tuberculin (purified protein derivative) is injected intradermally. A weak-strength solution (1:10,000) is used in testing a patient in whom active tuberculosis is probable (in order not to provoke a severe local tissue reaction). For routine testing of apparently non-tuberculous persons a 1:2000 solution of tuberculin is injected, and the skin reaction is read in 24 and again in 48 hours. The reaction is considered doubtful if there is slight erythema, and edema of less than 5 mm. in diameter; 1 plus if there is erythema, and edema of 5 to 10 mm. in diameter; 2 plus if there is erythema, and edema of 10 to 20 mm. in diameter; 3 plus if there is marked erythema, and edema that exceeds 20 mm. in diameter; and 4 plus if there is central necrosis in addition to erythema and edema. A positive tuberculin reaction indicates that the individual has at some time harbored a tuberculous infection, but does not necessarily mean that an active tuberculosis infection exists currently.

SEROLOGIC TESTS FOR SYPHILIS

Because it is impossible to culture Treponema pallidum from the blood of syphilitic patients, diagnosis of the disease usually must be made by demonstrating the presence of antibodies against that organism in the patient's serum. During a syphilitic infection, a syphilis reagin appears in the patient's serum which has the ability to combine with certain tissue lipids. There are several different serological tests for syphilis. The Kahn, Mazzini, and VDRL are flocculation tests, and depend upon the fact that the syphilitic reagin in the patient's serum will combine with particles of lipid-coated cholesterol (the antigen) to form a visible aggregation of particles. The Wassermann and Kolmer are complement fixation tests. Complement, a heat-sensitive substance which is present in the serum of all warm-blooded animals, must be present in order for certain antibody-antigen reactions (as the reaction of syphilis reagin with beef heart antigen) to occur. Thus, in order to determine whether syphilis reagin is present in a patient's serum, a measured quantity of the serum should be combined with a certain amount of active or heated complement (from fresh guinea pig serum) and a specified amount of antigen (beef heart extract). If syphilis reagin is present the complement will be "fixed" or removed from solution because it is bound up in the antigen-antibody reaction. Since this reaction is not visible an indicator test is then used to demonstrate whether, in fact, the complement has been used up in the reaction. The most frequently used indicator test consists of adding washed sheep red blood cells and an artificially produced sheep cell hemolysin. If free complement is present the hemolysin will cause the sheep red cells to rupture (a visible reaction). Thus, visible hemolysis during the indicator test signifies that syphilis reagin was not present in the patient's serum, since complement was not "fixed" in the first reaction and therefore was available to facilitate the combination of sheep red cells and hemolysin.

BLOOD CHEMISTRY STUDIES

Serum Glucose Determination

Determinations of the quantity of various biochemical components of the blood serum are usually performed on venous blood, preferably drawn after the patient has fasted for several hours or overnight. A standard battery of tests, sometimes referred to as the SMA, or sequential multiple analysis, is often done in large hospital laboratories. The individual tests making up this battery differ from institution to institution. The tests described here are those likely to be of principal importance to the nurse practitioner and her patients.

Normally, when a person has been without food for several hours, his serum glucose level ranges from 60 to 100 mg. per 100 ml. of blood. Following ingestion of carbohydrate the serum glucose level usually rises from 120 to 150 mg. per 100 ml. of blood by the end of 45 to 60 minutes but declines to the previous fasting level by the end of the second hour, as a result of the withdrawal of glucose from the blood and its storage as glycogen in liver and muscle. Normally, glucose in the blood is filtered through the glomerulus but, as mentioned previously, when the serum glucose level is 170 mg. per 100 ml. of blood or less, it is totally resorbed from the renal tubule.

Serum glucose levels tend to be elevated in diabetes mellitus, hyperthyroidism, Cushing's disease, pheochromocytoma, and hyperpituitarism. Serum glucose levels are decreased in hyperinsulinism and in starvation, and following surgical removal of liver tissue (as in treatment for blunt trauma to the liver).

As a screening test for diabetes mellitus a fasting blood glucose determination may be made (analysis of glucose level in a blood sample drawn early in the morning after the patient has fasted for twelve hours). A fasting blood glucose level higher than 110 mg. per 100 ml. of blood is highly suggestive of diabetes. An even more sensitive screening test is the two hour postprandial serum glucose determination, in which the patient fasts for twelve hours, is given a 100 gm. carbohydrate meal, then has blood samples drawn both one and two hours later for analysis. In a postprandial test a one hour serum glucose value higher than 170 mg. per 100 ml. or a two hour serum glucose value higher than 120 mg. per 100 ml. is suggestive of diabetes mellitus.

In some patients with a disturbance of glucose metabolism the fasting serum glucose level may fall within normal limits. Therefore, patients with glycosuria but without other symptoms of diabetes who have normal fasting blood glucose levels, and patients with family incidence of diabetes who are themselves symptom free should be given an oral or intravenous glucose tolerance test. In the oral glucose tolerance test the patient fasts for 12 hours, the fasting serum glucose and urine glucose levels are determined, he is given a mixture of 100 gm. of glucose in 500 ml. of flavored water to drink within 5 minutes, and samples of urine and whole blood are taken after 30 minutes, 1, 2, and 3 hours and tested for glucose content. In non-pregnant adults up to the age of 50 the following are normal serum glucose levels for the oral glucose tolerance test: fasting level, 110 mg. per 100 ml.; 1/2 hour, 170 mg. per 100 ml.; 1 hour, 170 mg. per 100 ml.; 2 hours, 120 mg. per 100 ml.; and 3 hours, 110 mg. per 100 ml. If both the fasting and three hour serum glucose levels or if any three of the glucose levels are elevated above these normals, the test results are considered to be abnormal. Glycosuria should not occur at any time during the glucose tolerance test. In patients with gastrointestinal disease an intravenous rather than an oral glucose tolerance test should be used. For this test 0.5 gm. of glucose per kg. of the patient's weight should be given in a 20 per cent solution intravenously over a 30 minute period. Blood samples are drawn just before the glucose is injected and 30 minutes, 1, 2, and 3 hours following injection. Normally, the fasting blood glucose level should fall below 110 mg. per 100 ml, the glucose level should not exceed 250 mg. per 100 ml in any specimen, and the blood glucose concentration should have returned to fasting level within two hours following injection of the glucose loading dose.

Serum Cholesterol Determination

Cholesterol is a fat-soluble alcohol, found in fats, oils, plant seeds, egg yolk, and brain tissue, which is capable of forming esters with fatty acids. Cholesterol is utilized in the production of such hormones as estrogen, testosterone, and adrenal steroid hormones. In addition to the dietary cholesterol which is absorbed from the small intestine, liver cells synthesize cholesterol and excrete it in the bile. In the United States, where dietary patterns involve ingestion of large amounts of animal fat, the normal range of serum cholesterol concentration is 150 to 250 mg. per 100 ml. of blood. Hypercholesterolemia may result from ingestion of a high fat diet, hypothyroidism, nephrotic syndrome, diabetes mellitus, familial hypercholesterolemia, and biliary tract obstruction. Hypocholesterolemia may result from hyperthyroidism and generalized liver cell damage. Sustained elevations of serum cholesterol are associated with atheromatosis and arteriosclerosis. A hereditary predisposition and a high intake of saturated fats tend to increased serum cholesterol levels. Substitution of polyunsaturated fats for the animal fats in the diet tends to decrease serum cholesterol levels.

Serum Electrolytes

In the lean man, approximately 66 percent, or 45 liters, of the total body weight is water. The intracellular compartment contains slightly less than 30 liters, or two thirds of the total body water, and the extracellular (blood and interstitial) spaces constitute about 15 liters of fluid, or one third of the total body water. The composition of fluids in these two main compartments is critical to normal metabolism.

Plasma, one component of extracellular fluid, contains cations (+) and anions (−) in the following concentrations, which represent the normal range of these substances as determined by the usual tests.

Cations			Anions		
Na^+	136–145	mEq/L	Cl^-	98–106	mEq/L
K^+	3.5–5	mEq/L	PO_4^{---}	3–4.5	mEq/L
Ca^+	4.5–5.5	mEq/L	SO_4^{--}	2–5	mEq/L
Mg^{++}	1.5–2.5	mEq/L	HCO_3^-	24–26	mEq/L

In contrast to the extracellular fluid, the intracellular fluid contains very little sodium (10 mEq/L) and a much higher concentration of potassium (150 mEq/L) and phosphate (150 mEq/L).

The regulatory mechanism of the body tends to maintain constancy in the composition of body fluids. Although the ionic concentrations of intracellular and extracellular fluid are different, the osmolality of the two fluid compartments is the same. By the processes of diffusion, osmosis, and active transport, solute and water move across the semipermeable membranes separating the body's fluid compartments so as to restore the isosmotic state where there has been a loss of water or ions from one or the other compartment.

Sodium (Na^+)

Sodium is the principal extracellular ion and, therefore, the chief contributor to the osmolality of the extracellular fluid. Hyponatremia (low Na^+ concentration in the serum) causes movement of water into cells, while hypernatremia causes movement of water from the cells. Thus, if the sodium concentration in the serum is normal (140 mEq/L) the volume of the intracellular fluid will also be normal.

Hypernatremia is not as common as hyponatremia but is of extreme importance because it is an early sign of cellular water depletion. The body's compensatory mechanisms for correction of hypernatremia include thirst, increased ADH secretion, low aldosterone secretion, high urinary output of sodium, and urine of low volume, high specific gravity, and high urea concentration. Patients with fever, diarrhea, brain injury, and hyperpnea, and those who are in the recovery phase of diabetic acidosis are prone to hypernatremia.

Hyponatremia due to sodium loss in excess of water loss, as occurs in acidosis, uremia, or severe diarrhea, is often accompanied by weakness, anorexia, and apathy. When the serum concentration of sodium is low, the concentration of chloride is usually also low. Hyponatremia can also occur if water is retained in excess of sodium, as results from excessive sweating, inadequate aldosterone secretion, and hypersecretion of ADH.

Potassium$^+$

Because potassium is a predominantly intracellular ion, measurement of serum potassium is not a good indicator of the total body concentration of the ion. The concentration of extracellular potassium influences the membrane potential of nerve and muscle cells. Hyperkalemia, or elevated concentration of potassium in the serum, is rare but can occur in acidosis, anoxia, or low glomerular filtration rate, or it can be iatrogenically induced by vigorous potassium replacement therapy. The chief clinical danger of hyperkalemia is cardiac arrest, because increasing the extracellular potassium concentration causes the myocardial muscle cells to remain depolarized (in diastole).

Hypokalemia may occur in (1) continued vomiting or diarrhea; (2) renal tubular failure; (3) excessive sodium retention in the glomerular filtrate; (4) deficient secretion of hydrogen ion in the distal tubule due to administration of a diuretic that inhibits carbonic anhydrase (as chlorothiazide, acetazolamide); or (5) any condition creating acidosis, such as diabetes mellitus. Low potassium concentration in the extracellular fluid interferes with neuromuscular impulse transmission and produces muscular weakness.

Calcium$^+$

Of the two forms in which calcium is found in the body only the ionized form (about half of total calcium) is physiologically active. Concentration of ionized calcium is controlled by the parathyroid hormone, which acts on bone to release calcium and phosphate ions and on the distal portions of the renal nephrons to excrete phosphate ions in the urine. Hypercalcemia results from elevated parathyroid hormone, elevated vitamin D, increased dietary intake of calcium, hyperproteinemia, and acidosis. Hypercalcemia can cause renal failure by causing precipitation of calcium phosphate ($Ca_3(PO_4)_2$) in the renal tubules. Hypercalcemia depresses neuromuscular excitability in several types of muscles: in smooth muscle of the gastrointestinal tract, causing constipation and abdominal pain; in skeletal muscle, causing poor muscle tone; and in cardiac muscle, leading to cardiac arrest.

Hypocalcemia causes increased neuromuscular activity, which may result in tetany. Low serum calcium levels also may result in cataract formation.

Calcium deficiency is called rickets in children and osteomalacia in adults. Hypocalcemia may be caused by hypoparathyroidism, malabsorption of calcium from the gut, or hypoalbuminemia.

A reciprocal relationship exists between calcium and phosphorus in the blood, and this relationship is important to the body's metabolism because calcium phosphate is highly insoluble at the pH of body fluids. Calcium absorption in the gastrointestinal tract is influenced by the amount of dietary calcium, the availability of vitamin D, and the presence of phosphate. Ingestion of a large quantity of phosphate interferes with calcium absorption by forming insoluble calcium phosphate ($Ca_3(PO_4)_2$).

Phosphate (PO_4^{---})

Most of the phosphate in the body is in combination with calcium in the bones. Phosphate has a key role in maintaining normal serum calcium concentration, normal pH, and adequate energy supplies in the form of adenosine triphosphate (ATP). Excessive phosphate is excreted in the feces and urine. Toxic symptoms of high phosphate concentration in the plasma are those of hypocalcemia because of the reciprocal relationship that exists between calcium and phosphorus. Secretion of parathyroid hormone, which tends to increase serum concentration of calcium ions, decreases serum phosphorus ion concentrations. Phosphate depletion may lead to a decrease in the ATP stores. Renal insufficiency results in elevated serum levels of phosphate, owing to the fact that phosphate ions must be combined with hydrogen ions in the renal tubule in order to be eliminated in the urine.

Magnesium (Mg^{++})

Magnesium is found in the body both intracellularly and extracellularly. Magnesium enters and leaves bone with calcium and moves in and out of cells with potassium and phosphate ions. Hypomagnesemia, like hypocalcemia, can cause tetany and occurs as a result of malabsorption, diarrhea, or diabetes. Hypermagnesemia results in muscular hypotonia and is caused by renal failure, hypothyroidism, or certain antacids.

Chloride (Cl^-)

Chloride, the most abundant anion in the body, is usually found in combination with sodium. Thus, when sodium is transported across a cell membrane, chloride passively follows. Plasma bicarbonate (HCO^-_3) and chloride concentrations are usually inversely related. Chloride depletion results in alkalosis by indirectly causing increased reabsorption of HCO^-_3 in the distal tubules of the nephron. As bicarbonate concentration increases, hydrogen ion is secreted into the tubules and an acid urine is excreted. Hyperchloremia has an opposite effect on the pH of the plasma; that is, it causes acidosis.

Serum Proteins

Plasma proteins have a variety of functions:

1. Maintenance of vascular fluid volume by creating the colloid osmotic pressure
2. Immune response (antibodies are proteins)

3. Plasma buffering (release or combine with hydrogen ions)
4. Blood clotting (fibrinogen and thromboplastin are proteins)
5. Metabolism (enzymes are proteins, and protein is a source of calories)
6. Transport (certain hormones, vitamins, and calcium are transported in the plasma in combination with proteins)

Five fractions of the serum proteins can be identified by zone electrophoresis. In this process an electric current flows through a serum-buffer solution. The individual protein fractions migrate in different directions and at different speeds, depending on their molecular size and electric charge. The fractions, and their normal range per 100 ml. of serum, are as follows:

Total protein	6.5–8.0 gm./100 ml.
Albumin	3.5–5.5 gm./100 ml.
α_1-Globulin	0.2–0.4 gm./100 ml.
α_2-Globulin	0.5–0.9 gm./100 ml.
β-Globulin	0.6–1.1 gm./100 ml.
γ-Globulin	0.7–1.7 gm./100 ml.

Disease states may specifically alter certain protein fractions. In a specific disease, change may be evident in all fractions or in only one of the five. An increase in all fractions is observed in dehydration, while a decrease in only the gamma fraction is evident in hypogammaglobulinemia. A specific pattern change in all protein fractions is seen in nephrotic syndrome. Non-specific changes often occur in plasma protein concentrations in conditions of tissue damage or inflammation.

The gamma globulin fraction is composed chiefly of the immunoglobulins which have antibody activity. Of the five classes of immunoglobulins the major ones are IgG, IgM, and IgA.

Blood Urea Nitrogen (BUN)

Urea, an end product of protein metabolism which is formed in the liver, is produced from the ammonia released from amino groups. Because urea diffuses freely through capillary walls and cell membranes, it is present in approximately equal concentrations in intra- and extracellular fluid. Urea is filtered through the glomerulus, and partially resorbed from the tubules. The normal range of urea nitrogen is 10 to 20 mg. per 100 ml. of blood. Urea nitrogen levels should be measured in the fasting state, since blood urea levels increase following ingestion of protein. Blood urea nitrogen levels are increased in dehydration, intestinal obstruction, gastrointestinal hemorrhage, chronic glomerulonephritis, chronic pyelonephritis, and prostatic hypertrophy. Blood urea nitrogen levels may be decreased in starvation or in cirrhosis (owing to inability of liver cells to break down amino acids).

Uric Acid Determination

Uric acid is a nitrogenous waste product that results from the breakdown of purines, the major constituent of nucleoproteins. The uric acid in blood serum derives both from the digestion and metabolism of exogenous protein and from endogenous production of uric acid.

Uric acid is totally filtered through the glomerulus, and most uric acid in the glomerular filtrate is resorbed from the tubules. In a healthy person, enough uric acid is then actively excreted by the tubular cells to maintain serum uric acid concentration at 1.5 to 8 mg. per 100 ml. of blood (normal level).

Since protein digestion and tissue catabolism continuously produce new uric acid, in the healthy person there is continuous excretion of uric acid in the urine. The serum level of uric acid may increase as a result of either overproduction or underexcretion. Overproduction of uric acid occurs in lymphoma and leukemia, as a result of rapid proliferation of cells in the bone marrow or lymph nodes. Underexcretion of uric acid occurs in gout, toxemia of pregnancy, and acute or chronic glomerulonephritis. In gout there is a tendency for uric acid crystals to be deposited in the first metatarsophalangeal joint, in the helix of the ear, and in the collecting tubules and pelvis of the kidney.

The serum uric acid level is rarely decreased, except following administration of allopurinol, a drug which inhibits uric acid production and is used in treating gout.

Creatinine

Creatinine is a breakdown product of creatine, a compound in muscle that constitutes a source of high energy phosphate bonds. Creatinine in the blood serum is both filtered through the glomerulus and secreted by the renal tubules. Since creatinine production is related to the mass of the body's muscle tissue rather than to the amount of protein in the diet, the amount of creatinine excreted daily in the urine is constant in a healthy individual. Normal serum creatinine concentration ranges from 0.7 to 1.5 mg. per 100 ml. of blood. Serum creatinine levels are increased in renal failure resulting from acute and chronic glomerulonephritis, nephrosis, and pyelonephritis. Although creatinine tends to increase in the same conditions that cause an increase in blood urea nitrogen and uric acid, the increase in creatinine lags behind the increase in the other two substances, so elevation of serum creatinine suggests a more serious prognosis.

Serum Bilirubin

Hemoglobin, which is released by the rupture of red blood cells, is broken down by cells of the reticuloendothelial system to form free or indirect bilirubin, which is transported in the blood to the liver, where it is extracted by the liver cells, conjugated with glucuronic acid to form conjugated or direct bilirubin, and excreted in the bile. This conjugated bilirubin gives bile its characteristic yellow color. In the bowel, bilirubin is converted by intestinal bacteria to urobilinogen, a small amount of which is absorbed into the blood and re-excreted by the liver, another small amount of which is excreted in the urine, and most of which is oxidized to urobilin and excreted in the feces.

In hemolytic jaundice excessive destruction of red blood cells causes increased concentration in the serum of free or indirect bilirubin because the liver cells are unable to remove the bilirubin from the blood as rapidly as it is being released from red cells. In obstructive jaundice there is increased concentration in the serum of conjugated or direct bilirubin because the free bilirubin is removed from the blood by the liver cells and conjugated with glucuronic acid; this conjugated bilirubin is then forced back into the blood by the increased pressure in the obstructed biliary tract. In hepatitis there may be an increase in both free (indirect) and conjugate (direct) bilirubin, since the damaged liver cells cannot remove bilirubin from the blood at the normal rate, and inflammation of the canaliculi obstructs normal bile flow from the liver, forcing conjugated bilirubin back into the blood. The upper limit of normal for conjugated bilirubin in the serum is 0.4 mg. per 100 ml., and the normal level of total bilirubin is 0.7 mg. per 100 ml. Thus, the difference between the two, or the indirect bilirubin, is usually about 0.3 mg. per 100 ml. Jaundice is usually apparent when the total serum bilirubin exceeds 2.5 mg. per 100 ml.

Protein-Bound Iodine

Iodine which is ingested is absorbed from the small intestine and "trapped" by the thyroid gland where, under the influence of thyroid stimulating hormone, it is oxidized and combined with thyroglobulin (a glycoprotein produced in thyroid cells) to form triiodothyronine and thyroxine, both of which hormones regulate the rate of oxygen utilization by tissue cells.

Because iodine is the principal component of thyroid hormone, the concentration of protein-bound iodine in the serum is an indicator of the amount of circulating thyroid hormone. The normal concentration of protein-bound iodine ranges from 3.5 to 8 μg. per 100 ml. of serum. In general, protein-bound iodine is decreased in hypothyroidism and increased in hyperthyroidism.

Serum Iron

The normal diet includes from 5 to 15 mg. of iron per day. Iron absorbed from the intestine is bound to transferrin, a serum globulin, for transportation to the liver and to various tissue cells. Normally, very little iron is excreted from the body. Rather, iron released from red cell breakdown is recycled and reused in the formation of new hemoglobin. Sixty-five per cent of iron in the body is a component of hemoglobin. The remainder of the body's iron stores exists in myoglobin, in cellular oxidative enzyme, and as hemosiderin (an insoluble storage form).

The organic form of iron in the blood, that is, in hemoglobin, constitutes about 52 μg. per 100 ml.; while the inorganic iron in the blood, or that bound to transferrin and carried in the serum, constitutes from 75 to 175 μg per 100 ml. The level of serum iron concentration is lowered in uremia, chronic infection, and malignant disease. Serum iron levels are increased in hemochromatosis, a rare disease which is characterized by increased iron absorption and deposition of iron in parenchymal cells of the liver, pancreas, heart, spleen and kidney.

PAPANICOLAOU SMEAR TEST FOR MALIGNANT CELLS

Cells of the lining of the uterine tubes, uterus, and vagina exfoliate and mix with cervical and vaginal secretions. Because the cervix is the most common site for cancer of the female reproductive tract, cervical carcinoma is most common between the ages of 30 and 50, and the survival rate of patients with cervical carcinoma is greatly increased by early treatment, all women over 35 years of age should have an annual pelvic examination and cytological study of cervical and vaginal secretions.

The technique for inserting the vaginal speculum was described in Chapter 3.

In Papanicolaou technique, cells are scraped from the cervix with a wooden Ayre spatula; the material thus removed is spread in a thin film on a clean glass slide, and the slide is placed immediately in a covered jar of fixative solution (equal parts of 95 per cent alcohol and ether) until the preparation can be stained and read by a trained cytologist.

A smear of vaginal secretions should then be obtained by compressing the bulb of a vaginal pipette, inserting the pipette into the vagina with an upward and backward motion so as to contact secretions from the posterior fornix, then releasing the bulb of the pipette so as to aspirate secretions. The pipette is then withdrawn from the vagina and the secretions expressed onto a clean slide and spread in a thin smear with the side of the pipette. This smear, like the other, should be placed immediately in a closed container of the ether and alcohol fixative. If slides of both smears are to be stored in one jar of fixative, a paper clip should be attached to the end of each slide to prevent the slides from rubbing together and damaging a smear. The bottles of fixative in which the smears are stored must not be placed near heat or flame, since the solution is flammable.

Each smear is classified by the cytologist in one of four categories: Class I, no abnormal cells are seen; Class II, atypical cells are seen which appear to be the result of inflammatory change; Class III, cells are seen which arouse suspicion of carcinoma; Class IV, carcinoma cells are definitely present. In the patient in whom there is no visible cervical lesion, but whose Papanicolaou smear is Class III or IV, Schiller's solution (an iodine preparation) is applied to the cervix to determine whether there are any non-staining areas, which would indicate a lack of glycogen in the cell. Since normal cervical epithelial cells contain glycogen, and carcinoma cells are void of glycogen, an area of tissue that does not stain with iodine should be biopsied.

STOOL EXAMINATION

The intestinal content is liquid when it reaches the cecum. As it passes through the large intestine, water is removed from the bolus so that the stool becomes semisolid in consistency in the transverse or descending colon. Normally, the feces contain undigested food elements (such as cellulose); intestinal secretions; bile; degenerated epithelial cells that have sloughed from the lining of the esophagus, stomach, and bowel; and bacteria, which inhabit the gastrointestinal tract. The normal brown color of stool is produced by certain food pigments and by breakdown products of bile. Bile that is poured into the duodenum is acted upon by intestinal bacteria to form biliverdin (green in color), which is further altered by the action of intestinal bacteria to form stercobilin (brown in color).

In obstructive jaundice, stools tend to be clay colored, owing to a lack of bile (and thus of stercobilin) and an excess of fat (improper fat absorption caused by a lack of bile). In pancreatitis the stool may also be clay colored and greasy owing to an excess of fat (improper fat digestion caused by a lack of pancreatic lipase). In diarrhea the stool may be green because the intestinal content is moved along too rapidly for the biliverdin to be converted to stercobilin. Ingestion of spinach may make the stool green; ingestion of chocolate may render the stool gray.

Hemorrhage high in the gastrointestinal tract, as in bleeding esophageal varices or bleeding peptic ulcer, renders the stool black, because of the effect of digestive juices on the constituents of the blood. Hemorrhage low in the intestinal tract, as in ulcerative colitis, diverticulitis, carcinoma of the sigmoid colon, or hemorrhoids, causes the stool to be streaked with bright or dark red blood.

Test for Occult Blood

There must be a blood loss of about 100 ml. from the upper gastrointestinal tract to produce black stool; for this reason, it is necessary to test for occult or hidden blood in the stool through the use of chemical tests, as the guaiac or benzidine test. For either test the patient should be directed to eat no red meat for 24 hours preceding the test. The guaiac test consists of streaking a small amount of stool on a piece of filter paper, then applying to the stool specimen first two drops of glacial acetic acid, then two drops of a saturated solution of gum guaiac in 95 per cent alcohol, then two drops of 3 per cent hydrogen peroxide. The appearance of a blue color, which can be graded in intensity from 1+ to 4+, indicates the presence of occult blood. Ingestion of oral iron tablets does not produce a positive reaction to a stool guaiac test. The benzidine test, which is more sensitive than the guaiac test, may yield a positive reaction to the hemoglobin in dietary meat for as long as three days following ingestion. Since it is difficult to arrange for a patient to refrain from eating red meat for three days preceding a stool examination, the less sensitive guaiac test for blood is more frequently used.

ROENTGENOGRAPHIC EXAMINATION

X-rays (roentgen rays) are high-energy electromagnetic waves capable of penetrating body tissues to varying degrees, depending on tissue density. When x-rays are passed through the body to focus on photographic film, tissue of low density, such as lung tissue or fat, interferes very little with electromagnetic wave transmission to underlying film, and substances of high density, such as bones or calculi, block wave transmission to underlying film. After development, areas of highly irradiated or exposed film will appear dark, and areas of less irradiated or exposed film will appear light. These contrasting areas of lightness and darkness on a particular film make it possible to determine the location, size, contour, and density of certain structures (heart, lung, stomach, bowel), to identify breaks in continuity of dense structures (bone), and to identify the presence of abnormal substances in certain body parts (calculi in the kidney or gall bladder, air in the peritoneal cavity, fluid in the pleural cavity).

Certain radiopaque substances can be used to outline hollow structures to more clearly visualize the size and shape of the cavity or the character of the cavity lining. For instance, a radiopaque, iodine-containing dye that can be given orally is absorbed from the bowel, carried to the liver, excreted in the bile, and concentrated in the gall bladder, thereby permitting visualization of the size and contour of that organ and outlining any non-radiopaque stones it may contain.

Another iodine-containing radiopaque substance that can be administered intravenously is filtered through the glomerulus, concentrated in the tubules, and when collected in the renal pelvis and excreted through the ureters to the bladder, outlines those structures in a way that reveals dilation of the kidney pelvis and dilation, narrowing, deflection, or tortuosity of the ureter. Barium sulfate solutions (also radiopaque) can be administered either orally or rectally to outline either the upper or lower gastrointestinal tract on x-ray, thereby visualizing such structural abnormalities as esophageal narrowing or displacement; gastric herniation (through a diaphragmatic defect), gastric ulcer, or gastric tumor; and tumor, ulceration, diverticulosis, dilation, narrowing, or displacement of the large bowel.

Chest X-ray

X-ray of the chest provides valuable information about the respiratory and circulatory systems. As part of routine physical examination and health workup it is customary to order a plain posterior-anterior (P-A) chest film (the x-rays or waves are directed through the patient's back toward a film placed in front of his chest). This film may reveal a chest abnormality in an asymptomatic person, may indicate pulmonary or cardiac involvement in someone who is ill but whose symptoms are limited to other body parts, or may corroborate a tentative diagnosis suggested by the patient's presenting respiratory or circulatory symptoms. A P-A chest film may, for instance, reveal lung tumor, pulmonary consolidation, pulmonary fibrosis, emphysema, pulmonary cavitation, pulmonary collapse, pleural effusion, calcified lymph nodes, mediastinal shift, cardiac enlargement, and aortic dilation.

When structural abnormalities are found on chest x-ray, the examiner should locate the patient's previous chest films and compare these with the current film to determine whether the present pathology is of long duration. Occasionally, the finding of abnormality on a plain chest film may suggest the need for more complex radiographic procedures, such as angiocardiography, bronchography, pulmonary radiophotoscanning, or laminography. Occasionally, too, such other diagnostic procedures as bronchoscopy, pleuroscopy, pulmonary function studies, or cardiac catheterization may be needed to further investigate findings made on plain chest films.

ELECTROCARDIOGRAM

An electrocardiogram is a graphic recording of the electrical currents generated by the depolarization and repolarization of different portions of heart muscle. Because these electrical currents are transmitted from the heart to the body surface they can be picked up by electrodes applied to the patient's skin and transmitted to a galvanometer and amplifier (the electrocardiograph), which measures the direction and amplitude of the electrical currents and records them on graph paper. Electrocardiographic leads are created by connecting two points on the body surface to which electrodes are attached. As an electrical impulse in the heart muscle moves toward a particular lead, a positive or upward deflection is produced in the electrographic recording. When an electrical impulse in the heart muscle moves away from a particular lead a negative or downward deflection is produced in the recording.

The standard 12-lead electrocardiogram is useful in diagnosing arrhythmias, myocardial damage, and cardiac strain. For this procedure the patient is relaxed and in a supine position; electrodes are strapped in place over the ventral aspect of both wrists and the medial aspect of both ankles, while the single chest lead is attached by a suction cup to first one and then another of several points on the chest.

In the electrocardiographic record the electrical events of the cardiac cycle are recorded as a sequence of five wave deflections. The P wave or first event in the cardiac cycle is a positive deflection that represents the spread of the impulse from the SA node throughout the atria. The Q wave is a short negative deflection; the R wave is a rather long positive deflection; and the S wave is a short negative deflection (Fig. 47).

The Q, R, and S waves are a complex representing the spread of the impulse throughout the ventricular muscle. Finally, the T wave, a positive

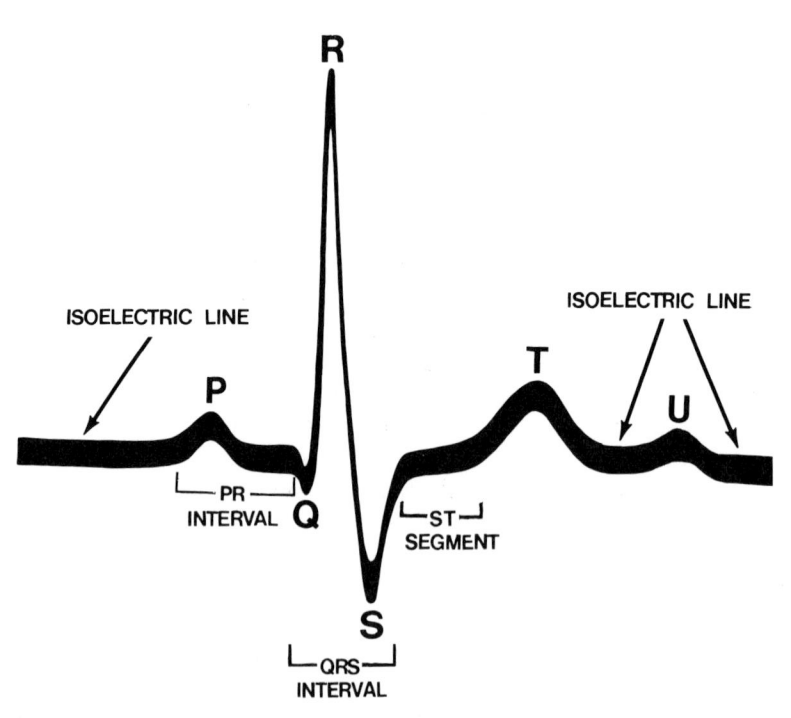

Figure 47. Electrocardiographic components of the cardiac cycle. (From Phillips, R. E., and Feeney, M. K.: *The Cardiac Rhythms.* Philadelphia, W. B. Saunders Co., 1973.)

deflection, represents repolarization of ventricular muscle. Because electrocardiographic paper is scored vertically and horizontally, it is possible to measure the force and duration of each wave in the cardiac cycle. (Each small vertical line on the graph paper represents 0.04 second, and each small horizontal line represents 0.1 millivolt.) Diagnostic implications can be derived from observing not only the direction, force, and duration of the P, Q, R, S, and T waves on the recording from a particular lead, but also the length of the interval between the P and R waves, and the character of the segment of the tracing between the S and T waves.

The details of electrocardiographic recording and interpretation will not be discussed here. For further information, see bibliography for appropriate sources.

BIBLIOGRAPHY: LABORATORY EXAMINATIONS

Davidsohn, I., and Henry, J. B., Eds.: *Todd-Sanford Clinical Diagnosis by Laboratory Methods.* 15th ed., Philadelphia, W. B. Saunders Co., 1974.
Eastham, R. D.: *A Laboratory Guide to Clinical Diagnosis.* Baltimore, Williams & Wilkins Co., 1973.
Goldberger, Emanuel: *A Primer of Water, Electrolyte and Acid-Base Syndromes.* 4th ed., Philadelphia, Lea and Febiger, 1970.
Goodale, R. H.: *Clinical Interpretation of Laboratory Tests.* 7th ed., Philadelphia, F. A. Davis Co., 1973.
Hoffman, W. S.: *The Biochemistry of Clinical Medicine.* 4th ed., Chicago, Year Book Medical Publishers, 1970.
Maxwell, Morton, and Kleeman, Charles, Eds.: *Clinical Disorders of Fluid and Electrolyte Metabolism.* 2nd ed., New York, McGraw-Hill Book Co., 1972.
Phillips, R. E., and Feeney, M. K.: *The Cardiac Rhythms.* Philadelphia, W. B. Saunders Co., 1973.
Reed, Gretchen Mayo, and Sheppard, Vincent: *Regulation of Fluid and Electrolyte Balance: A Programmed Institution in Physiology for Nurses.* Philadelphia, W. B. Saunders Co., 1971.
Schedl, H. P.: Water and electrolyte transport: Clinical aspects. Med. Clin. N. Amer., 58 (6): 1429–1448, 1974.
Turk, J. L.: *Immunology in Clinical Medicine.* 2nd ed., London, William Heinemann Medical Books, 1972.
Wallach, J.: *Interpretation of Diagnostic Tests: A Handbook Synopsis of Laboratory Medicine.* Boston, Little, Brown Co., 1970.
Zilva, J. F., and Pannall, P. R.: *Clinical Chemistry in Diagnosing and Treatment.* Chicago, Yearbook Medical Publishers, 1971.

5
PSYCHOSOCIAL ASSESSMENT AND INTERVENTION

The experience of illness is a complex physiological and psychological situation. To understand the response of a sick individual to the experience of illness, it is useful to consider how he responded during health to stressful situations, and to assess both his cognitive abilities and his socioeconomic situation. An accurate psychosocial assessment of the patient will enable the practitioner to anticipate his ability and willingness to cooperate in the treatment process.

PRELIMINARY ASSESSMENT

As the patient enters the examining room, his walk should be observed for stability, coordination, and speed. His general appearance and posture should also be noted, and attention should be given to how and where he sits. Sitting with head down, arms crossed, and legs motionless may indicate depression. Excessive nodding, smiling, gesturing, or talking may be ways of expressing anxiety. If the patient places his hand on his face several times during the interview the practitioner should note the topic of conversation which seems to provoke such gestures. An anxious person will often place his hand on his face in an attempt to comfort himself.

The facial expression can reveal much to the observer about a person's affect, mood, anxiety level and general health. Communication experts report that the majority of one's total communication is conveyed via facial expressions. The face reveals not only the emotion the person wishes to convey to others, but also less well controlled physiological information (such as that conveyed by flushing, sweating, pallor, tearing, or pupillary dilation).

Eye movements, the direction of gaze and blinking, are associated with emotional expressions and levels of anxiety. The practitioner can gain useful cues to the patient's emotional state by observing whether the patient blinks excessively, whether he looks at or away from the examiner, and whether his pupils are dilated or constricted. Persons usually make eye contact when they wish to interact, and look away when they want to avoid interaction or wish to increase psychological distance.

The tone of voice provides valuable cues about the verbal message the communicator wishes to send. In fact, the tonal cue is very often the primary message communicated, and the tonal message may or may not match the concomitant verbal message. The practitioner can obtain much information about a patient by noting the smoothness and rate of his word flow, the pitch and intensity of his speech, the hesitations or silences interspersed between words, and his verbal enunciation. Vocal cues should always be interpreted in conjunction with such other aspects of the patient's total communication as facial expression, dress, hair, body language, and words. The patient's tone of voice is especially useful in ascertaining such strong emotions as happiness, sadness, anger, or affection.

The words that the patient selects to describe his needs to the practitioner provide additional facts about him. The logic of his words, his grammar, diction, and accent should be noted, as they tend to reveal information about his education, intellect, memory, reality orientation, insight into his illness, reaction to illness, and race or national origin. It is also important to note how freely the patient talks and offers information about himself and his health status, for his ability in self-revelation has important consequences to the later success of the care relationship.

It is useful to the practitioner when she talks with the patient to determine his general satisfaction with the following key areas in his life: financial, sexual, housing, living arrangements, role in home, mode of transportation, and personal achievements. Appropriate questions are asked only as needed to gain the information that is required to help the patient meet his current needs. As the patient relates his problem, the practitioner should attempt to assess whether his reaction to his situation resembles the usual reactions of others to a similar stress.

To obtain information from which to judge the patient's ability to relate to other people, several questions should be asked about his educational and employment histories. For example, what types and amount of schooling has he had? Is he working in a job that is suited to his educational preparation? How frequently has he changed jobs? How recently has he been promoted? Does he like what he is doing? Is he satisfied with his salary? What does he do for recreation? With whom does he participate in social activities? Answers to these questions will indicate how well rounded he is, how able he is to cope with life's problems, and what social resources he can rely upon.

If the physical examination reveals signs of an acute or chronic illness, it is helpful to assess the patient's perception of that illness and the meaning of illness to the patient and his family at this time. To obtain this information, the practitioner should inquire whether the patient has changed jobs recently or anticipates a job change in the future, whether he has modified his long range career plans as a result of illness, and whether changes in his health have dictated changes in living arrangements, travel plans, or social relationships. If, in fact, the patient has not yet accepted his illness he may deny symptoms and not follow diagnostic or treatment instructions. If he has accepted his illness, but is to some extent regressed, he will tend to respond egocentrically to even minor discomforts or inconveniences. He may show unusual concern with certain of his body parts or body functions. Even when he has accepted his illness and is progressing toward a higher level of health, the patient may show some ambivalence about getting well and assuming his usual role and responsibilities.

ASSESSING HEALTH NEEDS AND STRENGTHS

Throughout the health assessment process the practitioner's objective should be to organize the data gained during the interview and examination, in order to see the logical relationships between the facts elicited to identify the patient's health needs, and to formulate a plan for care. A good method to use when organizing the assessment is to start by determining the patient's needs, and establishing with the patient's help those that have the highest priority. Next, the practitioner should decide at which levels of disease prevention the patient's needs can best be categorized. Finally, the practitioner should diagram, in the form of a balance, the stresses that the patient is currently experiencing and the supports that are currently available to him. At the fulcrum of the balance (the point of division between stresses and supports) the practitioner should list the patient's inner resources, such as defense mechanisms, ego strength, values, intelligence, and general level of physical health. Such inner strengths can only be surmised in an initial health screening situation, but in later interactions more data of this type will be forthcoming. In order that the health assessment process yield the most accurate information, it is important that throughout the entire interview and examination the practitioner not confuse her own judgment and insights with those of the patient.

An outline of Maslow's hierarchy of needs is given in Figure 48. Considering the base of the pyramid as the first or primary level of need and the apex as the sixth or final level of need, the need levels can be identified as follows:

Sixth — self-actualization needs
Fifth — esteem needs
Fourth — love needs
Third — safety needs
Second — physiological stimulation needs
First — physiological survival needs

An individual does not fulfill all needs at the first level and then move to the next, gratify all needs at that level and proceed in like fashion to the point at which one strives chiefly for self-actualization. Rather, a need at one level may govern behavior at a particular time while other needs at the same level, which are better satisfied, do not serve as significant motivators of behavior. Physiological survival needs do have a peculiar dominance over the other needs because, obviously, there are limits to the individual's ability to delay gratification of the need for air, water, elimination, rest and food, or to tolerate extremes of temperature or pain.

The practitioner can easily memorize this hierarchy of needs and, using it

```
                        Hierarchy of Needs
                        SELF-ACTUALIZATION
                 ESTEEM           SELF-ESTEEM
            LOVE            BELONGING            CLOSENESS
         SAFETY            SECURITY              PROTECTION
      SEX    ACTIVITY   EXPLORATION   MANIPULATION    NOVELTY
 FOOD   AIR   WATER   TEMPERATURE   ELIMINATION   REST   PAIN AVOIDANCE
```

Figure 48. Maslow's hierarchy of needs, as adapted by Kalish. (From Kalish, R. A.: *The Psychology of Human Behavior*. Belmont, CA, Wadsworth Publishing Co., 1966.)

as a model, identify the level in the hierarchy at which the patient's chief need exists. The need hierarchy is also useful in drawing up a problem list upon which to base a plan for care. It is advisable for the practitioner to ask the patient to identify his most pressing need. A question such as, "What do you think is the main cause of your trouble?" or, "What brought you here today?" will frequently help to identify the patient's impression of his chief need. Problems in treating the patient often occur when the practitioner and the patient differ in opinion as to the priority of the patient's needs and each is unaware of the other's opinion as to which of several problems is of paramount importance. Since an individual's needs change through time, evaluation of need gratification and reassessment of need priority must be repeated at intervals. The time between reassessments should be determined by the acuteness of the patient's illness.

Many of the needs included in Maslow's hierarchy are gratified through social interaction. Gratification of these needs is most likely to occur through interpersonal relationships that are sufficiently based upon trust to allow for reciprocal need gratification between two or more persons. Obviously, a person with limited ability to relate with other people will have fewer of his needs for love, closeness, sex, esteem, and security met than will a person who interacts with people more comfortably. The practitioner, of course, experiences the same human needs as all other individuals and gratifies some of her needs through interaction with her patients. However, it is frequently necessary for the practitioner to delay satisfaction of some of her needs in order that the patient's needs (which are presumably more urgent) can be met first. Of course, it is important to recognize that in many instances certain of the patient's social needs (such as the need for sexual activity, for love, or for belonging) cannot or should not be satisfied by members of the health team.

LEVELS OF PREVENTION OF ILLNESS

Primary, secondary, and tertiary levels of prevention are traditionally identified. After the special needs of the patient have been identified, it is helpful to consider, for each of his needs, the level of prevention that seems indicated. Often there will be some needs referable to each of the three levels. The functional definition of each level of prevention is as follows:

Primary Prevention: Preventing a temporary decompensation from becoming a permanent disability; that is, taking action to defer symptom formation.
Secondary Prevention: Recognizing symptoms of disease and providing specific treatment to remove the cause and/or interrupt progress of the disease.
Tertiary Prevention: Minimizing residual disabilities that have resulted from disease processes.

Primary Prevention

Primary prevention consists of undertaking certain actions to prevent the occurrence of specific illness (for example, immunizations) and of teaching the patient how to live in a way that will maintain and maximize his health. Primary disease prevention includes such activities as brushing the teeth regularly; eating a well-balanced diet; maintaining normal weight; resting adequately; reducing stress; avoiding unnecessary risk taking; obtaining appropriate immunizations; and maintaining a group of friends.

Although stress cannot be avoided in daily life, the healthy person manages to achieve a state of psychological and physiological equilibrium. In the healthy individual most alterations from normal balance are fairly quickly checked and adjustments made to regain equilibrium. Disorganization of psychological functioning tends to result 1) when the stressful event has a profound impact on the individual, 2) when the timing of the stress is such that the individual's perception of the stress is distorted, and 3) when the person's usual coping mechanisms and supportive resources are inadequate to restore equilibrium, Excessive stress, together with a decrease in coping ability, tends to change both the individual's view of himself and his relationship with others, the combination of which constitutes crisis. When the practitioner encounters a patient in crisis, her objective should be to help the patient to decrease the intensity of stress impinging on him, so as to prevent a temporary decompensation (in this case, a crisis) from becoming a permanent disability. Help is given to the patient by:

1. being a supportive resource who channels the patient's tension release
2. helping the patient to correct faulty perceptions or to gain new insights
3. mobilizing new coping methods in the patient
4. assisting the patient with goal redefinition
5. referring the patient to agencies or individuals that can give aid that is beyond the practitioner's ability
6. observing and listening intently to the patient's communications.

A psychological crisis is for some reason always resolved either in a constructive, dynamic way or in a destructive, limiting way.

Anticipatory guidance given by the practitioner to a person soon to experience loss can often prevent crisis development, and certainly can help abate anxiety once it is generated. Experience in observing human interpersonal relationships has shown that certain events often constitute crisis situations. Natural disaster, separation, divorce, death of a loved person, promotion, marriage, adolescence, physical illness, amputation, immobility and pregnancy are only a few of the events that can produce a psychological crisis in vulnerable individuals. When an individual experiences or is likely to experience severe loss or trauma of the aforementioned types, help should be freely offered to prevent psychological disequilibrium.

Secondary Prevention

Secondary prevention of illness consists of recognizing the symptoms of illness early in a disease process and providing treatment to remove etiologic factors and interrupt pathological processes. Early symptoms of psychological disequilibrium include excessive or prolonged anxiety, distortion of reality, failure to recognize reality, bizarre behavior, preoccupation with minutiae, inability to concentrate, inappropriate affect, and extremes of motor activity.

Assessing and treating physical signs and symptoms and, if possible, eradicating the cause of physical illness is an important part of the management of a patient with psychosocial illness. In many cases physical symptoms are aggravated or caused by emotional stress. Tissue cells of the body's physiological systems can be changed by emotional affect or feelings. When physical symptoms of illness are perceived by an individual, he devotes more time to thinking about or giving attention to the affected body part. If concentration on one's body is exaggerated, disorganization of daily activities results. A patient may not seek medical treatment for a physical symptom, either because he fears that he is seriously or fatally ill or because he fears that he will be told that he is imagining or exaggerating his symptoms. If, in treating a patient with psychosomatic disorder, the practitioner says, "This problem is all in your mind," the message that the patient receives is, "Your mind is not important." The patient often translates this message into "I'm not important." When the practitioner concludes that that patient's symptoms are of psychosomatic origin she might better say, "I can't figure out the cause of your symptoms. Tell me more about how and when they developed."

In an effort to ascertain the impact of disease and treatment upon an individual and his family, the following factors should be considered by the practitioner:

1. Any role changes in the home or at work which have been induced by the patient's illness.
2. Resistance on the part of any family member to relating the patient's symptoms and recognizing their meaning.
3. Satisfaction derived by various family members from the practice of their religious faith.
4. Recreational activities engaged in by individual family members and by the family as a whole.
5. Social relationships in the home, particularly in regard to decision making.
6. Degree to which the family residence is suited to the family's need at this time.
7. Reaction of various family members to accepting professional help with crisis resolution.

After assessing the patient's needs and obtaining a notion of the impact of his symptoms upon the family as a whole, the practitioner can begin to provide more comprehensive treatment.

Certain therapeutic interventions, such as preventing oral intake of food, confinement to bed, physical isolation from others, and attachment to monitoring machines, because they are mutilative, painful or inconvenient, cause anxiety, lowering of self-esteem, anger, insecurity, guilt, loneliness, regression, boredom and physiological disequilibrium. The person under stress tends to employ some or all of the following defense mechanisms in order to protect his ego (that is, his self-esteem, sexuality, or status) from disintegration: denial, withdrawal, aggression, repression, projection, sublimation, rationalization, verbosity and silence. Any of these defense mechanisms may be effective in protecting the ego against stress if the mechanism is not overused. For example, denial is often essential for psychological survival in situations of acute stress but may be detrimental when its use is prolonged for months or years. Also, a certain amount of anxiety may serve to marshal the individual's efforts to combat an external, reality-based threat, but extreme or prolonged anxiety can be seriously incapacitating; it may immobilize the individual so that he cannot respond at all effectively to external stimuli.

Tertiary Prevention

Tertiary prevention consists of minimizing residual disabilities and restoring maximal functioning. Many of the chronically ill patients whom the practitioner serves will have needs for tertiary disease prevention. The chronic diabetic, the hypertensive, the cardiac, the arthritic, and the alcoholic patient all have need for rehabilitation or tertiary disease prevention. Rehabilitation should be considered to include maximal parallel recovery from both physical limitation and psychological regression. However, for many patients, physical and psychological recovery do not proceed at the same rate. At certain times, each of the members of the patient's family may have reached a different stage of insight regarding the meaning of his illness, his capabilities, and his future potential than has the patient himself. Unless the practitioner recognizes this disparity between the patient's and the family's understandings and expectations, and somehow narrows the communication gap between the patient and those close to him, confusion and resentment are bound to develop. Through skillful interviewing and planned health teaching of both the patient and his family, the practitioner can facilitate clear understanding of the disabled person's abilities, strengths, and limitations, as well as help to formulate realistic goals in the following areas of his life: education, employment, housing, marriage, child rearing, traveling, recreation.

UTILIZING THE HEALTH BALANCE

Diagramming the balance of the patient's stresses, supports, and inner resources will help the practitioner to summarize her psychological assessment of the patient and will suggest a more comprehensive plan for psychological intervention and support than might be constructed without reference to such a diagram (Figure 49). If the balance is worked out mentally, rather than

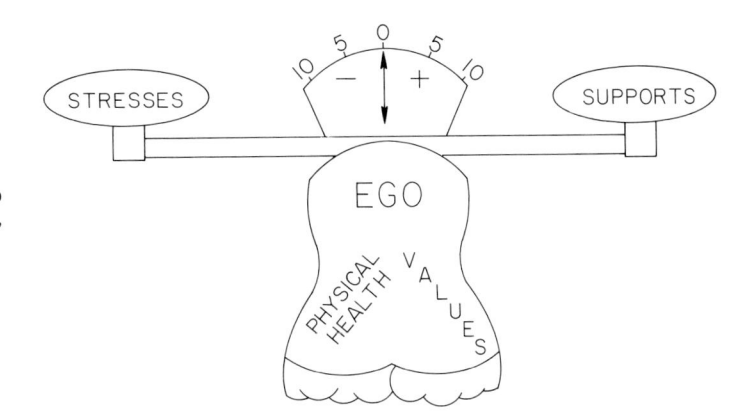

Figure 49. Health balance to assess an individual's stresses, supports, and inner strengths.

on paper, the plan is often not acted upon or periodically evaluated. The construction of a problem list (à la problem-oriented charting) does provide a record of the patient's chief stresses or needs, but neglects consideration of an important aspect of intervention; that is, strengthening his existing supports or eliciting new ones.

Once the patient's stresses and supports are listed and his inner strengths (ego strength, intelligence, values, physical health) enumerated, the practitioner can better visualize ways in which available supports can be mobilized or current stresses reduced or removed. Mobilization of support for the patient is facilitated by the fact that the human mind and body have an inherent drive toward health. As a result of this drive, patients employ selective attention in maintaining or restoring psychological balance; that is, the individual tends to concentrate on manageable or supportive thoughts and to temporarily or permanently blot out those thoughts that are painful or incapacitating. This selective attention in the handling of psychological stress is akin to the physiologic shunting or shift mechanisms that serve to maintain homeostasis. For instance, during stress the sympathetic nervous system is stimulated and the parasympathetic system is inhibited. As a consequence, blood is supplied to such critical tissues as brain, heart, and muscle and shunted from such less critical areas as skin, splanchnic, and renal tissues.

Ideally, the practitioner should aim to help patients and their families maintain a balance of stresses and supports while at the same time building their ego strength. Usually, this is accomplished by 1) increasing the available supports, 2) decreasing the stresses or converting a stress into a support, 3) improving or maintaining physical health, 4) allowing the patient and his family to express their preferences and to make as many decisions about their lives as is feasible. Occasionally, the main intervention is to increase stress in order that the patient matures psychologically or seeks needed physiological treatment.

In summary, psychosocial assessment requires that the practitioner invest considerable time with a patient and his family in order to obtain the data needed for planning effective psychological interventions. The patient's psychological needs should be assessed and placed in order of priority. Each need should then be analyzed to determine which level of disease prevention is called for. Finally, the patient's psychological stresses, supports, and inner

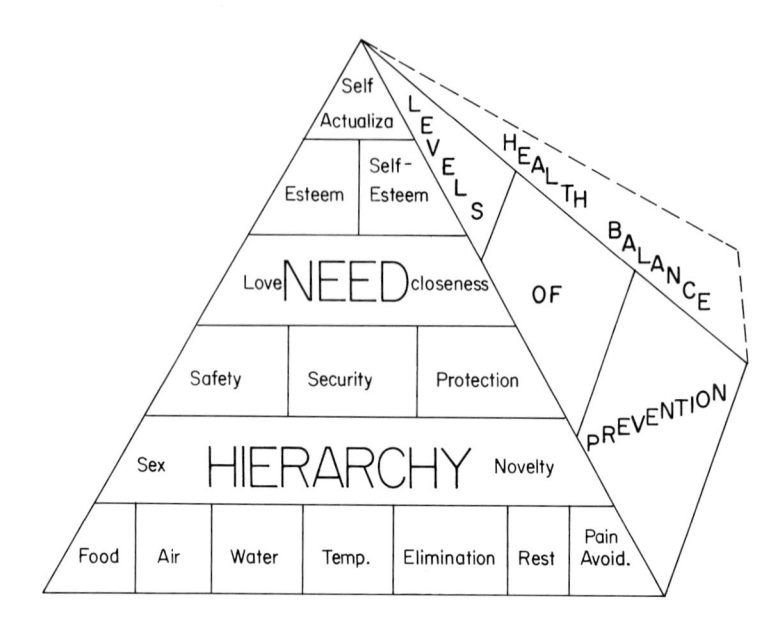

Figure 50. Pyramidal view of assessments to be made by the nurse practitioner.

strengths should be weighed on a so-called "health balance": The diagram in Figure 50 demonstrates that consideration of this "health balance," and determination of the level of disease prevention required by the patient is as vital a part of his health assessment as is identification of his lacks according to Maslow's need hierarchy.

BIBLIOGRAPHY: PSYCHOSOCIAL ASSESSMENT

Beiser, M., et al.: Assets and affects, a study of positive mental health. *Arch. Gen. Psychiat.* 27:545–549, October, 1972.
Braceland, F. J.: The mental hygiene of aging: a present day view. *J. Amer. Geriat. Soc.* 20:467–472, October, 1972.
Keezer, William: *Mental Health and Human Behavior.* 3rd ed., Dubuque, William C. Brown, 1971.
Knapp, Mark: *Nonverbal Communication in Human Interaction.* New York, Holt, Rinehart, Winston, 1972.
Lewis, Howard, and Lewis, Martha: *Psychosomatics.* New York, Viking Press, 1972.
Milne, J. S., et al.: The design and testing of a questionnaire and examination to assess physical and mental health in older people using a staff nurse as the observer. *J. Chron. Dis.* 25:385–405, 1972.
Roeske, Nancy: *Examination of the Personality.* Philadelphia, Lea & Febiger, 1972.

6
RECORDING DATA AND PLANNING CARE

The patient's medical history and the findings on physical examination should be recorded in the medical record as soon as the physical examination is concluded to ensure that vital information is not forgotten and that needed data are immediately available to members of the health team.

As was mentioned earlier, the nurse should not write extensive notes while taking the patient's medical history, since he will talk freely and candidly only if he feels that he has her undivided attention. Likewise, the nurse should not interrupt the routine of the physical examination to record lengthy notes, since by thus extending the examination she might tire the patient or otherwise cause him discomfort. In both situations, however, the nurse may need to jot down certain key dates, symptom clusters, physicians' names, vital signs, and the like for later reference when she records her findings in the medical record.

PURPOSE AND NATURE OF DATA RECORDING

The practitioner's writeup of the patient's history and physical findings should be a rich source of information for her own and others' use in diagnosing the patient's illness and prescribing treatment. The patient's medical record is a legal document that may be used as evidence in a court of law or as source material for filing insurance claims. For both of these reasons, the record must be scrupulously factual and should be written in sufficient detail and so organized as to reveal significant relationships among different categories of data. For diagnostic and legal use, the exact dates and chronology of significant medical events in the patient's past life must be recorded. For diagnostic, therapeutic, and legal reasons, the time relationships between certain treatment measures and symptom changes must be specified exactly. For purposes of insurance adjustment, detailed descriptions of traumatic events and resulting dysfunction are necessary.

Most medical schools, hospitals, and clinics have developed standard outlines that physicians and nurse practitioners are expected to follow in recording data obtained by interviewing and examining the patient. It is reasoned that if all practitioners record data in the same sequence, it will be easier for each care giver to quickly find needed information in the patient's record.

A suggested outline for organizing and recording the patient's medical history was given in Chapter 2; an outline for recording the physical findings was developed in Chapter 3. In using each outline, the nurse should record normal as well as abnormal findings, since some diseases are characterized by the appearance of a particular normal finding in conjunction with one or two other findings that are abnormal. Further, in following each outline, the nurse should carefully qualify and quantify each symptom or unusual physical finding. If the patient has pain, his discomfort should be specified as to type, using any descriptive adjectives or adverbs employed by the patient in telling about his problem. The nurse should also quantify the pain, indicating its intensity (perhaps by noting whether and to what degree it interferes with the patient's normal activities), its frequency, its duration, and the amount of analgesic required to relieve it. If the patient has diarrhea, the nurse should record the quality of diarrhea by describing the color, consistency, and character of the stool, and should quantify the symptom by recording the number of stools per day and the duration of diarrhea.

Both records, that of the medical history and that of the physical examination, should be dated and followed by the nurse's signature and title, so that later readers of the record can easily distinguish findings obtained by the nurse practitioner from those obtained by medical students or physicians in those situations where the patient has been examined by more than one caregiver.

THE PROBLEM-ORIENTED MEDICAL RECORD

Since the advent of Medicare there has been increasing pressure from within and without the health care professions to increase the physician's and nurse's accountability for the quality of their patient care. In order to acquire a reliable data base from which to evaluate the quality of care given a particular patient, a Problem Oriented Patient Record System has been developed by Dr. Lawrence Weed.* This system, which can be modified to suit the special needs and conditions of a particular hospital, clinic, or ambulatory care facility, is roughly patterned after the scientific method of inquiry. The scientific method consists of making observations, formulating a hypothesis to explain the observations made, designing an experiment under controlled conditions to test the validity of the hypothesis, analyzing data obtained through experimentation and, finally, utilizing conclusions drawn from the data to explain initial observations and to expand or modify knowledge.

---

* Weed, L.: Medical records, medical education, and patient care: The problem-oriented record as a basic tool. Cleveland, Case-Western Reserve Press, 1969.

The steps in the problem-oriented system of patient record keeping parallel these steps of observing, hypothesizing, experimenting, analyzing, and theory building. First the practitioner gathers information about the patient so as to acquire a data base about him and his problems. From that data base the practitioner identifies certain problems with which the patient is currently confronted. Since some of these problems can be identified and understood only imperfectly, that is as symptoms rather than as specific tissue pathology of known cause, diagnostic tests are ordered to refine the diagnosis. At the same time, treatment is prescribed to relieve symptoms or to counteract etiologic forces where these are known. Results of diagnostic tests and responses to therapy are recorded in the form of progress notes.

The *data base,* or that information obtained about the patient through history, physical examination, and laboratory tests, should be recorded as soon as it has been obtained, should be given in considerable detail, and should be organized so as to enable care givers to see the relationship among interdependent variables. It is expected that the practitioner will include information about the patient's family, home, job, social interests, religious affiliation, and economic situation as well as about his present illness and past medical history. The nurse practitioner should use the same outline in recording her findings on history and physical examination as that used by physicians in the same institution, in order to facilitate comparison of the findings of the two different types of care givers in those situations where the patient is examined by both. In many institutions, in fact, the physician and the nurse record their findings on the same forms.

The *problem list* is a carefully constructed list of problems that have been identified from the data base (Figure 51), and includes social, economic, and demographic as well as medical and psychiatric problems. Not all problems on the list will be described with the same degree of specificity. That is, available data may make it possible to list one problem in the form of a specific diagnosis, such as rheumatoid arthritis, while another can be designated only as a symptom, such as elevated diastolic blood pressure, a pathophysiologic state, such as congestive heart failure, or an abnormal laboratory test finding, such as fasting blood glucose level of 200 mg per 100 ml.

As each problem is added to the list, it is given a number and the date of entry is recorded. Earlier problems, which are now inactive but which might be significant to the patient's future health management, such as a previous episode of rheumatic fever or a previous gastrectomy, should be included on the problem list. In order to keep the problem list to manageable length, temporary and self-limited problems (such as upper respiratory infection, skin laceration, or vaginal discharge) which are not significant to the patient's overall health management should not be included on the regular, numbered problem list. Rather, such acute, short-term problems should be recorded on a second, lettered list. Again the date on which the temporary problem is identified should be recorded, as well as the date on which the problem is resolved. If there are repeated occurrences of a temporary condition, as for instance serial episodes of cystitis, the problem should then be added to the numbered problem list as a chronic, recurrent condition.

Occasionally, as additional diagnostic tests are performed and the patient's response to treatment is observed, it becomes obvious that several separately listed problems are really different manifestations of the same problem; for example, tachycardia, chest rales, and hepatomegaly may all be

PROBLEM LIST

	ACTIVE			INACTIVE	
Date Onset	Problem No.	Problem-Active	Date Onset	Problem-Resolved	Date Resolved
10/3/75	1	Hypertension			
10/3/75	2	Obesity			
10/3/75	3	Anemia			
10/3/75	4	Cardiomegaly			
10/3/75	5	Alcoholic Husband			
			1970	Hysterectomy	1970
			1972	Pneumonia	1972

Figure 51. Problem list of a patient with hypertension, obesity, anemia, and cardiomegaly.

manifestations of congestive heart failure. In such case the problem "tachycardia," if it appears first on the problem list, should be renamed "congestive heart failure," and "chest rales" and "hepatomegaly" should be dropped from the problem list.

The therapeutic scheme should include a specific *plan* for further diagnosis and management of each problem listed. Each plan should include, in addition to the problem number and title to which it relates, the diagnostic or management objectives to be sought, the diagnostic tests to be performed, the treatment to be undertaken, the patient education to be given, the referrals to be made, and a schedule for followup care.

The *progress notes* should include new information relative to the patient's problems that becomes available during treatment or as a result of additional diagnostic tests. Each progress note should be headed by the problem number and title to which it relates and should contain four different types of information. These types are often abbreviated by the designation SOAP.

1. Subjective data: what the patient says about the problem, using whenever possible the patient's own language in describing his experiences.

2. Objective data: observations made by the practitioner and the results obtained from laboratory tests.

3. Assessment of the data: the practitioner's analysis of the subjective and objective data as it relates to the etiology of the problem, the adequacy of treatment response, and the probable outcome of the problem.

4. Plan for solving the problem: the practitioner's intentions regarding additional diagnostic tests to be done, future treatment to be followed, and additional patient education to be given.

Not only are diagnostic test results and responses to treatment recorded in the progress notes, they are analyzed in relation to what is already known regarding the patient (his history and physical findings), and the conclusions derived from such analysis are used to expand the original data base and to refine or expand the problem list. The relationship of these activities may be diagrammed thus:*

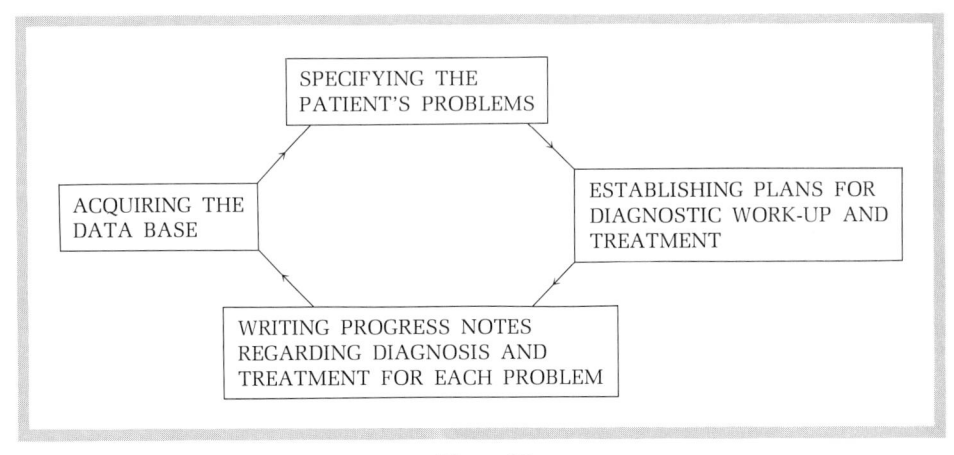

Figure 52.

---

* From Weed, Lawrence L., Medical Records, Medical Education, and Patient Care. Cleveland, Case Western Reserve University Press, 1969.

PLANNING PATIENT CARE

If the problem-oriented method of record-keeping is in effect in the institution or agency with which the nurse practitioner is affiliated, it may be that her care plan can be incorporated into the general record. However, she still may find it desirable to structure her care of patients according to the framework of the nursing process. The usual steps in the nursing process are assessment, planning, intervention, and evaluation. The first five chapters of this book have dealt with the assessment aspects of patient care. The construction of a nursing care plan will be dealt with here.

There are two reasons why the patient care plan should be written. First, a written plan is likely to be more specific and detailed than one the nurse carries about in her head. Francis Bacon noted in 1625 that "Writing maketh an exact man." Thus, in the process of committing her care plan to paper the nurse is encouraged to think through the significance of the patient's historical and physical findings and to consider relationships between his needs and available treatment modalities.

Second, the nurse practitioner's plan for the patient's care should be communicated to all other health workers who serve him in order to maximize their support of her efforts on his behalf. A written plan can be more easily and consistently communicated than one that is unwritten. The care plan should, probably, be appended to the patient's chart so that it is readily available to all persons having contact with him (physicians, other nurses, aides, clerks, dietitian, social worker, and therapists of various types).

The first step in preparing a care plan should be the construction of short, intermediate, and long-range goals for management of the patient and his problems. Short-range goals are those changes in the patient's condition or situation which it is hoped will occur within a period of hours, days, or a few weeks. Long-range goals are those changes which it would be desirable to effect within several weeks or months. Intermediate objectives aim at a point between these two extremes.

As one means of motivating the patient toward recovery, the nurse should involve the patient in establishing objectives for his care. The first step in so doing consists of identifying the patient's chief complaint or reasons for seeking care (one of the first items of information sought in the health history). As indicated in Chapter 2, the nurse can discern which of several existing problems is of greatest present concern to the patient by asking some such question as: "What caused you to come to the clinic (hospital) today?" or, "Can you tell me something about why you came here today for care?"

Further information about the patient's major fears and worries can be gained during history taking by asking, "Can you describe how this problem (illness, symptom) has brought about changes in your usual way of life?" The answer to this query may reveal certain discomforts, inconveniences, incapacitations, or problems which the patient attributes to his illness and which he hopes to be relieved of by treatment.

Further insights into the patient's goals for care may be obtained near the end of the health interview by asking, "What results do you expect from the care that you will receive here?" Sometimes a patient's expectations of treatment are so unrealistic as to be incapable of attainment. If, however, his expectations are completely ignored in setting care goals, if he is not encouraged to verbalize his expectations and helped to modify any completely unreasonable expectations he may hold, he will certainly be disappointed with the care he receives, however successful it is in reversing pathophysiology or relieving symptoms.

Having thus obtained the patient's assistance in identifying desirable goals for care, the nurse can determine, on the basis of her own past experience in managing patients with similar problems and in line with the protocols established by her physician colleague, what objectives she should strive for in treating the patient. The objectives chosen to direct patient care should be realistic in both number and content so as to be capable of attainment in the time available and under existing circumstances (the patient's present condition, the support systems that are available to him, and the efficacy of existing drugs and other treatments).

All objectives, both long and short range, should be clearly stated in behavioral terms. That is, each objective should describe a specific behavior that the nurse hopes to observe in the patient as a result of care. A well-written nursing care objective is characterized by the fact that easily observable behavior is described in such terms that any two nurses attending the patient would agree as to whether or not the desired behavior has been displayed. Further, whenever possible, the desired behavior should be quantified and the conditions under which the behavior is to occur should be specified.

Following is a short-range objective for a patient in whom long-term dietary indiscretions have led to obesity.

After one hour of dietary instruction on each of three successive days, the patient will, without referral to a diet manual, write out a week's menu which yields the recommended daily allowances of the basic four food groups.

Here the observable behavior is writing the names and amounts of foods to be included in each meal. Quantification consists of specifying both the three hours of instruction the patient is to receive and the 21 menus he is to construct. The condition under which the behavior is to occur is also described: the patient is to construct the week's menus without referral to a diet manual; that is, by remembering what he has been taught about which foods fall into each of the four food groups.

Following is a short-range objective for a patient whose long-term use of a night-time sedative–hypnotic should be broken:

After practicing progressive relaxation techniques three times each day for three days, the patient will fall asleep, without sedation, within twenty minutes after retiring.

Here the falling asleep behavior could be observed by the patient's spouse. Quantification includes both specification of nine practice sessions and achievement of sleep within twenty minutes. The condition under which the behavior is to occur is also indicated: no sedative medication is to be given.

An intermediate-range goal for a patient who is recuperating following a cerebrovascular accident might be

After six sessions with a physiotherapist, the patient will, without assistance, move himself from bed to wheelchair and back again each morning, afternoon, and evening.

Here again, the behavior in question can be observed by a relative; quantification consists of specifying the number of physiotherapy sessions and the number of bed to wheelchair and wheelchair to bed transfers; and the condition under which the behavior is to occur (without assistance) is delineated.

An intermediate goal for a patient with chronic arteriosclerotic heart disease in mild congestive failure might be:

At the end of the patient's second clinic visit he will, on request, and from memory, write the names of twenty foods which should be eliminated from a 1 gram sodium diet.

In this objective the behavior to be observed is the writing of the names of foods; the quantity of names to be written is set at twenty; and the condition given is that the list should be written from memory.

A long-term goal for a patient with hypertension might be:

After two months of treatment, the patient's daily systolic blood pressure reading will not exceed 140 mm. Hg and his daily diastolic blood pressure reading will not exceed 90 mm. Hg even if the patient should by then have returned to full-time employment.

This objective illustrates that the behavior sought may be a physiologic phenomenon instead of an overt motor activity. Blood pressure is, of course, a measurable and thus observable phenomenon (either the patient or his relative can be taught to take his blood pressure daily); the acceptable upper levels of both systolic and diastolic pressure are established; and the conditions under which the patient's pressure is to remain under 140/90 mm. Hg. are to include his return to work.

After short-, intermediate-, and long-range goals for care have been clearly, specifically, and behaviorally stated, a plan of care should be constructed which includes diagnostic tests to be performed, drugs and treatments to be given, referrals to be made, instructions to be given the patient and his family, limitations to be imposed on his daily activities, and schedules for later followup visits.

Because the patient's condition will change through time, as a consequence of either the natural progression of his disease or the effects of treatment, the plan for his care will need to be modified in accord with these changes. Each addition to or modification in the care plan should be dated. If space allows, it would be helpful to indicate, in connection with each modification, the subjective or objective findings which necessitated a change in the care plan. Because the plan will be used over an extended period of time (many of the nurse practitioner's clients will be long-term, chronically ill patients), because it may undergo repeated revisions or alterations, and because a chronological record of these revisions may be useful in later evaluation of the quality of patient care given, the care plan should be recorded on a card or heavy paper form which, when appended to the chart, can be handled repeatedly without rolling or tearing.

The actual design of the form on which the nursing care plan is recorded will vary considerably from one clinic or hospital to another. In each institution, representative nurse practitioners from each clinic and/or hospital service area to which practitioners are assigned should cooperate in designing the form on which care plans are to be recorded. Physicians and other employees who will refer to the care plan should then be asked to criticize the form and to suggest improvements. Finally, the form should be subjected to trial use in a restricted area for a few months, evaluated, and revised before final adoption as an official chart form.

As mentioned previously, in some agencies the nursing care plan may be integrated with the patient's problem list, being developed from the original data base and undergoing serial revisions as additional data accumulate in the regular progress notes.

BIBLIOGRAPHY: RECORDING AND MAINTAINING THE DATA

Aronson, M. D.: The problem oriented record, a two column modification. J.A.M.A., 225:716–717, 1973.

Berni, R., and Ready, H.: *Problem-Oriented Medical Record Implementation.* St. Louis, The C. V. Mosby Co., 1974.

Bjorn, John: What problem oriented records can do for your practice. Med. Times 100:205–225, 1972.

Bjorn, John, and Cross, Harold: *The Problem Oriented Private Practice of Medicine.* Chicago, Modern Hospital Press, 1970.

Hurst, J. Willis, and Walker, H. Kenneth, Eds.: *The Problem Oriented System.* New York, Medcom, 1972.

Weed, Lawrence: *Medical Records, Medical Education, and Patient Care: the Problem Oriented Record as a Basic Tool.* Cleveland, Case–Western Reserve Press, 1969.

Woolley, F. R., Warnick, M. W., Kane, R. L., and Dyer, E. D.: *Problem-Oriented Nursing.* New York. Springer, 1974.

7
MANAGEMENT OF THE PATIENT WITH HYPERTENSION

Hypertension, or prolonged elevation of blood pressure over normal levels, is a serious disease which is responsible for about 15 per cent of deaths in persons over 50 years of age. Elevation of the systolic pressure alone has less far reaching consequences than elevation of the diastolic pressure alone or of both systolic and diastolic pressure.

PATHOPHYSIOLOGY

The factors that are chiefly responsible for determining the level of arterial blood pressure are the pumping action of the heart, the volume of circulating blood, and the degree of constriction of the arteriolar bed (peripheral resistance). Predominant elevation of the systolic pressure is largely due to increased cardiac output. Predominant elevation of the diastolic pressure is the result of increased peripheral resistance.

In order to understand the several mechanisms by which the arterial blood pressure may be elevated, it is helpful to consider the equation $P = QR$, where P, the arterial blood pressure, is the product of Q, or blood flow, times R, the peripheral resistance. In this equation Q, is approximately equal to cardiac output, which in turn is the product of stroke volume times cardiac rate. Thus, blood pressure increases with an increase in stroke volume, cardiac rate, arteriolar constriction, or any combination of the three.

As indicated in Figure 53, the arterial blood pressure can be elevated through several mechanisms. In so-called "renal" hypertension, renal ischemia (due to a reduction in renal blood flow) causes the production of the enzyme renin by certain cells in the renal tubule. Renin itself has no effect on blood vessels but it acts upon a plasma protein to form angiotensin I, which, in turn, is converted by another plasma enzyme to angiotensin II. This sub-

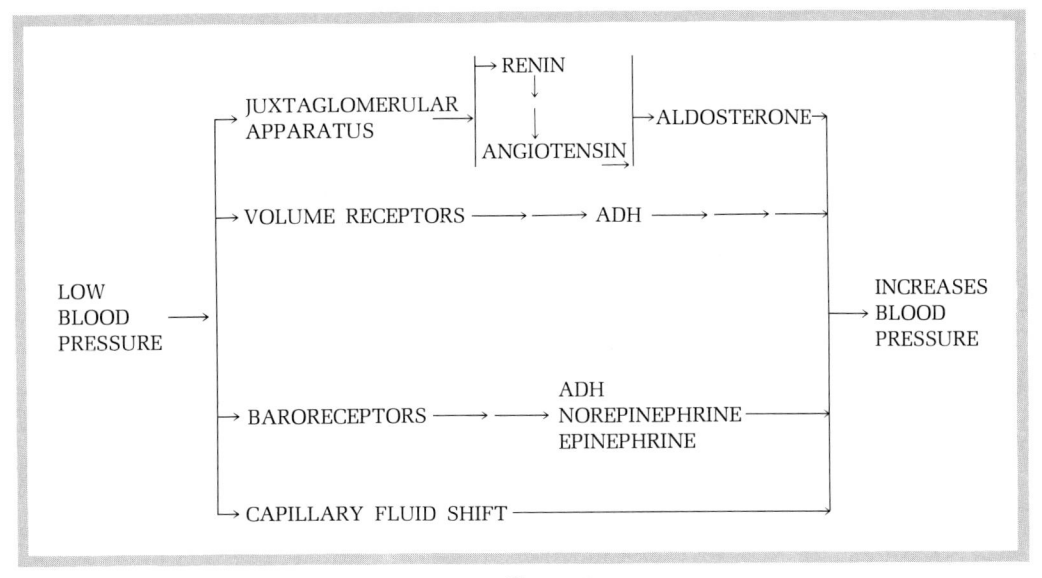

Figure 53.

stance raises blood pressure either by direct vasoconstriction or by stimulating the adrenal cortex to increased production of aldosterone, which increases the resorption of sodium ion in the distal tubule. The results are fluid retention and an increase in circulating blood volume.

When the blood pressure falls below normal levels, pressure receptors are stimulated in the walls of the left and right atria, the carotid artery, and the aortic arch. Impulses from these baroreceptors stimulate the hypothalamic production of increased amounts of antidiuretic hormone which, when released from storage in the posterior pituitary gland, cause increased water resorption in the distal tubule, with consequent increase in blood volume and blood pressure. Impulses from the baroreceptors in the carotid artery and aortic arch also stimulate the cardiac and vasomotor centers in the medulla oblongata, producing an increase in cardiac output (through an increase in heart rate) and an increase in peripheral resistance, which together raise the blood pressure.

A pheochromocytoma, or tumor of the adrenal medulla, secretes excessive amounts of epinephrine and norepinephrine into the circulation, which by increasing both cardiac output and peripheral resistance produce an increase in blood pressure. In hyperthyroidism, the increased cardiac output produced by an increased heart rate causes an increased systolic blood pressure. In adrenal cortex hypersecretion, the increased production of aldosterone causes increased sodium retention by renal tubular cells, with consequent increase in circulating blood volume and blood pressure.

Finally, it is thought by some that severe emotional stress can, through strong stimulation of the sympathetic nervous system, produce marked vasoconstriction and an acute elevation of blood pressure.

DEFINITIONS

The American Heart Association defines hypertension as a sustained elevation of systolic pressure above 140 mm. Hg and a sustained elevation of diastolic pressure above 90 mm. Hg.

The term "essential" hypertension is applied to those conditions of sustained arterial blood pressure for which no specific renal, endocrine, or neurogenic cause can be found. All cases of hypertension, whether "essential" or resulting from specifically identified causes, can be classified as either "benign" or "malignant." In benign hypertension the blood pressure elevates slowly and progressively over a period of years and complications of the disease develop somewhat insidiously. In malignant hypertension the vasoconstriction is often so rapid and severe as to be associated with arteriolar necrosis, especially in the kidney.

THE EFFECTS OF HYPERTENSION

In most hypertensive patients there are no signs or symptoms that derive directly from the increased systolic and/or diastolic blood pressure. However, prolonged elevation of diastolic pressure, particularly, causes permanent damage to the heart and arteries. When the heart must pump blood through the vessels against a greatly increased head of pressure, the left ventricular muscle hypertrophies to compensate for the increased cardiac work load. With progressive cardiac hypertrophy, the increase in muscle mass eventually outstrips the oxygen-carrying capacity of the coronary system, leading to diffuse myocardial fibrosis and eventual myocardial decompensation.

Elevation of blood pressure, whether benign or malignant, will eventually produce thickening and narrowing of arterioles and small arteries throughout the body (arteriosclerosis). In hypertensive patients, increased intravascular pressure causes injury to the medial layer of the arterial wall, at which point lipids and calcium salts tend to be deposited, further narrowing the vascular lumen and roughening the intimal lining so as to predispose to thrombus formation. Arteriosclerosis of coronary arteries may lead to coronary thrombosis and myocardial infarction. Arteriosclerosis of cerebral vessels predisposes to cerebrovascular thrombosis or hemorrhage. Arteriosclerosis of renal vessels may, through thrombosis or vascular rupture, produce renal ischemia, which by triggering renin → angiotensin I → angiotensin II production further elevates blood pressure.

DIAGNOSIS

Both the medical history and the physical examination can yield information which is helpful in establishing a diagnosis of hypertension. Hypertensive patients often report having been troubled with morning occipital headaches, occasional palpitations, epistaxis, and frequent light-headedness. Many patients with essential hypertension indicate that their grandparents, parents, siblings, or children have been diagnosed as having hypertension. Other hypertensive patients give a history of chronic renal disease; that is, previous bouts of glomerulonephritis (oliguria, hematuria, proteinuria, fatigue, facial edema, convulsions) or repeated urinary tract infections (fever, chills, dysuria, urgency, frequency, and pyuria). Patients with hypertension of several years' duration often have a history of angina, myocardial infarction, or congestive heart failure. Patients whose hypertension is secondary to an endocrine disorder may relate symptoms of thyrotoxicosis, diabetes mellitus, or adrenal cortical hypersecretion.

Physical examination of all patients should include taking the blood pressure in the supine, sitting, and standing position, since the pressure in the patient on antitensive medications may drop sharply when he changes from horizontal to vertical position. If the patient has an elevated blood pressure or a high pulse pressure, his blood pressure should be taken in both arms, since in aortic aneurysm and mediastinal tumor the blood pressure is unequal in the two extremities. Whenever an elevated blood pressure reading is obtained, the blood pressure should be rechecked after an interval of time. In tense, hyperreactive patients the blood pressure is often elevated during the early stages of the examination but returns to normal levels as the investigation proceeds and the patient develops greater confidence in the examiner. In order to eliminate possible sources of error in blood pressure determination the patient should be physically and emotionally relaxed, the arm should be at the level of the patient's heart, and the blood pressure cuff should be fully deflated and then wrapped firmly and smoothly around the arm about 2 cm. above the antecubital fossa.

Findings of an enlarged boot-shaped heart and rales in the lung bases, especially when accompanied by cough, dyspnea, and insomnia, suggest decompensation of the left ventricle, as may result from severe or prolonged hypertension. Exaggeration of the second heart sound over the aortic area (second intercostal space at the right sternal border) may result from increased systemic arterial pressure. Funduscopic findings of papilledema, hemorrhages, exudates, increased light reflex, segmental arteriolar constriction, and arteriovenous nicking give direct evidence of the vascular narrowing and degeneration that is characteristic of hypertension. In long-standing hypertension with secondary arteriosclerosis there may be diminished or absent carotid, femoral, posterior tibial, or dorsalis pedis pulses.

The diagnostic workup for the hypertensive patient should include a PA chest x-ray, to evaluate the size and shape of the cardiac outline and to look for evidence of pulmonary edema and pleural effusion secondary to congestive heart failure. On x-ray, the hypertensive heart is often large and boot-shaped owing to the disproportionate hypertrophy of the left ventricle, the chamber most burdened by increased systemic blood pressure. On x-ray, pulmonary edema usually reveals itself as increased density distributed diffusely throughout both lung fields, and pleural effusion presents as blunting of the normally sharp costodiaphragmatic angle. Urinalysis may reveal gross or microscopic hematuria in the patient whose hypertension is secondary to glomerulonephritis, or bacteria and pus cells in the patient whose hypertension results from chronic pyelonephritis. A fixed, low specific gravity reveals renal tubular damage which may have resulted from nephritis, nephrosis, infection, or nephrosclerosis. A history of facial edema and urinary symptoms, together with abnormal findings on urinalysis, suggests the need for such measures of renal function as intravenous pyelogram, concentration and dilution tests, phenylsulfonphthalein test, and urea clearance test.

A 12-lead electrocardiogram should be part of the workup of the hypertensive patient in order to check for evidences of cardiac strain, arrhythmias, and previous myocardial infarction.

Biochemical examinations of the hypertensive patient may reveal abnormally high levels of serum sodium or potassium in the patient with impaired renal function, or abnormally low levels of serum potassium in the patient on thiazide diuretics. The blood urea nitrogen, creatinine, and uric acid concentrations tend to be elevated in the patient whose hypertension is secondary to chronic renal disease.

If it is suspected that the patient's hypertension is of the secondary variety it may be necessary to order additional diagnostic tests. Analysis of 17-ketosteroids in the urine may be helpful in diagnosing adrenocortical hypersecretion. An LE preparation will help to identify lupus nephritis. Measurement of urinary vanillylmandelic acid (VMA) or metanephrine is useful in diagnosing pheochromocytoma. Palpation of femoral pulses and comparison of blood pressures in upper and lower extremities are helpful in diagnosing coarctation of the aorta.

TREATMENT

There is fairly general agreement that a patient whose diastolic blood pressure persistently exceeds 90 mm. Hg or whose systolic pressure persistently exceeds 140 mm. Hg should be considered to be hypertensive and should be treated so as to lower the blood pressure.

The objective in managing the hypertensive patient should be to achieve as nearly normal a standing blood pressure as is possible without producing undesirable side effects. To achieve this goal, it is frequently necessary to employ a combination of general hygienic measures and specific drug therapy. The general hygienic measures that have proved helpful in reducing blood pressure are weight control, restriction of sodium intake, a balanced program of exercise and relaxation, modification of life style so as to decrease stress, and cessation of smoking. Those hypertensive patients who are overweight should decrease their caloric intake so as to lose weight gradually and steadily to the point of ideal weight for their age and body build. In some cases, it may be helpful for the nurse to refer the patient to an organization like Weight Watchers or to enroll other members of the patient's family in a weight reduction program in order to provide the patient with social and emotional support in changing his dietary habits.

The hypertensive patient should be taught to decrease his sodium intake by avoiding both the use of salt in the preparation of food and the addition of salt to food as it is eaten. It is often helpful for the patient to eliminate the salt shaker from his table setting and to substitute lemon juice or vinegar as seasoning for those foods which he has been in the habit of salting.

If the hypertensive patient's cardiac status and general condition permit, he should be encouraged to engage in a half-hour to an hour of mild exercise daily. Such activities as walking, golfing, bowling, and swimming are well tolerated by many patients and provide avenues for the discharge of pent-up feelings of hostility. To balance this motor activity the patient should be encouraged to rest at regular periods throughout the day. Either by temperament or as a result of health worries, many hypertensive patients are tense, anxious individuals who tend to overreact to irritations and frustrations. If the hypertensive patient has difficulty in relaxing, he should be taught the techniques of progressive muscle relaxation so that he can realize the greatest possible advantage from daily rest periods.

Because emotional stress tends to increase blood pressure in persons with essential hypertension, such patients should be advised to adjust their daily schedules and living arrangements to avoid highly pressurized social, emotional, and work situations. Through non-directive counseling, the nurse can help the patient to accept the need to avoid hurry, competitive activities, upsetting social contacts, or unusually demanding work assignments. He may need encouragement, too, to develop relaxing hobbies to fill leisure hours previously devoted to work or worry.

Since smoking has been shown to produce vasoconstriction, the hypertensive patient should be urged to stop smoking. For those persons who are strongly habituated to tobacco, group therapy and conditioning techniques may be helpful in breaking the smoking habit.

Drug Treatment

The patient who requires drug therapy to lower his blood pressure should have his blood pressure measured at home on a regular basis by a family member whose ability to measure blood pressure accurately has been determined by the practitioner. The specific drug to be given the patient, as well as the drug dosage, will depend on the cause and severity of hypertension, but, in general, it is best to begin treatment by administering a small dose of a single drug, then either increasing the drug dosage or adding or substituting other drugs as needed to lower the blood pressure the desired amount while producing minimal side effects. If the patient must take several doses of medicine each day and has difficulty remembering to take his medicine, it may be helpful for him to place all doses of prescribed medication for the entire day in a pillbox on first arising. In this way he can carry his medicine with him throughout the day and can, by checking the container on a regular basis (as at mealtime), quickly and accurately determine whether he has taken all scheduled doses of prescribed medication.

Several different types of drugs are useful in decreasing arterial blood pressure. Some, such as reserpine, act by depressing the vasomotor center in the medulla oblongata. Some, such as Veratrum viride, act reflexly by stimulating the pressure receptors in the carotid sinus. Some, such as pentolinium tartrate, act by blocking impulse transmission through autonomic ganglia. Some, such as phentolamine, act by counteracting the effect of norepinephrine on the blood vessels. And some, such as hydralazine, directly depress smooth muscle fibers in the arterial wall.

The severity of the patient's hypertension is determined both by the level of his diastolic pressure and the evidence of such secondary effects as changes in the ocular fundi, cardiac enlargement or failure, cerebral dysfunction, or abnormal urinary findings.

For treatment of *mild* hypertension (diastolic pressure under 110 mm. of Hg and no evidence of secondary changes in brain, ocular fundi, heart, or kidneys) a mild oral diuretic such as the thiazides or chlorthalidone is usually ordered. These drugs block resorption of sodium and water by renal tubular cells, leading to a decrease in extracellular fluid volume and a decrease in blood pressure. The mild hypertensive should be started on a small dose of drug once daily (perhaps 25 mg. of hydrochlorothiazide), and then the dosage should be slowly increased to a level that will control his pressure with minimum side effects (perhaps 25–50 mg. of hydrochlorothiazide b.i.d.; or 50 mg. of chlorthalidone once daily). Possible toxic effects of the thiazides and related diuretics are hypokalemia, dizziness, dermatitis, gastroenteritis, increased blood urea nitrogen, leukopenia, and thrombocytopenia. To combat hypokalemia, the patient should be given potassium chloride syrup 10%, 1–2 teaspoonfuls b.i.d., or should be encouraged to eat an orange or banana daily.

Treatment of *moderate* hypertension (diastolic pressure of 110 to 125 mm. Hg and some evidence of secondary changes in brain, ocular fundi, heart, or kidneys) may begin with administration of a thiazide diuretic, but usually includes administration of an adrenergic inhibitor such as reserpine, which blocks sympathetic outflow from the vasomotor center in the medulla; or methyldopa, which interferes with biosynthesis of norepinephrine. The usual dosage of reserpine is 25 mg. daily and the possible side effects are drowsiness, postural hypotension, sleep disturbances, impotence, and hemolytic anemia. The effective dose of methyldopa is highly individualized, and the drug may cause drowsiness, dry mouth, and liver damage.

Treatment of *severe* hypertension (diastolic pressure over 125 mm. Hg) usually requires administration of a sedative, a diuretic, and an adrenergic inhibitor. Phenobarbital 16 mg. b.i.d., or reserpine 0.25 mg. once daily are the most commonly used sedatives. When the thiazide diuretics are not effective in treating severe hypertensives, especially those with some renal impairment, then furosemide or ethacrynic acid may be useful. The effective dosage of either furosemide or ethacrynic acid is highly individualized and the toxic effects are the same as for the thiazides. Guanethidine, a stronger adrenergic inhibitor than methyldopa, may be needed to reduce arterial pressure in severe hypertension. Guanethidine, which blocks impulse transmission in sympathetic postganglionic fibers, is usually given in doses of 10–20 mg. and may produce such toxic effects as lassitude, postural hypotension, nasal congestion, and diarrhea. In some severe hypertensives the sedative drug may be omitted and the patient given hydralazine, which decreases peripheral resistance by directly depressing smooth muscle fibers in the arterial wall. The usual dosage of hydralazine is 25 mg. b.i.d. The drug may cause tachycardia, palpitation, angina, headache, and gastrointestinal symptoms. Spironolactone is a steroid-like substance which is used to treat hypertension resulting from primary aldosteronism.

Because of their greater susceptibility to complications, patients with severe hypertension should generally be treated by a physician rather than by a nurse practitioner.

BIBLIOGRAPHY: MANAGEMENT OF THE PATIENT WITH HYPERTENSION

Barondess, Jeremiah: Systemic arterial hypertension. In Barondess, J., Ed.: *Diagnostic Approaches to Presenting Syndromes.* Baltimore, Williams & Wilkins, 1971, pp. 102–132.
Beeson, Paul, and McDermott, Walsh, Eds.: *Cecil–Loeb Textbook of Medicine.* 14th ed., Philadelphia, W. B. Saunders Co., 1975.

Burr, Helen, Ed.: *Psychological Functioning of Older People*. 3rd ed., Springfield, Charles C Thomas Co., 1971.
Conn, Howard, Ed.: *Current Therapy 1975*. Philadelphia, W. B. Saunders Co., 1975.
Eisdorfer, Carl, and Lawton, M. Powell, Eds.: *The Psychology of Adult Development and Aging*. Washington, D.C., American Psychological Association, 1973.
Laragh, John, Ed.: *Hypertension Manual*. New York, Dun–Donnelley, 1974.
Merck Sharp and Dohme: *The Hypertension Handbook*. West Point, Pennsylvania, Merck Sharp and Dohme, 1974.
Onesti, Gaddo, Kim, Kwan, and Moyer, John, Eds.: *Hypertension, Mechanisms and Management*. New York, Grune and Stratton, 1973.
Page, Lot, and Sidd, James: *Medical Management of Primary Hypertension*. Boston, Little, Brown, and Co., 1973.
Poe, Ro, Lowell, F. M., and Fox, H. M.: Depression: Study of 100 cases in a general hospital, *J.A.M.A.* 195:345–350, January, 1966.
Reiser, M., Rosenbaum, M., and Ferris, E.: Psychologic mechanisms in malignant hypertension. In *Psychosomatic Classics*. Basel, S. Karger, 1972, pp. 56–72.
Wintrobe, Maxwell, Thorn, G., Adams, R., Bennett, I., Braunwald, E., Isselbacher, K., and Petersdorf, R., Eds.: *Harrison's Principles of Internal Medicine*. 6th ed. New York, McGraw-Hill Book Co., 1970.

8
MANAGEMENT OF THE PATIENT WITH DIABETES MELLITUS

Diabetes mellitus, an incurable metabolic disorder, may produce a variety of acute and chronic clinical problems. Complications of the disease can be minimized by diet therapy and weight reduction in conjunction with insulin administration.

PATHOPHYSIOLOGY

Degeneration of the islet cells of the pancreas results in underproduction of insulin which, in turn, has numerous and varied metabolic consequences. Lack of insulin in the plasma leads to decreased glucose entry into and utilization by tissue cells. Since glucose cannot be directly used as fuel in body metabolism, fat and protein are catabolized to free fatty acids and amino acids, respectively. These free fatty acids and amino acids are converted to glucose by the process of gluconeogenesis, producing hyperglycemia. Since in the absence of insulin, glucose can enter only brain and liver cells, excess glucose is excreted in the urine (glycosuria). High concentration of glucose in the renal tubule produces an osmotic diuresis with excessive loss of water, potassium, and sodium. If such fluid loss is prolonged, intracellular dehydration results (Fig. 54).

Catabolism of protein increases the plasma concentration of amino acids and accelerates the process of gluconeogenesis. Increased gluconeogenesis may produce a negative nitrogen balance, a condition in which more protein is catabolized than is ingested or laid down in the tissues.

In severe insulin lack, breakdown of lipids into free fatty acids results in the formation of ketone bodies. As the concentration of these acids (ace-

```
                        INSULIN LACK
                             │
                             ▼
                  Decreased glucose utilization
                       │           │
                       ▼           ▼
              Increased lipolysis    Increased protein catabolism
                       │                      │
                       ▼                      ▼
Increased ketone bodies ◀── Increased free fatty acids    Increased amino acids
         │                      │                    ╱
         ▼                      ▼                   ╱
    Ketonuria                                      ╱
       and                                        ╱
     acidosis        Increased gluconeogenesis ──────▶ Negative
                             │                         nitrogen
                             ▼                         balance
                       Hyperglycemia
                             │
                             ▼
                  Glycosuria—osmotic diuresis
                             │
                             ▼
                   Renal loss of water, Na, K
                             │
                             ▼
                    Intracellular dehydration
```

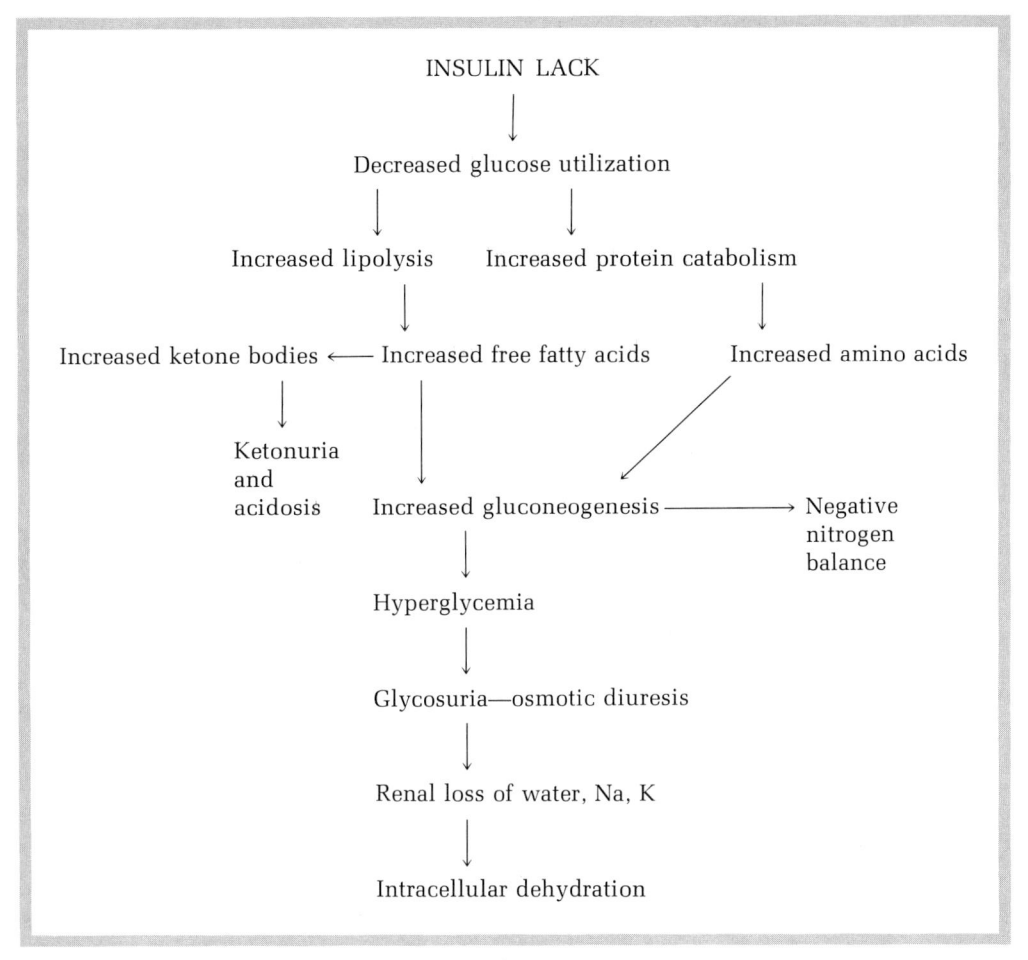

Figure 54.

toacetic acid and beta-hydroxybutyric acid) increases in the body, acidosis results. As the kidney tries to neutralize these acidic substances, potassium ions, sodium ions, and body bases are excreted in the urine, causing the serum bicarbonate content to decrease. After body base has been thus depleted, the carbon dioxide concentration of the serum begins to increase and this, in turn, causes hyperventilation (Fig. 55). At the same time, as fatty acids are catabolized, some of the excess acetyl CoA is converted to cholesterol. The hypercholesterolemia resulting from this conversion contributes to atherosclerosis, a frequent complication in diabetic patients.

Symptoms and Signs

In the diabetic patient, diuresis and intracellular dehydration (both of which result from the hyperglycemia) cause thirst (polydipsia), weakness, and dry, itchy skin. Weight loss and excessive hunger (polyphagia) occur because, even if carbohydrate intake is high, glucose cannot enter tissue cells and be metabolized because there is insufficient insulin to mediate these reactions.

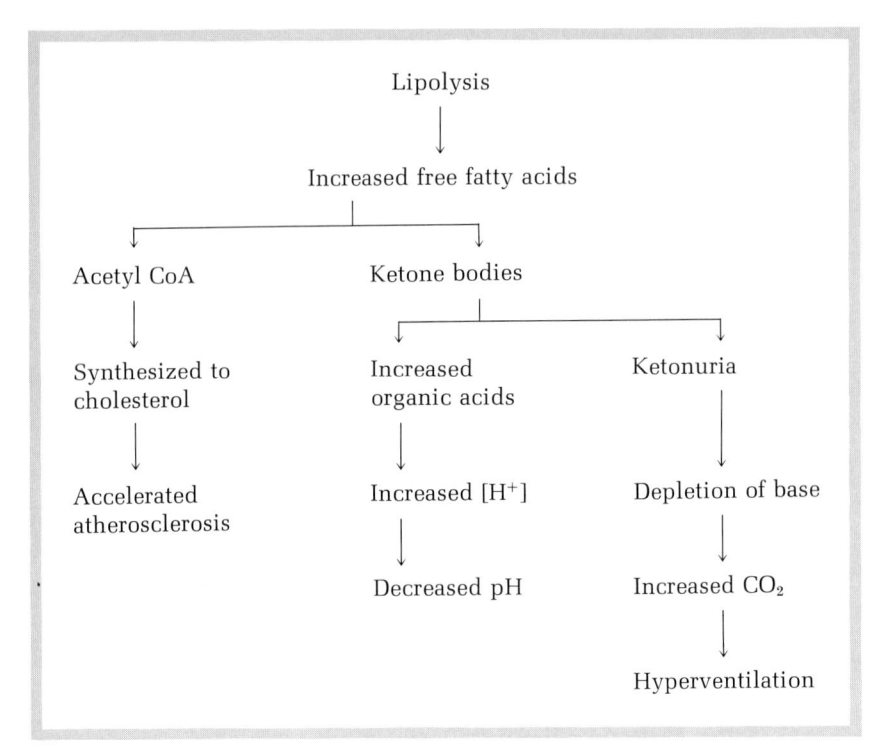

```
                        Lipolysis
                            ↓
                Increased free fatty acids
                  ┌─────────┴─────────┐
                  ↓                   ↓
            Acetyl CoA           Ketone bodies
                  ↓              ┌──────┴──────┐
          Synthesized to      Increased      Ketonuria
            cholesterol      organic acids       ↓
                  ↓                ↓         Depletion of base
           Accelerated        Increased [H⁺]      ↓
          atherosclerosis          ↓         Increased CO₂
                               Decreased pH       ↓
                                            Hyperventilation
```

Figure 55.

The negative nitrogen balance produced by increased tissue catabolism results in muscle weakness and weight loss; therefore, the specific diagnostic signs of diabetes are hyperglycemia, hypercholesterolemia, glycosuria, and ketonuria.

Typically, early symptoms of diabetes mellitus are minimal and constitute little physical stress; therefore, treatment is usually not sought during the early stages of the disease. Since early diagnosis and treatment tend to lessen the complications of diabetes, practitioners should be alert to early symptoms of the disease in high risk patients in order to initiate appropriate diagnostic procedures where indicated.

Persons with a family history of diabetes mellitus, the obese, the aged, and women who have delivered a very large baby should all receive periodic screening tests for diabetes mellitus, since incidence of the disease is high in these groups.

Diagnosis

A tentative diagnosis of diabetes mellitus can be made on the basis of a history of polyuria, polydipsia, polyphagia, weakness, and weight loss. The diagnosis is confirmed by the clinical findings of hyperglycemia, glycosuria, and ketonuria. Although glycosuria may indicate the presence of diabetes, it may also result from aging, pregnancy, stress, or chronic renal disease.

Fasting blood glucose, postprandial blood glucose, or glucose tolerance tests can be used to confirm a diagnosis of diabetes mellitus when ketonuria is not present. The techniques and normal values for these tests are discussed in Chapter 5.

PATIENT ASSESSMENT, EDUCATION, AND DIET

Diet therapy and weight control are crucial to effective health management of patients with diabetes mellitus. Because obesity greatly increases insulin requirements, it is advisable for the diabetic to be of normal weight. Ideal weight in women of medium frame is 100 pounds for 5 feet of height, and 5 pounds additional weight for each inch over 5 feet. Ideal weight in men of medium frame is 106 pounds for 5 feet of height and 6 pounds additional weight for each inch over 5 feet. Weekly weight measurement is indicated during the initial treatment period for the diabetic patient and most patients can be relied upon to keep an accurate record of their weight.

Prior to initiation of diet-control for the treatment of diabetes the patient's urine should be tested q.i.d. for glucose, and his blood glucose level measured at a couple of different times during the day. Information about the efficiency of glucose utilization (as indicated by unusually high or low values at certain times during the day) is useful in regulating the patient's diet and in determining his need for insulin.

In calculating the proper diet for the diabetic patient, consideration must be given to 1) the total number of calories to be ingested per day, 2) the percentage of total calories to be given at each meal or in snack feedings, and 3) the partition of total caloric intake into the number of calories to be ingested as carbohydrate (150–250 gm.), protein (50–90 gm.), or fat (70–120 gm.).

For the individual of normal weight, the basic caloric requirement is roughly determined by multiplying the ideal body weight in pounds by 10. Another method used to calculate caloric requirement is to allow 30 Cal/Kg (1 Kg = 2.2 pounds) of body weight per day. The caloric prescription is then adjusted in relation to activity, age, obesity, or malnutrition. For example, a weight loss of 1 pound per week occurs with a daily caloric deficit of 500 calories. The prescribed daily caloric intake should be distributed among the several daily feedings in such manner as to accommodate the patient's routines, his eating habits, the severity of his glucose intolerance, and the type of insulin he receives. Typically, the calories are divided into three meals and one bedtime snack in the following ratio: 3/10, 3/10, 3/10, 1/10. If, on the prescribed treatment regimen, hypoglycemia occurs before a meal, a snack should be added or additional food ingested at the previous meal. Patients receiving insulin usually require a bedtime snack to prevent hypoglycemia during nighttime hours. The amount of carbohydrate, protein, and fat to be included in the diet is the amount of each that will provide an adequate number of calories while at the same time providing a well-balanced diet. It is recommended that the carbohydrate intake be 1 gram per pound of ideal body weight and that the protein intake be 0.5 gram per pound of body weight. Fat intake is then prescribed according to the number of additional calories needed to reach the suggested total daily intake. Some practitioners simply advise 150 to 250 Gm. per day of carbohydrate, 60 to 100 Gm. per day of protein, and 70 to 120 Gm. per day of fat.

The caloric value of carbohydrate and protein is 4 Cal. per gram, while metabolism of each gram of fat yields 9 Cal. Since fat has a high caloric value and, also, contributes to development of atherosclerosis, it is advisable to minimize the fat intake in the diabetic diet and to supply most of the fat that is given in the form of unsaturated fatty acids.

After determining the patient's ideal body weight, the number of calories required per day to achieve or maintain this weight, the amount of the total caloric allowance that should be given as carbohydrates, protein, and fat, and the number of calories of each of these that should be given in each meal, the practitioner should decide how many of each of the following six types of food exchanges should be given for each meal: 1) milk exchange; 2) A and B vegetables; 3) fruit exchanges; 4) bread exchanges; 5) meat exchanges; and 6) fat exchanges. In discussing his prescribed diet with the diabetic patient it is useful to determine whether or not all of the six food exchanges will be available to the patient. (Patients on limited income may not be able to afford meat daily; patients without refrigeration will not be able to store milk.) Booklets on meal planning with diabetic exchange lists are available from the American Diabetes Association, 18 East 48th Street, New York, New York 10017. The patient should be helped to interpret his diet prescription (that is, shown how to use the exchange lists), and be taught the importance of diet management in disease control. Achievement and maintenance of optimum weight, glucose and acetone-free urine, reduction of blood glucose levels, and freedom from symptoms of hypoglycemia indicate that the patient's caloric intake is adequate for his needs.

Oral Hypoglycemic Agents

Many clinicians now agree that oral hypoglycemic agents have serious cardiovascular side effects and should only be prescribed for diabetic patients who are poorly controlled by diet and who are unable to take insulin. Tolbutamide (Orinase, 500 mg., b.i.d.) is the most widely prescribed oral hypoglycemic agent but has been found to significantly increase cardiovascular mortality. Oral hypoglycemic drugs should be used only with the informed consent of the patient.

Insulin

Seven different types of insulin are available, in four different strengths (U 40, U 80, U 100, U 500). The most commonly used types of insulin are crystalline, N.P.H., and Lente insulin. Crystalline insulin, the most rapid acting, is rarely used alone except in treatment of acute hyperglycemia, acidosis (complications for which the patient would be treated by a physician), trauma or infection. An intermediate-acting insulin (N.P.H. or Lente), injected before breakfast, is adequate to control hyperglycemia in the majority of diabetic patients. Crystalline insulin has an onset of action within two to three hours after injection, and has a six-hour duration of action. N.P.H. and Lente have an onset of action within eight to 10 hours after administration and a 24 hour duration of action. It is, of course, essential that the patient and his family know which type of and how much insulin is to be administered, how to aseptically prepare the proper dose for injection, how to prepare the injection sites, and the proper technique for injection. The diabetic patient and his family must also know how to handle and store the insulin vials in order to prevent deterioration and contamination.

The object of insulin therapy is to maintain a normal glycemic state in those patients who are hyperglycemic on diet therapy alone. The type, dose, and time of insulin injection required to maintain normal blood glucose concentration must be determined for each patient.

Typically, crystalline insulin is used to treat acute diabetic acidosis according to the following schedule: 20 units is administered for a 4+ glycosuria, 15 units for a 3+ glycosuria, and 10 units for a 2+ glycosuria. After the acute episode of acidosis has been successfully treated, 10 to 20 units of N.P.H. or Lente insulin per day may be ordered and the dosage increased if the patient requires additional insulin to maintain normoglycemia. The blood glucose concentration is checked daily, before breakfast and supper, during the initial phases of treatment. After the patient is found to be in good diabetic control, blood glucose determinations can be done infrequently, but are still needed on a regular basis to monitor the patient's progress.

Diabetic patients must know how and when to test their urine for glucose and acetone and what adjustments of insulin dosage they are to make in the event of glycosuria or insulin reaction. Patients should know, for example, that exercise increases glucose utilization and decreases the need for insulin, while stress may increase the body's glucose concentration, producing hyperglycemia and glycosuria.

Complications of Insulin Therapy

Insulin reaction and insulin shock are names for the hypoglycemia and accompanying symptoms that occur when there is excess insulin in the plasma. Severe hypoglycemia is dangerous and can result in bizarre behavior, brain damage, or death. The usual symptoms of insulin excess are drowsiness, nausea, anxiety, irritability, restlessness, perspiration, pallor, hunger, headache, and mental confusion. The onset of reaction to excessive dosage of crystalline insulin is abrupt. When crystalline insulin is taken before breakfast, hyperglycemic reactions are most likely to occur about noon. Onset of reaction to intermediate insulin is gradual. When N.P.H. or Lente insulin is injected before breakfast, hyperglycemic reactions are most likely to occur about 4 or 5 P.M. Diabetics learn to recognize the symptoms of hypoglycemia and to take sugar or candy to prevent or relieve such symptoms. Following an insulin reaction, rebound hyperglycemia often occurs. Rebound hyperglycemia should not be treated with insulin but rather by reducing the patient's insulin dosage.

All persons with diabetes should carry a card or wear a medallion identifying them as diabetic in order that they may be properly diagnosed and treated during episodes of diabetic acidosis or insulin shock, which may render them confused or unconscious.

Tissue reactions at the site of insulin injection are common during the initial phase of therapy. Urticaria, redness, and pain may occur as a part of such reactions but usually disappear in a few days or weeks without treatment. Patients should be taught to rotate the site of insulin injection, as hypertrophy or atrophy of the subcutaneous adipose tissue tends to occur at a site used for repeated injections.

Complications of Diabetes

The most common acute complication of diabetes mellitus is ketoacidosis (hyperglycemic or hyperosmolar coma), which may be precipitated by severe infection, trauma or emergency surgery. With proper health management most diabetic patients can withstand surgery and pregnancy without serious complications. Adult onset diabetics experience ketoacidosis less frequently than do childhood onset diabetics because of the former group's tendency to maintain a higher insulin concentration in the plasma.

Chronic complications of diabetes mellitus include retinopathy, nephropathy, arteriopathy, gangrene of the feet, and neuropathy. Optimal control of diabetes and maintenance of ideal body weight delay onset and progress of these complications, even though no treatment program has been found that will prevent development of vascular and neural degenerative changes in diabetic patients. The patient who understands the relationship between dietary management, insulin administration, good personal hygiene, and diabetic control is, of course, less prone to acute episodes of ketoacidosis and insulin shock, both of which are threatening in themselves and, if not fatal, predispose the patient to serious circulatory and nervous system complications. Retinopathy, once it develops, is an irreversible process which is first evident as microaneurysms, hemorrhages, and/or yellowish exudates on the posterior fundus near the macula. Such vascular damage may give rise to retinal edema and/or detachment, causing decreased vision or blindness.

Nephropathy is common in diabetics and may consist of several different types of pathology. The initial clinical sign of glomerulosclerosis (atheromatous narrowing of renal arteries and arterioles) is proteinuria. If the degree of sclerosis is great, renal insufficiency can develop.

The tendency toward generalized arteriopathy predisposes the diabetic patient to such cardiovascular problems as coronary atherosclerosis, myocardial infarction, hypertension, and occlusive atherosclerosis of the cerebral arteries and arteries of the lower extremities.

Obliterative atherosclerosis of the lower extremities contributes to the development of infections, ulcers, gangrene and, eventually, to the need for amputation. Patients are instructed to exercise daily foot care and to seek immediate treatment of any foot or leg lesion.

In the diabetic, nervous tissue degeneration chiefly occurs in the peripheral nerves but may involve any part of the nervous system. Therefore, diabetic neuropathy is typically characterized by multiple clinical signs: loss of vibratory sense, paresthesias, weakness, paralysis, diminished or absent tendon reflexes, pupillary changes, gastric atony, sexual impotence, bladder atony, orthostatic hypotension, Charcot joints, and skin ulcers. With prolonged normoglycemia (one to two years) and good diabetic management, neuropathic changes may be reversed in many diabetic patients.

Careful evaluation of the diabetic patient's eyes, skin, renal functioning, and neurological and cardiovascular status will provide the practitioner baseline data against which to compare any future change as complications of the patient's disease occur. The eyes should be examined for microaneurysms, which appear as sharply outlined red spots occurring around the macula. The patient's skin is inspected for dryness, reddened areas, ulcers, or necrosis. The color and temperature of the extremities should be noted as indices of the adequacy of peripheral arterial circulation, and tests of renal functioning are conducted to determine the adequacy of renal circulation.

Evaluation of the diabetic patient's cardiovascular status should include an electrocardiogram, blood pressure determination, and bilateral palpation of arteries to determine whether pulse volumes are equal and whether vessels are thickened or tortuous. Chest x-rays are used to determine whether the diabetic patient's lowered resistance to infection has led to bronchial or pulmonary infection. Urinalysis and 24 hour urine cultures are helpful in detecting urinary infection as well as in determining the degree of glycosuria present. Depending on how long the patient has been diabetic and the efficacy of disease control, medical history relating to nervous system functioning may reveal impotence, poor digestion, weakness, visual changes, and limitations of movement. Neurological signs frequently found in diabetic patients include joint deformity without pain, decreased tendon reflexes, paresthesias, pupillary changes, decreased ocular movements, orthostatic hypotension, loss of vibratory sense, and muscle weakness or paralysis.

BIBLIOGRAPHY: MANAGEMENT OF THE PATIENT WITH DIABETES MELLITUS

Beeson, Paul, and McDermott, Walsh, Eds.: *Cecil–Loeb Textbook of Medicine*. 14th ed., Philadelphia, W. B. Saunders Co., 1975.
Bloodworth, J. M.: Diabetes mellitus and vascular disease. *Postgrad. Med.*, 53:84–89, 1973.
Boggie, A., et al.: Ambulatory management of the new diabetic. *Canad. Med. Assoc. J.* 107:660–663, 1972.
Conn, Howard, Ed.: *Current Therapy 1975*. Philadelphia, W. B. Saunders, 1975.
Damron, J. J., et al.: Tape recorded instruction for patients with diabetes. J. Amer. Diet. Assoc., 62:426–427, 1973.
Danowski, T. S., Ed.: Diabetes Mellitus: Diagnosis and Treatment, New York, American Diabetes Association, 1964, Vol. 1.
Ellenberg, Max, and Rifkin, Harold, Eds.: *Diabetes Mellitus, Theory and Practice*. New York, McGraw-Hill Book Co., 1970.
Fajans, Stefan, and Sussman, Karl, Eds.: *Diabetes Mellitus, Diagnosis and Treatment*. New York, American Diabetes Association, 1971.
Fusaro, R. M., and Goetz, F. C.: Common cutaneous manifestations and problems of diabetes mellitus. *Postgrad. Med.*, 49:84–90, 1971.
Gibbons, Euell, and Gibbons, Joe: *Feast on a Diabetic Diet*. New York, David McKay Co., 1969.
Gormican, Annette: *Controlling Diabetes With Diet*. Springfield, Charles C Thomas, 1971.
Hamwi, George, and Danowski, T. S.: *Diabetes Mellitus: Diagnosis and Treatment*. New York, American Diabetes Association, 1967 Vol. II.
Kimura, Samuel, and Caygill, Wayne, Eds.: *Vascular Complications of Diabetes Mellitus*. St. Louis, C. V. Mosby Co., 1967.
Power, Lawrence, Bakker, Doris, and Cooper, Marilyn: *Diabetes Outpatient Care Through Physician Assistants*. Springfield, Charles C Thomas, 1973.
Trayser, L. M. A teaching Program for diabetics. *Amer. J. Nurs.*, 73:92–93, 1973.
Whitehouse, F. W.: Infections that hospitalize the diabetic. *Geriatrics*, 28:97–99, 1973.

9
MANAGEMENT OF THE PATIENT WITH CHRONIC ARTHRITIS

Arthritis, or inflammation of joint structures, may be caused by infection (gonococcal, syphilitic, or tuberculous arthritis), hypersensitivity (arthritis associated with rheumatic fever or drug reaction), degenerative change (osteoarthritis) or inflammatory reaction of unknown cause (rheumatoid arthritis or the arthritis associated with systemic lupus erythematosus).

Between six and seven million Americans suffer from arthritis. The two most common types, osteoarthritis and rheumatoid arthritis, are chronic disabling diseases the effects of which can be minimized by early diagnosis and judicious treatment. Patients with osteoarthritis and rheumatoid arthritis are frequently referred to the nurse practitioner for workup and health management.

OSTEOARTHRITIS

Osteoarthritis, the most common of all joint disorders, could more correctly be referred to as degenerative osteoarthropathy, since it is a noninflammatory joint disease characterized by deterioration of the articular surfaces within the joint and formation of new bone at the joint margins. Since osteoarthritic joint destruction results from the wear and tear of use, the incidence of the disease increases with age, and the large weight-bearing joints (hip, knee, spine) and the finger joints are those most frequently involved. When osteoarthritis occurs in younger persons it is usually a result of joint injury or malalignment, as in congenital subluxation of the hip or slipped femoral epiphysis. Obesity and repeated percussive joint trauma, such as that caused by typing or the use of a pneumatic hammer, contribute to development of degenerative osteoarthropathy.

The pathological changes that occur in osteoarthritis include: softening and rupture of the articular cartilage; rarefaction, erosion, and roughening of the articular surface of the bone; formation of bony "spurs" at the margins of the articular cartilage; and, occasionally, fibrosis and thickening of the synovial membrane. Where articular cartilage is thinned, underlying bone shows increased density and new bone formation. Where the articular cartilage is completely eroded, directly opposing bone surfaces become thickened and highly polished (eburnation).

Osteoarthritic changes occur slowly and insidiously, developing over a period of years. Typically, only one or a few joints are involved, though in an occasional patient diffuse polyarthropathy is seen. The primary symptoms of the disease are joint pain, stiffness, crepitus, joint enlargement, and limitation of motion. Joint pain, which is aching in character and typically located over points of synovial thickening or bony spur formation, at first occurs on use of the involved joint and is relieved by rest. As the disease progresses, pain may occur even with limited motion or at rest and may waken the patient from sleep. Frequently osteoarthritic joint pain is increased by changes in the weather.

Joint stiffness is generally most marked on awakening in the morning or after periods of prolonged inactivity. Typically, such stiffness disappears within a few minutes if the joint is moved.

Crepitus, a grating sensation that is provoked by joint movement, results from the rubbing together of irregular joint surfaces.

Joints are enlarged in osteoarthritis, owing to either thickening of the synovial membrane or proliferation of bony tissue at the joint margins. The pattern of joint enlargement is often diagnostically significant. For instance, Heberden's nodes, or cartilaginous and bony enlargement of the distal interphalangeal joints of the fingers, are often seen in osteoarthritic women. Similar nodes may be seen at the proximal interphalangeal joints (Bouchard's nodes) but are less common.

Limitation of joint motion, which becomes more pronounced as deterioration of joint structures progresses, is primarily due to capsular fibrosis, irregularity of joint surfaces, and muscle spasm and contracture.

During physical examination of the patient with joint symptoms all joints should be carefully examined for swelling, heat, tenderness, discoloration, deformity, crepitus, and limitation of motion, for a patient with polyarthropathy may limit his complaints to the one or two joints that cause him the greatest discomfort. Also during the physical examination the functional capacity of each of the diseased joints should be evaluated. That is, can the patient with osteoarthropathy of the hip, ankle, or knee climb stairs, sit, rise from a chair, and rise from a recumbent position without difficulty? Can the patient with osteoarthropathy of the hands tie his laces, open a screwtop jar, and button his clothes?

Degenerative osteoarthropathy can be differentiated from other types of arthritis by means of careful history and physical examination, X-ray of the involved joints, and a few specific laboratory tests. Osteoarthritis differs from most other arthritides in that the former engenders no systemic symptoms, thereby limiting findings to joint structures alone. Patients with infectious arthritis are usually febrile, complain of malaise, and may give a history of an antecedent venereal, respiratory, skin, or other infection. Acute rheumatic fever has a sudden acute onset, and is characterized by migratory polyarthritis, which is often accompanied by fever, malaise, skin lesions, subcutaneous nodules, cardiac murmurs, and cardiomegaly. Patients with rheumatoid arthritis typically exhibit subcutaneous nodules on the extensor surface of the forearm, muscular atrophy, and atrophy or bronzing of the skin, as well as more marked and more rapidly progressive joint damage than that seen in osteoarthritis. Patients with gouty arthritis often demonstrate tophi in the helix of the ear, the olecranon or prepatellar bursae, or the tendons of the fingers and toes. Patients with gout may also demonstrate albuminuria, urinary stones, or other signs of renal dysfunction. The patient with lupus erythematosus is likely to have symptoms referable to several organ systems and may demonstrate either a butterfly-shaped discoloration over the malar area or other skin lesions.

In osteoarthritis the differential white cell count and red cell sedimentation rate are normal (the former would typically be elevated in infectious arthritis, and the latter is usually elevated in acute rheumatic fever), and the serology tests, L. E. preparation, and latex fixation test are negative.

X-ray findings in osteoarthritis may include narrowing of the joint space, due to erosion of articular cartilage; increased density of articulating bone surfaces, due to deposition of new bone; and bony spur formation at the joint margin.

Treatment of osteoarthritis should include reassurance, rest, reduction of joint stress, physiotherapy, and administration of analgesic drugs.

The patient with osteoarthritis will be reassured to learn that since his disease is not the "crippling" arthritis which leads to severe deformity, his symptoms will probably be limited to a few joints, and his discomfort can be alleviated by a combination of physical and pharmaceutical agents.

The patient should be advised to take several 20- to 30-minute rest periods at intervals throughout the day. Whenever possible, he should rest in a recumbent position on a flat, hard surface. The patient should get eight hours of sleep each night and his bed should be fitted with a firm mattress and a bedboard in order to ensure good body alignment. Total bedrest is to be avoided, for it would rapidly lead to muscle atrophy and increased debility.

The osteoarthritic patient who is obese should be encouraged to lose weight in order to decrease trauma to the large, weight-bearing joints. Specially constructed orthopedic shoes may, by shifting the body weight slightly, decrease the strain on a damaged joint.

The patient who has an osteoarthritic knee or hip may find that using a cane or a crutch on the side opposite the diseased joint will alleviate joint stress and decrease discomfort.

Local heat, applied by means of a heating pad, may be used to decrease muscle spasm, either to relieve discomfort or to enable the patient to cooperate more fully with rehabilitation exercises. Both passive and active exercises should be used to maintain as nearly as possible full range of motion both in the involved joint and in the joints proximal and distal to it. Active resistive exercises will be needed to prevent muscle atrophy, since muscle weakness alone will cause joint instability and would lead to further mechanical strain in an osteoarthritic joint.

When muscle spasm is severe in osteoarthritis of the hip, traction may be needed to relax hypertonic muscles. A cervical collar during the day and a small neck pillow at night may help to overcome muscle spasm in the patient with cervical osteoarthritis.

In most osteoarthritic patients who are treated with rest periods, activity control, local heat, and range of motion exercise, aspirin, 0.6 Gm. t.i.d. or q.i.d., is effective in controlling joint pain. Occasionally a tranquilizer such as diazepam, 2 to 5 mg. t.i.d., or meprobamate, 400 mg. t.i.d., may be given for a brief period in order to relax the patient and encourage physical rest.

The osteoarthritic patient who fails to improve with rest, physiotherapy, and analgesics should be referred to a physician for continuing workup and modification of the treatment plan.

RHEUMATOID ARTHRITIS

Rheumatoid arthritis, or arthritis deformans, is a constitutional disease of unknown cause that is characterized by widespread inflammatory change in connective tissue. Rheumatoid arthritis is most common in damp, temperate climates, is more likely to affect women than men, most often develops during the fourth decade of life, and is especially likely to occur in persons with a familial incidence of the disease.

Although the cause of rheumatoid arthritis has not been identified, the disease is often precipitated by an episode of severe physical or psychic stress. Although in a few patients rheumatoid arthritis has an acute and fulminating onset, the disease usually begins slowly and insidiously with fatigue, malaise, anorexia, and weight loss, followed shortly by the development of joint pain, swelling, redness, heat, deformity, and limitation of motion.

The pathological changes of rheumatoid arthritis include edema, congestion, capillary proliferation, and thickening of the synovial membrane; effusion of synovial fluid into the joint space; formation of a layer of granulation tissue, or pannus, which causes erosion of articular cartilage; inflammation and destruction (osteolysis) of subchondral bone; formation of adhesive fibrous tissue bands between opposing surfaces of denuded, inflamed, and lysed bone; and joint ankylosis.

The joints most commonly affected in rheumatoid arthritis are those of the hands, feet, and knees, though the hip, spinal joints, elbow, shoulder, and even the temporomandibular joint are involved in some patients. Typically, the patient notes pain and stiffness of one joint which persists or worsens as the same symptoms begin to appear in other joints. Often there is symmetry of joint involvement, with inflammatory changes occurring in both knees, both hands, or both feet.

While at first rheumatoid joint pain occurs only on motion, as the disease progresses and cartilaginous and bony destruction take place, the patient often experiences rest pain as well. Muscle aching and tenderness usually accompany joint pain, and prolonged morning joint stiffness is a common feature of the disease. Joint swelling is fusiform, or spindle-shaped, and, together with pain, causes severe limitation of joint motion. The skin over the affected joint is often warm to the touch.

Severe muscle wasting frequently occurs in the area surrounding an inflamed joint, and firm, non-tender subcutaneous nodules may develop on the extensor surface of the forearm or over other pressure points in the rheumatoid patient. The skin over the involved joints is usually thin, taut, pale, and shiny. The patient often complains of such vasomotor symptoms as periodic coldness, flushing, numbness, or tingling of the hands and feet.

Some patients with rheumatoid arthritis, especially those with rheumatoid spondylitis, develop associated ocular lesions, such as keratoconjunctivitis, uveitis, and scleritis. Patients with such lesions should, of course, be promptly referred to an ophthalmologist for treatment.

Rheumatoid arthritis is diagnosed on the basis of the history of the illness, x-ray evidence, and certain laboratory tests. The insidious onset of polyarticular arthritis affecting small as well as large joints, with accompanying fatigue, malaise, anorexia, and weight loss, and with periodic remissions and exacerbations leading to progressive joint damage, suggests a diagnosis of rheumatoid arthritis. The proximal interphalangeal joints of the hand are frequently affected, showing fusiform swelling early in the disease and severe angulation and deformity in later stages. Destruction of the metacarpophalangeal joints produces ulnar deviation of the hand. Destruction of interphalangeal and wrist joints produces flexion deformities of the fingers and wrist. Muscular weakness and atrophy, skin atrophy and discoloration, and subcutaneous nodules frequently occur in association with the joint changes. Prolonged morning stiffness of involved joints is a cardinal symptom. An episode of severe physical or psychological stress often antedates the onset of both the malaise and the joint symptoms.

Early in the disease, x-rays of the affected joints may show only soft tissue swelling. Within months or a few years after onset, roentgenographic findings include first, osteoporosis of juxta-articular bone (perhaps the result of pain-induced immobility); followed by narrowing of involved joint spaces (due to destruction of articular cartilage); destructive erosion of denuded bone surfaces; and finally, subluxations, ankylosis, and malalignment.

The majority of patients with rheumatoid arthritis present with a normocytic, hypochromic anemia that fails to respond to treatment with iron salts. Such patients may also demonstrate a moderate leukocytosis (12,000–20,000/ml^3), with a disproportionate increase in immature white cells. The erythrocyte sedimentation rate is usually elevated in rheumatoid arthritis, and the amount of its elevation is a rough index of the degree of inflammatory activity in joint tissue. The red cell sedimentation rate is increased when there is a greater than normal tendency for rouleaux formation. Increased concentrations of plasma fibrinogen and globulins foster rouleaux formation. Since in inflammatory conditions the liver is stimulated to produce excess fibrinogen, and lymphoid tissue is stimulated to produce excess globulins, increased rouleaux formation and elevated red cell sedimentation rates are common in inflammatory disease. The abnormal C-reactive protein, which appears in the serum during certain acute infections and inflammatory conditions, is present in rheumatoid arthritis. Certain abnormal macroglobulins, called "rheumatoid factors," are also present in the serum of patients with rheumatoid arthritis and can be detected through an agglutination test. This latter test has prognostic as well as diagnostic significance, since patients who consistently demonstrate the presence of the rheumatoid factor on repeated tests usually pursue a progressively unfavorable course, with rapid development of severe joint damage.

In making a definitive diagnosis of rheumatoid arthritis it may be necessary to rule out a number of other diseases which present similar findings. The patient with rheumatic fever will probably demonstrate cardiac symptoms, and on subsidence of his joint symptoms there will be no residual damage to joint structures. The patient with lupus erythematosus may demonstrate a butterfly-shaped rash over the malar eminences and will usually demonstrate disturbed functioning of many organ systems. The patient with gout may develop urate deposits (tophi) in the ear lobe or on the hands and feet. His first metatarsophalangeal joint is most apt to be involved, and his joint symptoms will be relieved by the administration of colchicine. The patient with degenerative arthritis or osteoarthritis typically has involvement of the distal rather than the proximal interphalangeal joint, has no constitutional symptoms, and his joint symptoms are relieved by rest, heat, and aspirin. In Reiter's syndrome, which usually occurs in young men, the patient suffers urethritis and conjunctivitis as well as arthritis.

Treatment for rheumatoid arthritis should be aimed at reducing inflammation, relieving pain, preserving function, and preventing deformity. These objectives can best be achieved by a combination of rest, physiotherapy, and analgesic and anti-inflammatory drugs.

The patient who is febrile and who has acutely inflamed and painful joints should be kept at bedrest until the joint symptoms are relieved and his temperature has returned to normal. If he is afebrile and his joint symptoms are less severe, he should be advised to obtain at least eight hours of sleep at night and to take three to four hour-long naps during the day. His bed should be fitted with a firm mattress and a bedboard and only a small head pillow should be used in order that his spine be kept in proper alignment during the prescribed rest periods. Occasionally, during acute episodes of arthritic symptoms, the patient may require mild sedatives to achieve needed rest. Phenobarbital, 30 mg. t.i.d., or pentobarbital sodium 90 mg. h.s., may be used for this purpose but should be discontinued as soon as the acute arthritic episode has subsided.

An acutely inflamed and painful joint should be supported and immobilized with a posterior plaster or aluminum splint. Because the weight of the bed linen may prevent proper alignment of the legs and feet, the upper linen should be supported by a bed cradle; the feet of the patient with lower extremity involvement should be supported with a footboard.

Just as joint rest is needed to foster subsidence of inflammatory joint changes and to reduce mechanical trauma to inflamed synovia, cartilage and bone, moderate joint exercise is needed to restore muscle tone and to maintain joint mobility. Accordingly, all joints, including those involved in the rheumatoid process, should be put through full range of motion twice daily. During the acute phase of joint involvement, passive exercises should be used and the inflamed joints should be moved to, but not beyond, the point of pain. After the acute joint symptoms have subsided, the patient should be taught to perform active range of motion exercises and should be supervised to ensure that he carries out the exercises as prescribed.

Either acetylsalicylic acid (aspirin) or sodium salicylate is usually effective in relieving inflammatory joint pain and stiffness. The patient should be started on a dosage of 0.6 Gm. q.i.d.; if the symptoms are not relieved, the dosage should be increased to 0.9 or 1.2 Gm. q.i.d. Enteric coated preparations of salicylate should be used to prevent gastrointestinal irritation, and the patient should be watched for symptoms of salicylism (nausea, vomiting, skin rash, gastric bleeding, diplopia, dizziness, and tinnitus) which, if severe, would require reduction of drug dosage or use of a different medication. Because aspirin decreases the prothrombin level it should not be given to patients on anticoagulant therapy.

Patients whose joint symptoms cannot be controlled by the salicylates may respond to phenylbutazone (Butazolidin), adrenocorticosteroids, chloroquine (Aralen), or gold salts. The patient should be referred to a physician for reassessment before treatment with any of these drugs is undertaken.

Phenylbutazone is given in dosages of 100 mg. t.i.d. and should be taken with food or milk to prevent gastric irritation. Because the drug tends to depress hemopoietic tissue, frequent blood counts must be taken. The drug should be discontinued if beneficial effects are not obtained within two weeks of treatment.

Adrenocorticoids should not be used to treat rheumatoid arthritis except in those patients who do not respond to salicylate or phenylbutazone therapy. If corticoids are to be used, prednisone, 2.5 mg., is given two or three times daily, and at the same time the patient is continued on his previous salicylate, rest, and physiotherapy regimen.

The patient must be observed for such toxic drug effects as excessive fluid retention, peptic ulcer, osteoporosis, diabetes mellitus, and increased susceptibility to infection. As soon as the acute joint symptoms have been controlled, the dosage of prednisone should be gradually reduced and the drug discontinued.

Although the exact mechanism of action is not known, it has been observed that in some rheumatoid patients who are unresponsive to salicylates and cannot for some reason be given adrenocorticoids, chloroquine 250 mg. daily over a period of several weeks will gradually relieve joint symptoms. Toxic effects of the drug include nausea, vomiting, diarrhea, headache, and skin rash.

Occasionally, the physician will treat a patient who does not respond to any of the aforementioned drugs with injections of gold salts. Gold sodium thiomalate or thioglucose is injected intramuscularly once weekly in first 10 mg., then 25 mg., then 50 mg. doses, and the patient is observed for such evidence of toxic effects as skin rash, gastrointestinal bleeding, proteinuria, anemia, leukopenia, and thrombocytopenia. The appearance of any of these complications would dictate discontinuation of gold therapy.

Those patients with chronic rheumatoid arthritis in whom repeated exacerbations of joint inflammation have produced severe deformity are sometimes referred for surgical correction of malalignment. Obviously such patients must be carefully evaluated to determine their ability to profit from surgical intervention, and the patient must be carefully counseled preoperatively so that he does not expect greater improvement in his condition than the surgical procedure can effect.

BIBLIOGRAPHY: MANAGEMENT OF THE PATIENT WITH CHRONIC ARTHRITIS

Beeson, Paul, and McDermott, Walsh, Eds.: *Cecil-Loeb Textbook of Medicine.* 14th ed. Philadelphia, W. B. Saunders Co., 1975.
Boyle, James, and Buchanan, W.: *Clinical Rheumatology.* Oxford, Blackwell Scientific Publications, 1971.
Conn, Howard, Ed.: *Current Therapy 1975.* Philadelphia, W. B. Saunders Co., 1975.
Conservative management of osteoarthrosis. Drug Therapeut. Bull. 11:29–30, 1973.
Ehrlich, George, Ed.: *Total Management of the Arthritic Patient.* Philadelphia, J. B. Lippincott Co., 1973.
Hollander, Joseph, and McCarty, Daniel, Eds.: *Arthritis and Allied Conditions.* 8th ed. Philadelphia, Lea & Febiger, 1972.
Moskowitz, R. W.: Osteoarthritis: A new look at an old disease. Geriatrics, 28:121–128, 1973.

10
MANAGEMENT OF THE PATIENT IN CHRONIC CONGESTIVE HEART FAILURE

Heart failure can be defined as that condition in which cardiac output is insufficient to meet tissue oxygen demands. Cardiac failure can be classified as acute or chronic failure, as high output or low output failure, as left sided or right sided failure, or as forward or backward failure. In acute heart failure, symptoms of circulatory congestion and tissue ischemia develop quickly over a period of a few hours in a patient previously without apparent cardiac dysfunction. In chronic heart failure, symptoms of congestion and inadequate tissue perfusion develop slowly and insidiously over a period of weeks or months while the patient becomes progressively debilitated. The nurse practitioner will frequently be called upon to care for patients of this latter type, often elderly persons with arteriosclerotic heart disease, in whom progressive obstruction of the coronary arteries gradually decreases myocardial efficiency until finally the heart is unable to pump out enough blood to meet the metabolic needs of body tissues.

High output failure is that form of cardiac failure in which, despite normal and even increased cardiac output, symptoms of congestion and inadequate tissue oxygenation develop. High output failure is not, then, failure of the heart as a pump, but overloading of the heart with excessive venous return flow. High output failure may occur as a consequence of hyperthyroidism (in which tissue oxygen demand is greatly increased), anemia (in which cardiac rate and stroke volume increase to compensate for decreased oxygen-carrying capacity of the blood), or arteriovenous fistula (in which the resultant decrease in systemic vascular resistance increases first venous return and then cardiac output). Low output failure, on the other hand, which is characterized by a subnormal cardiac output, is the consequence of such cardiac stresses as rheumatic valvular damage, the increased peripheral resistance of hypertension, and the myocardial ischemia resulting from coronary arteriosclerosis.

In left heart failure an abnormally heavy work load is imposed on the left ventricle by some factor such as hypertension or aortic valvular insufficiency, and excess fluid accumulates in that part of the circulatory system immediately behind the overburdened ventricle (the pulmonary circulation). In right heart failure the right ventricle is unusually burdened, as from diffuse pulmonary fibrosis or pulmonary valve stenosis, and excess fluid accumulates in that part of the circulation preceding the right heart (systemic venous circulation). Because blood moves in a circuit throughout the body, such localization of congestion does not persist for long; that is, the pulmonary congestion resulting from left heart failure constitutes an increased burden for the right ventricle. Therefore, left heart failure, if it persists long enough, will lead to right heart failure. Likewise, systemic venous congestion increases the work load of the left ventricle by obstructing the flow of blood through, first, the capillary circulation and, beyond that, the systemic arterial circulation. Thus, right heart failure, if it persists long enough, will lead to left heart failure.

The term "backward heart failure" refers to the inability of a diseased or overburdened ventricle to empty with each contraction, resulting in the accumulation of excess fluid and elevation of pressure in the damaged chamber and in that portion of the circulation immediately preceding it. Thus, dysfunction and symptomatology are referred backward through the blood circuit. The term "forward heart failure" signifies that as the heart becomes unable to pump effectively it fails to deliver adequate amounts of blood to peripheral tissues, and symptoms of cerebral, renal, hepatic, muscular, or other dysfunction develop.

There are many possible causes for cardiac failure. Intracardiac causes include congenital cardiac defects, such as pulmonary valve stenosis or interventricular septal defect, inflammatory valvular distortion due to rheumatic fever, reduction of myocardial blood supply due to coronary arteriosclerosis, and myocarditis secondary to severe thiamine deficiency. Extracardiac causes include the prolonged increase in peripheral resistance that occurs in hypertension; the widening of the ascending aorta and aortic valvular insufficiency caused by luetic aortitis; extreme anemia, which causes an increase in stroke volume and heart rate; the increase in pulmonary arterial pressure caused by pulmonary embolism; and hypersecretion of thyroxine, which causes an increase in cardiac output.

The increased circulatory demands imposed by infection or pregnancy and the impairment of pumping efficiency by cardiac arrhythmias may cause a stressed but previously compensated heart to fail, either suddenly or gradually.

The mechanism of chronic cardiac failure is generally the same regardless of the specific cause of dysfunction. The usual chain of events is as follows: When pericardial, myocardial, or endocardial disease decreases the pumping efficiency of the heart or increased tissue needs for oxygen and nutrients demand increased cardiac output, the heart first compensates by hypertrophy and elongation of myocardial fibers. Myocardial hypertrophy, or an increase in the diameter of the individual cardiac muscle fibers, enables each cardiac muscle cell to contact more strongly. Elongation of the myocardial fibers also effects more forceful contraction because a slightly stretched myocardial fiber contracts more strongly than one of normal length (Starling's Law). Tachycardia is another compensatory mechanism by which the heart under stress temporarily increases cardiac output (cardiac output = stroke volume × cardiac rate). Unfortunately, all three compensatory mechanisms—myocardial hypertrophy, myocardial dilatation, and tachycardia—have only limited effectiveness in increasing circulatory efficiency in the face of persistent or increasing cardiac stress. If the underlying cause of cardiac inefficiency or increased circulatory demand is not removed, the cardiac reserve, or the ability of the heart to compensate for an increased work load, will eventually be exceeded and the heart will fail. At this point the previously thickened or hypertrophied heart wall will become thin and lax, the cardiac chambers will dilate and fail to empty with each contraction, pressure will increase in the cardiac chambers and be referred backward in the blood circuit, and symptoms of pulmonary and/or systemic venous congestion will ensue.

The symptoms of heart failure derive from both the forward and backward aspects of failure. When the left ventricle fails, cardiac output is reduced to a point at which certain vital tissues receive insufficient oxygen and nutrients to support normal metabolic needs. Compensatory redistribution of blood flow through sympathetic vasoconstriction results in maintenance of a near-normal blood supply to the brain and myocardium at the cost of a marked reduction in the volume of blood flow to the kidneys, digestive organs, and skeletal muscles. Decreased blood flow to skeletal muscles produces weakness and fatigue. Decreased blood flow to the digestive organs leads to indigestion and anorexia. Decreased renal blood flow produces decreased glomerular filtration pressure. In heart failure there is also increased secretion of aldosterone by the adrenal cortex. This combination of reduced glomerular filtration, together with the effect of aldosterone in increasing tubular resorption of sodium, leads to excessive accumulation of extracellular fluid in the body.

At the same time that the inadequate cardiac output of forward failure leads to decreased glomerular filtration and increased intravascular fluid volume, backward failure, or the inability of the heart to readily accept returning venous blood, gives rise to symptoms of venous congestion. In predominantly left ventricular failure, pressure is increased in pulmonary veins and capillaries. Fluid escapes from engorged, distended pulmonary capillaries into pulmonary interstitial spaces and into the alveoli themselves. Interstitial pulmonary edema interferes with lung expansion on inspiration. The presence of transudate in alveoli reduces the available cross-sectional area for oxygen–carbon dioxide exchange. Consequently, the patient experiences dyspnea or breathlessness, and may demonstrate cyanosis as a result of increased concentration of reduced hemoglobin, tachypnea as a reflex response to hypercapnia, and cough as a reflex response to the presence of fluid in the alveoli.

In mild heart failure, dyspnea is often observed only on exertion. As failure persists and increases in degree, dyspnea develops with progressively less activity. In severe failure the patient will be dyspneic even at complete rest. Orthopnea, or dyspnea in the recumbent position, is also seen in more severe cardiac failure. Orthopnea results from redistribution of edema fluid from dependent portions of the body to the lungs when the patient changes from vertical to horizontal position.

Paroxysmal nocturnal dyspnea, or attacks of severe shortness of breath, may wake the heart failure patient from sleep. Typically, the patient wakes with a start, experiencing cough, wheezing, and a feeling of suffocation. He must then sit or stand for several minutes, often before an open window, to catch his breath before being able to fall asleep again. Occasionally such an attack will lead to an episode of acute pulmonary edema.

If congestive failure becomes very severe the patient may develop Cheyne-Stokes or cyclical respirations, in which periods of rapid, deep breathing alternate with periods of apnea lasting as long as a minute. Cheyne-Stokes respirations are the result of insensitivity of the respiratory center due to reduced blood supply to the brain.

The cough associated with left ventricular failure is usually productive of thin and watery or frothy, blood-tinged sputum.

Occasionally in congestive failure, pleural effusion develops as a result of transudation of fluid into the pleural space from engorged and dilated pleural capillaries. Effusion is more apt to occur in the right pleural cavity than the left and, if severe, will further increase respiratory difficulty.

The passage of air through transudate in the alveoli gives rise to moist inspiratory rales, which are most marked over the dependent portions of the lung. The presence of large amounts of transudate in the alveoli and interstitial spaces will also produce dullness on percussion. Again, gravitational effects on fluid distribution will make dullness to percussion most marked over the dependent portions of the lung.

In predominantly right ventricular failure congestion is most marked in the systemic venous circulation. Increased pressure in hepatic sinusoids leads to an enlarged and tender liver. Engorgement of peritoneal capillaries allows transudate to accumulate in the peritoneal cavity (ascites). Escape of fluid from capillaries in the lower extremities leads to pitting edema of the feet and legs of the upright patient.

The third heart sound, a brief, low-pitched sound occurring slightly after the second heart sound, is frequently heard in congestive heart failure. The third heart sound is produced when the rapid inflow of blood during diastole causes overdistention of a diseased ventricle (the wall of which has decreased compliance). The resulting triple rhythm, because it sounds like the canter of a horse, is called gallop rhythm. In left ventricular failure the third sound is most audible over the apex of the heart. In right ventricular failure it is best heard over the left lower sternal border. The pathologic third heart sound can be differentiated from the physiologic third heart sound, which is heard in many children and young adults, by the fact that the physiologic third sound usually disappears following a change to the upright position and the pathologic third sound does not.

Sometimes in congestive heart failure a fourth heart sound can be heard. The fourth heart sound is also brief and low-pitched, and occurs following the third heart sound or shortly before the first heart sound. The fourth heart sound results when the atrium contracts, forcing blood into a ventricle with decreased compliance. It is best heard between the apex and left lower sternal border.

In congestive heart failure the pulse is typically rapid and weak. Pulsus alternans, or a regular pulse with alternating strong and weak beats, is characteristic of left ventricular failure. If the patient has a cardiac arrhythmia, his pulse may be irregular. It may be regularly irregular in atrial flutter with associated heart block. It will be irregularly irregular with atrial fibrillation, premature atrial contractions, and premature ventricular contractions. With complete heart block the pulse rate will usually be less than 40 beats per minute. Distention of the neck veins in the sitting position, a large tender liver, and a positive hepatojugular reflux are characteristic of right ventricular failure.

The heart dilates in failure. Therefore, the point of maximum impulse is displaced to the left of the midclavicular line and below the fifth intercostal space. With dilation of the right ventricle as well, percussion may reveal cardiac dullness to the right of the right lower sternal border.

Chest x-ray is useful in diagnosing congestive heart failure. For this purpose, both a posteroanterior and a lateral view of the chest are required. Chest x-rays will reveal not only overall cardiac enlargement, but disproportionate increase in the size of one chamber. This information may be useful in identifying or confirming the underlying cause of heart failure. For instance, a greatly enlarged left ventricle is a typical finding when heart failure is the result of severe hypertension or luetic aortitis and aortic valve insufficiency. A greatly enlarged right ventricle is characteristic of heart failure due to rheumatic mitral stenosis or to chronic obstructive pulmonary disease. In heart failure the chest x-ray will also reveal dilation of the pulmonary vessels, with the result that the hilar areas of the lung show increased opacity. If pulmonary edema exists, a mottled density will extend outward through the lungs from the hilar region. If pleural effusion is present there will be obliteration of the normally sharp costophrenic angle.

Treatment for congestive heart failure should be directed toward removing the factor that precipitated heart failure, relieving the underlying cause of heart failure when possible, reducing cardiac work load, improving myocardial contractility, eliminating excess fluid retention, and preventing complications.

As has been indicated earlier, there are several acute stresses which when imposed on a previously overburdened but compensated heart can precipitate congestive failure. Thus, pneumonia, acute bacterial endocarditis, pulmonary embolism, thyrotoxicosis, acute blood loss, pregnancy, cardiac arrhythmia, myocardial infarction, and extreme emotional stress may all precipitate failure in a diseased heart. A carefully detailed medical history and a complete physical examination will frequently reveal in the heart failure patient findings other than the classical signs and symptoms of failure. Such findings, together with specific laboratory tests, will often identify the precipitating cause of failure. Thus, an elevated temperature, together with a history of chills, chest pain, and productive cough, and x-ray evidence of either a lobar or bronchial pattern of pulmonary consolidation indicates pneumonia. Fever, chills, petechiae, positive blood culture, and a changing heart murmur add up to bacterial endocarditis. Sudden dyspnea, oppressive chest pain, hemoptysis, syncope, and abnormal radiolucency of peripheral lung areas suggest pulmonary embolism. Nervousness, fine tremor, heat intolerance, palpitations, weight loss, and exophthalmos are characteristic of hyperthyroidism. Crushing substernal pain, severe weakness, dyspnea, dizziness, and syncope are suggestive of myocardial infarction. A patient whose congestive heart failure seems to have been precipitated by one of the foregoing conditions should be referred immediately to a physician for treatment of that condition.

In contrast with the precipitating cause of failure, which is often an acute or episodic process, the underlying cause of heart failure is often a chronic condition, which treatment cannot remove but may be able to alleviate. For instance, elevated blood pressure may be lowered, myocardial ischemia may be relieved by vasodilators or surgery, and rheumatic reactivation can be prevented with prophylactic antibiotics. Many patients with chronic arteriosclerotic heart disease in congestive failure who will be treated by the nurse practitioner will require drug treatment for chronic hypertension. A discussion of antitensive drugs and dosage regimens was given in Chapter 7.

Reduction of the cardiac work load is accomplished chiefly by mental and physical rest. The patient may require complete bedrest for a short time at the outset of treatment but can and should be allowed out of bed for increasing periods of time as he responds to treatment. The patient in mild failure can usually be adequately managed by decreasing his motor activity, getting more hours of rest each night, and taking naps two or three times during the day. Reduction of motor activity may require that the patient take a leave of absence from work, work fewer hours each day, reorganize household tasks so they can be performed while sitting rather than standing, or employ someone to take over certain housework, yard work, or other responsibilities.

Since the patient must achieve a certain degree of emotional equanimity in order to achieve adequate physical rest, some means must be found to relieve the anxiety which inevitably accompanies knowledge that one's heart is not functioning properly. Knowledge of cardiac weakness produces strong fears of disability, powerlessness, and death. The practitioner can help to dissipate such fears through non-directive counseling, in which she encourages the patient to express his worries openly, to test the validity of his concerns, and to explore means of minimizing certain outcomes of illness.

Cardiac work load can be reduced by eating several small meals rather than three large meals each day. The patient's long-term treatment plan for the obese patient should include a decrease in caloric intake, since reduction of body weight will also reduce cardiac work load. Constipation should be avoided by providing ample dietary roughage or by administering mild laxatives, since straining at stool both increases cardiac work load and interferes with venous return flow to the heart by increasing intrathoracic pressure.

In chronic heart failure myocardial contractility can be improved by the administration of some form of digitalis. The effect of digitalis is to increase the force and to decrease the rate of myocardial contraction, decrease the speed of impulse transmission through the myocardium, and increase the excitability of the myocardium. As a result of the first two of these actions, digitalis can be used to treat congestive heart failure resulting from several causes, such as hypertension, valvular damage, and arteriosclerosis. Because of its effects on impulse transmission and myocardial excitability, digitalis is contraindicated in patients with ventricular tachycardia and myocardial infarction (in whom the heart muscle is already hyperirritable).

Powdered digitalis leaf has been largely replaced by the purified glycosides digoxin and digitoxin in the treatment of heart failure. Because digitalis preparations have a cumulative effect, i.e. they are excreted more slowly than they are absorbed, a large initial, or digitalizing, dose is given to achieve the desired therapeutic effect and then a smaller maintenance dose is sufficient to perpetuate the therapeutic effect achieved. The average digitalizing dose of digoxin is 4.5 mg., which is usually given as an initial dose of 1.5 mg. followed by 0.75 mg. q. 6 h. for four doses, by which time cardiac contraction will usually be considerably slower and stronger. The patient is then continued on a maintenance dose of digoxin of about 0.5 mg. per day. The average digitalizing dose of digitoxin is 2 mg. given as an initial dose of 0.6 mg., followed in six hours by another 0.6 mg., then 0.2 mg. q. 6 h. for four doses. The average maintenance dose of digitoxin is 0.15 mg. per day. Toxic effects of digitalis include anorexia, nausea, vomiting, atrioventricular block, and premature ventricular contractions. These effects are especially apt to develop in patients receiving thiazides, furosemide, and ethacrynic acid, since the hypokalemia produced by these drugs fosters digitalis toxicity.

If symptoms of digitalis intoxication develop, the drug should be immediately discontinued and the patient referred to a physician for treatment. In cases of mild toxicity the physician will usually order that digitalis be withheld for several days, then administration of the drug resumed with a low maintenance dosage. If serious arrhythmias have developed, potassium, diphenylhydantoin, procainamide, propranolol, quinidine, or lidocaine may be required to restore normal rhythm.

Excess fluid accumulation is best prevented by a low sodium diet and by administration of diuretics. When reduction of physical activity, reduction of sodium intake, and administration of digitalis will relieve symptoms of failure, diuretics should be avoided because their use produces many undesirable side effects. However, if sodium and activity regulation and digitalis dosage do not control failure, diuretics will be necessary.

To ensure low sodium intake, the patient should be advised to avoid salted foods and to refrain from adding salt to foods either during cooking or at table. If elimination of salt makes meals unpalatable, the patient may season his food with lemon, vinegar, or a salt substitute to enhance its flavor. Unfortunately, many patients find that the salt substitutes produce a metallic aftertaste.

The diuretics most often used to relieve the edema of congestive heart failure are hydrochlorothiazide (Hydrodiuril), furosemide (Lasix), ethacrynic acid (Edacrin), and spironolactone (Aldactone).

The thiazides act on the ascending limb of the loop of Henle and on the distal convoluted tubule to increase the excretion of sodium ions, chloride ions, potassium ions, and water. The usual dose of hydrochlorothiazide is 50 mg. q. A.M. The chief toxic effects of the thiazides are hypokalemia, hyperuricemia, hyperglycemia, and skin rash. Hypokalemia can be avoided by oral administration of potassium salts, but these are unpalatable and can be dangerous in patients with renal failure (hyperkalemia has an even more deleterious effect than hypokalemia on myocardial functioning).

Furosemide and ethacrynic acid both act on the ascending limb of the loop of Henle to decrease sodium absorption, and both are effective in the presence of electrolyte imbalance or renal failure. When either is given orally, diuretic action begins within 30 minutes and lasts for eight hours. The usual oral dose of furosemide is 50 mg. per day; the usual dose of ethacrynic acid is 100 mg. per day. Either drug can produce hyponatremia, hypokalemia, hypochloremic alkalosis, hyperuricemia, or hyperglycemia. In addition, ethacrynic acid can produce vertigo, tinnitus, and acute hearing loss.

Spironolactone antagonizes aldosterone, thereby increasing the excretion of sodium and the retention of potassium in the distal renal tubule. Spironolactone is rarely given alone but may be used with hydrochlorothiazide, furosemide, or ethacrynic acid to offset their tendency to produce hypokalemia. The usual dose of spironolactone is 25 mg. t.i.d. Because of its potassium-saving effect, spironolactone must never be given to a patient with renal failure.

Common complications of congestive heart failure are intravascular thrombosis of the deep veins of the leg, hypostatic pneumonia, and acute pulmonary edema. The first two of these problems are provoked by immobility, hence even the bedridden patient in congestive heart failure requires passive, then active, motion of his extremities and regular changes of position. There is no way to prevent acute pulmonary edema except by treating congestive heart failure itself and alleviating the patient's anxiety over his illness. The development of acute pulmonary edema constitutes a medical emergency for which the patient should be referred at once to a physician for vigorous treatment, which usually includes administration of morphine to relieve anxiety and decrease respiratory effort, administration of oxygen under positive pressure to improve oxygenation of the blood and to decrease transudation of fluid into the alveoli, administration of aminophylline intravenously to decrease bronchospasm, and administration of furosemide or ethacrynic acid intravenously to promote rapid diuresis.

Finally, proper management of the patient in chronic congestive failure requires that the patient be informed of both the underlying and precipitating causes of his heart failure; that he be helped to accept whatever modifications of activity and diet are necessary to his recovery; that he be instructed concerning foods to be avoided on a low sodium diet; and that he be taught the purpose, ordered dose, and toxic effects of all prescribed medications. Since the patient will require support from his family in order to make the changes in life style that are required by his illness and treatment, members of his family should be included in the teaching sessions in which the foregoing content is presented and discussed.

BIBLIOGRAPHY: MANAGEMENT OF THE PATIENT IN CHRONIC CONGESTIVE HEART FAILURE

Beeson, Paul, and McDermott, Walsh, Eds.: *Cecil–Loeb Textbook of Medicine*, 14th ed. Philadelphia, W. B. Saunders, 1975.
Chunk, E. K.: Controlling cardiovascular problems, prescribing digitalis, procedures and pitfalls. *Geriatrics*, 28:79–83, March, 1973.
Conn, Howard, Ed.: *Current Therapy 1975*. Philadelphia, W. B. Saunders Co., 1975.
Edwards, Jesse: *An Atlas of Acquired Diseases of the Heart and Great Vessels*. Philadelphia, W. B. Saunders, 1961, Vol. II.
Eisendorfer, Carl, and Lawton, M. Powell, Eds.: *The Psychology of Adult Development and Aging*. Washington, D. C., American Psychological Association, 1973.
Friedberg, Charles: *Diseases of the Heart*. 3rd ed., Philadelphia, W. B. Saunders Co., 1966.
Gazes, Peter: Treatment of heart failure. *Postgrad. Med.* 51:209–323, 1972.
Harris, Alfred: Management of patients with chronic congestive heart failure. *Modern Treatment* 2:247–269, 1965.
Hay, D. R.: Treatment of heart failure. *Drugs*, 5:318–331, 1973.
Kirsten, E., et al.: Digoxin in the aged. *Geriatrics*, 28:95–101, 1973.
Lewis, Edith, Ed.: *Nursing in Cardiovascular Diseases*. New York, American Journal of Nursing Company, 1971.
Meyers, Sheridan, and Brandfonbrener, M.: Treatment of edema of heart failure. *Modern Treatment* 9:61–76, 1972.
Phibbs, Brendan, et al.: *The Human Heart, A Guide to Heart Disease*. 2nd ed., St. Louis, C. V. Mosby Co., 1971.
Wedgwood, J.: Heart failure in old age. *Postgrad. Med.*, 52:179–183, 1972.

11
MANAGEMENT OF THE PATIENT WITH OBESITY

Obesity is the excessive accumulation of fat in the body with the result that body weight exceeds that desirable for the individual's height, age, and bone structure. Excessive fat accumulation results from eating more food than that required to meet the body's energy needs. Most cases of obesity are the result of the patient's eating more calories (energy input) than are used in his daily activities (energy output).

An individual who weighs as much as 15 per cent more than his ideal body weight is considered obese. Obesity is a serious public health problem, as evidenced by the fact that by the foregoing definition more than one half of the people in this nation are obese.

ETIOLOGY OF OBESITY

In most individuals obesity probably results from both physiological and psychological causes. A hereditary tendency toward obesity may be due to such factors as defective enzyme production with consequent increased fat synthesis, abnormal functioning of the hunger and satiety centers in the hypothalamus, resulting in overeating, or decreased inclination to exercise with consequent low caloric (energy) expenditure.

In addition to overeating, overdrinking, and under-exercising, which are exogenous causes, obesity may also be caused by intrinsic factors such as constitutional tendency, hypothalamic involvement, cranial trauma, hypothyroidism, adrenal cortical overactivity, hyperpituitarism, or gonadal deficiency. Even so, scientific studies have not identified many subjects with "nonalimentary" obesity. Research has shown that when parents are obese there is increased likelihood that their children will also be obese. Such obesity could be the result of both genetic and social factors.

Social and psychological factors contribute both to development and to maintenance of obesity. Exposure to cultural influences that encourage the overeating of carbohydrate often leads to obesity. In some cultures, individuals are encouraged to eat when not hungry, in order to be polite. In many cultures there is pressure to overeat brought about by exposure to television food commercials and by constant contact with food while preparing family meals. In some groups there is pressure to clean up leftover food in order to be thrifty. In others, women are encouraged to overeat because plumpness is valued as an aspect of feminine beauty. In some cultures, women are expected to gain weight after pregnancy, because a buxom appearance is associated with the maternal role.

In any culture many women fail to lose, following delivery, all the weight that was gained during the pregnancy, so they gradually increase in weight from one pregnancy to the next. A baby who is fed excessively during the first year of life will have a permanent increase in the number of adipose cells in his body, and will retain this tendency toward obesity throughout life.

Some psychological factors that contribute to overeating and corpulence are boredom, insecurity, depression, and anxiety. The individual who eats when he is not hungry in order to fulfill his need for affection ingests excess carbohydrate, which is then stored in the body as fat. These people overeat to solve or camouflage problems, or they find certain advantages in obesity. For instance, to some, a large body gives the feeling of power and strength. To some, obesity is equated with good health and affluence. Because excessive fat is ugly and unattractive, the obese person is a less effective competitor in jobs, sports, sex, and love, and thus has a ready excuse for failure in any of these endeavors. Finally, obesity is sometimes a passive-aggressive maneuver to retaliate against one's parents or oneself for past disappointments.

The obese individual is frequently reproached for his adiposity by relatives and friends. Many people perceive the obese person as ugly, greedy, and lacking in will power or self-control. In reality, obesity is a state of equilibrium in which the individual has effected some sort of compromise between his needs and need-gratification.

In summary, food intake > energy expenditure $\Rightarrow$ obesity.

There are many physiological and psychological factors which bring about excess food intake and decreased ability or desire to exercise.

DETERMINATION OF THE DEGREE OF OBESITY

Measurement of body weight alone is an inaccurate way to determine the amount of excess body fat. Estimation of total body water, specific gravity of the totally immersed body, total exchangeable potassium (K^{40}), and skin-fold thickness have all been used to determine body composition or the amount of total body fat. Measurement of skin-fold thickness and of the circumference of the arms, legs, and waist is easily accomplished and can provide baseline data with which to estimate the amount of an individual's obesity or muscle hypertrophy. (Overweight may also be due to muscle hypertrophy or fluid retention rather than to excess fat accumulation.)

Measurement of skin-fold thickness at the mid-triceps area, below the scapula, on the abdomen, and at the mid-thigh point is accomplished by grasping the skin between the thumb and index finger and measuring the thickness with a caliper. The caliper should be placed about one centimeter from the finger and thumb. Normal skin-fold thickness is approximately one inch (2.54 centimeters). Determination of the mid-triceps skin-fold thickness is the single best measure of the degree of obesity.

Weight gain up to a 10 per cent increase over ideal body weight can usually be masked by the clothing normally worn indoors. In fact, the only early sign of a trend toward obesity may be an expanding waist line. Thus, regular measurement of waist circumference will provide useful data for monitoring the patient's weight gain or loss over a period of time.

HAZARDS OF OBESITY

Devouring more food than is required to maintain the body's need for energy results in metabolic changes that can be extremely detrimental to health. Included in the complications of obesity are the following.

1. Coronary artery disease, which results from increased intake of simple sugars leading to hyperlipemia.
2. Hypertension, which results from decreased renal blood flow, increased plasma levels of ADH, and arterial changes.
3. Dyspnea, which results from the increased work required for the lung to expand against a fat thorax and the interference with diaphragmatic contraction produced by a fat abdomen. These same problems increase the anesthetic risk and the tendency to pneumonia in the obese patient.
4. Liver disease, in those patients in whom obesity is in part due to excess alcohol intake.
5. Diabetes, which results from altered carbohydrate metabolism.
6. Joint strain, pain, and arthritis, due to increased weight bearing.
7. Increased surgical risk, with consequent greater postoperative mortality.
8. Decreased ability to exercise, which gives rise to the hazards of immobility.
9. Decreased ability to defend or protect oneself.
10. Decreased self-esteem and decreased positive interaction with people.
11. Decreased ability to reproduce, because obesity is often associated with amenorrhea.
12. Shortened life span, since the mortality rate is increased nearly 50 per cent in extremely obese individuals.

METABOLIC CHANGES IN OBESITY

Since the basal metabolic rate for obese individuals is the same as for normal-weight individuals, other metabolic changes must account for the development and maintenance of obesity. In fact, obese people require fewer calories to maintain a constant weight than do normal individuals because obesity leads to less activity and less energy output. It is, therefore, highly likely that obese people do actually eat fewer calories than do normal persons of comparable age and body build and yet remain overweight.

The thermic response to eating is enhanced by even mild exercise after meals. The obese person who fails to engage in walking or other mild activity after eating does not enhance his thermic response to eating. Specific dynamic action of food (thermic response) is probably decreased in obese people; that is, the rate of oxygen consumption does not increase as much postprandially in obese people as it does in thin people.

In obesity, a layer of subcutaneous fat with few blood vessels is deposited between the obese body and its environment. This adipose layer provides insulation against the cold but prevents the normal increase in metabolic rate or increase in lipolysis following cold exposure.

MANAGEMENT OF OBESITY

Obesity is an easily diagnosed syndrome, the treatment of which aims at upsetting the equilibrium sought by ingesting food in excess of the body's need for energy. The cause for and the risk of obesity will vary from person to person, so treatment must be individually outlined after baseline assessments are made.

Assessments should be made in regard to the duration of the obesity, the reason for wanting to lose weight; the amount of motivation for dieting, eating preferences and habits, the frequency and type of exercise, a family history of obesity, and the contribution of psychological factors to the development of the obesity.

Obesity developed by age 12 and maintained into adulthood is called juvenile-onset obesity and has several unique features which adult onset obesity (onset after 20 years of age) does not have. Obese adults with juvenile onset of obesity have increased numbers of adipose cells (hyperplasia), while individuals with adult onset obesity have increased fat in their adipose cells (hypertrophy) but no increase in cell number. Individuals with juvenile onset obesity show a disturbance in body image, a distortion of time perception, and some affective changes (depression, anxiety, fatigue). All individuals with adult onset obesity do not manifest these same disturbances. The importance of knowing the onset and duration of the obesity is obvious. It is usually difficult for the person with juvenile onset obesity to remain on a diet because dieting frequently makes him irritable, nervous, and more depressed.

Obese people who keep their weight constant over time are said to have passive obesity. Those individuals in active-state obesity are continually gaining weight. The distinction between active and passive obesity is important because passive obese individuals usually eat less than normal-weight individuals and do not lose weight. Thus, they are prone to becoming discouraged or depressed by their obesity and difficulty in weight reduction.

Knowledge of the client's reason for wanting to lose weight helps the practitioner to estimate the strength of his motivation to lose weight. Generally, persons who believe that they must either lose weight or lose their life or health tend to remain on their diets. Psychologically healthy persons with intrinsic reasons for dieting tend to successfully lose weight. However, if the advantages of obesity are great, the obese person may lack sufficient motivation for weight reduction. Previous failures to reduce may make obese people reluctant to resume dieting and risk another failure.

Assessment of the contribution of psychological factors to the obese state is essential, because persons who eat to compensate for their feelings of inferiority or insecurity tend not to be successful in weight reduction. If the obese person states that he is not now happy and never has been truly happy, or if he is coping poorly with his current problems, referral for psychological counseling or group psychotherapy will be a helpful adjunct to treatment for obesity. The practitioner should remember that the obese state is an attempt at adjustment, and that dieting upsets the patient's existing physiological and psychological homeostasis.

Assessment of the patient's family history for obesity and eating habits of relatives is useful because there is great likelihood that the children of obese parents will also be obese. If the family's eating pattern consists of two or three large meals a day, between-meal snacking, and pre-bedtime eating, it is likely that obesity exists or will develop. The amount of family members' alcohol intake, preference for sweet foods, foods eaten for snacks, and indulgence in eating when worried or bored should be specifically assessed. It is useful to determine when groceries are brought and which family member usually does the shopping.

In addition to determining the family's eating patterns, the type and level of activity of family members should be evaluated. The following questions will help the practitioner assess the patient's and his family's exercise and activity level: Where do individual members work? What type of work do they routinely engage in? How does each individual travel to work and/or to shopping? How much walking is done each day? How many stairs are climbed each day? How and where is leisure time spent? Does each family member have a hobby or engage in activities outside the home?

In addition to the assessment described above, the practitioner should perform a complete physical examination of the obese person, although this is often very difficult because large amounts of subcutaneous fat interfere with palpation of internal organs and with thoracic and abdominal auscultation and percussion. The practitioner should determine the patient's weight, height, blood pressure, and skin-fold thickness, and the circumference of the waist, upper arm, thigh, and calf, and should estimate the size of the bony skeleton (large, medium, or small). All baseline data, together with the patient's ideal body weight, should be noted on the patient's record to be used as a measure of his progress in weight reduction.

Laboratory tests should be used to identify any pathophysiological functioning in the several body systems. The following tests are especially helpful: glucose tolerance, concentration of protein bound iodine, complete blood count, plasma cholesterol, and triglyceride concentration.

The practitioner's treatment of the obese patient should include satisfaction of his needs for knowledge, insight, or referral. Patients who are emotionally stable but have little information about food values and engage in poor eating habits need knowledge. Patients who use food to allay fears, insecurity, and anxiety need insight. Patients who use obesity as the best or only available way of coping with their emotional problems need referral for psychological counseling.

The practitioner's treatment plan for disrupting the obesity cycle should include:

1. Developing a positive, nonpunitive *attitude* toward the obese patient.
2. Selecting the type and style of *diet* best suited to the individual patient's needs and life style.
3. Outlining a program of *exercise* appropriate to the obese person's ability and interest.
4. Recommending *drugs* only when they are a necessary adjunct to treatment.

The practitioner's attitude toward and expectations of the obese individual should be consciously examined. A judgmental attitude by a thin practitioner toward an obese patient is not a helpful basis upon which to begin treatment. A more helpful attitude is recognition that the obese person is as frustrated by his obesity as the practitioner is, and, indeed, is perhaps repelled by it. Understanding of when, how, and why the patient's obesity developed, and why it was maintained, will enable the practitioner to acquire realistic expectations of the patient's ability to lose weight. The practitioner should help the patient to achieve realistic expectations of the ways in which a loss of weight would benefit him. It can be dangerous to place undue emphasis on the external or social rewards of dieting, because the obese person may then develop the unrealistic expectations that all of his problems will disappear when he becomes thin. When he finds that this is not true, disappointment develops and his frustration may lead to overeating. The practitioner should be aware of both her own attitude toward obesity and unsuccessful dieting and the patient's family members' attitude toward the obese person and his failure to lose weight, if she is to understand the social pressure which will influence his response to treatment.

A no sugar, low carbohydrate, low fat, high protein diet is commonly advised for the obese patient. The Prudent Diet,* which is used by the New York Anti-Coronary Club for weight reduction and lowering serum cholesterol levels, is also popular to insure health. The diet should meet the individual's daily nutritional needs and be low in calories (about 1200 for women, and 1600 for men). Frequently patients can be successful dieters when given general instructions about the food categories that are freely allowed (vegetables, lean meat, fish, poultry) or to be avoided (alcohol, sugar), but some obese individuals require a detailed, specific diet outlining what to eat at each meal. Some prefer counting total calories, while others count carbohydrate intake.

If there is a familial tendency toward obesity, young patients should be instructed to curtail excessive food intake, to eat several (3 to 5) smaller meals a day, to engage in light exercise for 30 to 60 minutes after eating, and to avoid a large, late evening meal. All these have been shown to aid the body in its metabolism of sugar and fat so that food is efficiently used and not stored as adipose tissue. A gradual weight loss of about two pounds per week is recommended. The patient should be instructed to weigh daily at the same time on the same scale while wearing the same amount of clothing.

Before placing an obese patient on a rigid weight reduction regime, the

---

* From Jolliffe, N.: Reduce and Stay Reduced on the Prudent Diet. Simon and Shuster, 1964.

practitioner should assess the likelihood that he will maintain a lower body weight after weight reduction, since it is probable that it is during periods of marked weight change (both decrease and increase) that subintimal cholesterol deposition will be greatest. In other words, the patient who alternates between bouts of overeating and crash dieting may experience more rapid and severe arterial damage than the patient who, once obese, maintains himself at constant food intake and weight for many years.

Since decreasing the food intake removes oral gratification which may be required by the obese person for anxiety reduction, other types of need fulfillment could be discussed. At times, dieting becomes monotonous, so various changes in the dietary pattern, such as occasionally introducing liquid diet preparations, might be helpful to maintain motivation. Dieting and "watching one's weight" are not momentary gestures; careful evaluation of what one eats must continue for years.

After dieting has been tried and evaluated, the practitioner may suggest the use of drugs to enhance weight loss and supplement vitamin and mineral intake. Diuretics, appetite suppressants, hormones (especially thyroid), and mood elevators have been successfully employed in treating some obese patients but, if used at all, should be used with caution. Diuretics are seldom used in long-term treatment of obesity because they have many undesirable side effects, and the anorectic sympathomimetic amines frequently are only effective for two to three months of therapy.

Exercise is an essential part of weight reduction because most obese persons tend to underexercise. The movement pattern of most obese persons is typically slower than that of persons of normal weight. The prescribed exercise level should be adjusted to the patient's physiological and psychological ability and should be planned to be a part of his regular daily routine. Exercise for one hour after meals is thought to enhance the metabolism of food into heat rather than fat. Walking three or more miles each day, or using an exercise bicycle for 45 minutes each day will usually result in a weight loss of about three pounds a month.

A final consideration in the management of obesity is the use of behavior modification techniques to help the patient lose weight. These techniques can be extremely helpful in facilitating the patient's effort to lose weight. Many obese persons do not return to the practitioner for additional help in weight reduction because they are ashamed of their lack of weight reduction and fear that they will be chastised for their failure.

The patient's weight loss and adjustment to dieting should be evaluated at least every two weeks during the initial phases of management. Later, monthly consultations may be sufficient until the weight reduction curve levels off and weight becomes constant. At this point, patient and practitioner should together re-evaluate the patient's motivation and further need for weight loss.

BIBLIOGRAPHY: MANAGEMENT OF THE PATIENT
WITH OBESITY

Alstead, Stanley, MacGregor, Alastair, and Girdwood, Ronald, Eds.: *Textbook of Medical Treatment.* 12th ed. Edinburgh, Churchill, Livingstone, 1971.
Beeson, Paul, and McDermott, Walsh, Eds.: *Cecil–Loeb Textbook of Medicine* 14th ed. Philadelphia, W. B. Saunders Co., 1975.

Conn, Howard, Ed.: *Current Therapy 1975.* Philadelphia, W. B. Saunders Co., 1975.
Cormier, A.: Group versus individual dietary instruction in the treatment of obesity. *Canad. J. Pub. Health,* 63:327–332, July–August, 1972.
Court, J. M.: The management of obesity. *Drugs,* 4:411–418, 1972.
Craft, C. A.: Body image and obesity. *Nurs. Clin. N. Amer.* 7:677–685, 1972.
Crisp, A. H.: Psychological aspects of some disorders of weight. In Hill, O., Ed.: *Modern Trends in Psychosomatic Medicine 2.* London, Butterworth, 1970.
Gordon, T., et al.: The effects of overweight on cardiovascular diseases. *Geriatrics,* 28: 80–88, August, 1973.
Grinker, J.: Behavioral and metabolic consequences of weight reduction. *J. Amer. Dietet. Assoc.,* 62:30–34, January, 1973.
Kemp, R.: The over-all picture of obesity. *Practitioner,* 209:654–660, November, 1972.
Levitz, L. S.: Behavior therapy in treating obesity. *J. Amer. Dietet. Assoc.,* 62:22–26, January, 1973.
McCombs, Robert: *Fundamentals of Internal Medicine.* 4th ed. Chicago, Year Book Medical Publishers, 1971.
Reichsman, F., Ed.: *Hunger and Satiety in Health and Disease, Vol. 7 in Advances in Psychosomatic Medicine.* New York, S. Karger, 1972.
Shumway, S., et al.: The group way to weight loss. *Amer. J. Nurs.,* 73:269–276, 1973.
Stillman, Irwin, and Baker, Samm: *The Doctor's Quick Weight Loss Diet Cookbook.* New York, David McKay Co., 1972.
Wintrobe, Maxwell, et al., Eds.: *Harrison's Principles of Internal Medicine.* 6th ed. New York, McGraw-Hill Book Co., 1970.

12
MANAGEMENT OF THE PATIENT WITH ALCOHOLISM

Ethyl alcohol is a drug that has the ability to depress selected functions of the central system. It is for this reason that most individuals drink alcohol. Large doses of alcohol can be consumed over a prolonged period of time without producing a significant degree of disease, because the human organism can build up both metabolic and tissue tolerances to alcohol. However, if alcoholic consumption is great enough or long enough, serious impairment of the drinker's physiological and psychosocial functioning will result. Excessive alcohol intake causes physical impairment, decreased productivity, disturbed interpersonal relationships, and impairment of personal growth (self actualization).

Alcohol dependence is a chronic disease for which there is no simple cure. As in any chronic disease, the patient needs prolonged treatment, cannot recover alone, and tends to experience periods of remission (abstinence) and exacerbation (bouts of excessive or prolonged drinking). Since alcoholic dependence is a disease, the chief responsibility for managing the alcoholic patient should lie with the health professions rather than with the police or clergy. Alcoholism can be viewed in much the same terms as another chronic disease, diabetes mellitus. That is, in both diseases there are different degrees of severity of illness, various stages in disease process, different ages of onset, and different treatment approaches.

The social impact of alcoholism is profound. It is estimated that nine million United States residents are alcoholics, that one half of all automobile fatalities involve a drinking driver, that one third of all delinquent youth come from families in which there is excessive alcohol consumption, that one third of all family problems are related to excessive drinking, and that the monetary cost of alcoholic dependence to industry is considerable and is rising steadily.

PSYCHOLOGICAL ASPECTS

Alcohol dependence has on different occasions been labeled a psychological disease, a crime, a sin, and a physiological disease, but no one etiology or alcoholic personality has been delineated. In the alcoholic patient, the practitioner can usually identify a general pattern of events that parallel development of alcohol dependence. These events begin with oral craving or thwarted dependency needs. The frustration resulting from the thwarted dependency needs then leads first to anger and then to depression. As dependence on alcohol and feelings of guilt increase, the individual tends to deny the magnitude and consequences of his drinking.

No one drinks without a reason. Ethyl alcohol is a mind altering drug which is consumed for that very effect. In the prealcoholic, alcohol intake rapidly (alcohol can be detected in the blood 5 minutes after ingestion) results in a degree of relief from the tension or loneliness which prompted the drinking. After years of drinking, psychological changes occur within the alcohol dependent individual. He alibis for his drinking, covers up the quantity of his drinking, hides his drinking from others, defends his drinking, and finally spends most of his time thinking about drinking. The alcoholic patient has a low frustration tolerance and low self-esteem, and is fearful.

The stigma associated with alcoholism is great and results in part from recognition that alcoholism is self-inflicted. Rejection of the out-of-control drinker may be initiated by the very same people who encouraged him to drink alcohol socially. The alcoholic tendency to neglect the normal details of daily life, such as grooming or social amenities, leads to further rejection and increased thwarting of dependency needs.

PHYSIOLOGICAL ASPECTS

The behavioral effects of alcohol are unpredictable and vary with the patient's social and emotional environment. However, the action of alcohol on the brain frequently results in impairment of judgment, removal of inhibitions, loss of self-control, impairment of sensorimotor function (inability to write, speech disturbance, unsteadiness of movement), lack of memory, and dulling of attentiveness. As the percentage of alcohol in the blood increases, double vision, distortion of perception, apathy, and even shock and death may result.

Chronic alcohol intoxication results in hypoglycemia and malnutrition secondary to failure to eat a proper diet while drinking. Although alcohol initially causes diuresis, overhydration is a frequent complication of alcohol intoxication, because as the blood alcohol concentration is stabilized or decreases, water is retained in the body. The water diuresis following alcohol consumption is associated with urinary excretion of Na, K, Cl ions, leading to extracellular hypertonicity. Additionally, the hematocrit decreases because alcohol intoxication inhibits erythropoiesis. Leukopenia may occur and render the alcoholic prone to infection. Anemia may result from iron deficiency as a result of the gastric bleeding that occurs in alcoholic gastritis. Pancreatitis and intestinal malabsorption may also occur in chronic alcoholism.

In addition to the fatty infiltration and necrosis of the liver parenchymal cells, which is usually seen following chronic alcohol ingestion, hepatic inflammation without necrosis may be observed in some patients. Hepatic inflammation can be diagnosed by serum determination of ICD (isocitric dehydrogenase). Alcohol ingestion also depletes hepatic glycogen and impairs gluconeogenesis.

Chronic alcoholism may cause skeletal muscle aching, tenderness, edema, or weakness, which is usually accompanied by elevation of serum CPK (creatinine phosphokinase). Chronic alcohol intoxication may also produce a general myocardiopathy characterized by myocardial lipid infiltration and decreased contractility. Tachycardia with extra systoles and prolongation of the S-T segment is typical of the condition. Owing to the cardiotoxic effects of alcohol, patients with cardiovascular disease should not drink alcohol.

MANAGEMENT OF ALCOHOL DEPENDENCE

Because alcohol dependence is a chronic disease, a carefully detailed history including a drinking history, a complete physical examination, and appropriate laboratory data are needed to confirm the diagnosis. The approach to treatment should be holistic and symptomatic.

The objective of the drinking history should be to determine the importance of alcohol to the patient. Factual information may be difficult to elicit, since the alcoholic patient attempts to conceal how much and how often he drinks. At times, the practitioner's own drinking pattern may influence the questions he asks the patient and the information that he records relative to the patient's drinking. What one practitioner considers "social drinking" another may consider excessive consumption of alcohol. It will be helpful to the practitioner in history taking to remember that alcohol is a tranquilizing (depressant) drug and is ingested for this effect.

In ascertaining the history of alcohol dependence, the practitioner should seek information about changes in work performance, family living, or ability to tolerate stress without undue anxiety or depression. Frequently, alertness to small changes in behavior patterns are cues to an excessive alcohol intake. Concrete answers to questions, such as the ones that follow, concerning the patient's drinking are of value.

When did he first begin drinking?
Who in his family drinks?
How much and how frequently does he drink?
Where does his drinking usually take place?
What type of alcohol is consumed?
Is tolerance to the drug developing?
Is any of his behavior inappropriate when drinking?
Can details of events while drinking be subsequently recalled?

The physical examination should focus on the pathophysiology usually found as a consequence of chronic alcohol ingestion. The physical signs that are typically found in an alcohol-dependent person who is neither intoxicated nor in acute withdrawal at the time of examination are as follows: facial telangiectasia, periorbital edema, premature arcus senilis, pale conjunctiva;

bronchitis, evidence of chronic obstructive pulmonary disease, hypertrophy of mammary tissue in males; tachycardia, premature systoles, hypertension without major funduscopic changes; hepatomegaly, epigastric tenderness, right upper quadrant tenderness; mild dependent edema; hyperactive tendon reflexes, and cerebellar ataxia.

Abnormal laboratory findings which are frequently associated with but are not necessarily diagnostic of alcohol abuse include anemia (normochromic-normocytic or hypochromic-microcytic), reticulocytopenia, leukopenia, thrombocytopenia, elevated serum ICD and serum GOT, elevated BSP retention, elevated serum cholesterol, elevated serum uric acid, and hypoglycemia.

If alcohol abuse is extensive and of long duration, physiological and psychological addiction results and a complex of symptoms occurs upon acute withdrawal of alcohol. These withdrawal symptoms include tremor, hallucinations, illusions, and delirium. The severity of the withdrawal symptoms is directly related to the amount and duration of alcohol ingestion. Withdrawal symptoms must be distinguished from the symptoms of acute alcohol intoxication, which include staggering gait, slurred speech, uninhibited behavior, stupor, and coma.

Treatment of *acute* withdrawal from alcohol should include:

1. Sedation—accomplished by administration of hydroxyzine (Vistaril), chlordiazepoxide hydrochloride (Librium), or diazepam (Valium).
2. Diuretics—furosemide (Lasix) may be given if overhydration exists, but intravenous fluids should be administered if the patient is dehydrated.
3. Glucose or fructose is administered intravenously to correct hypoglycemia.
4. Antibiotics are given if infections of the pulmonary and genitourinary system are evident.
5. Symptomatic treatment is initiated for associated trauma, anemia, gastritis, pancreatitis, and/or peripheral neuropathy.

About two weeks after the acute phase of alcohol withdrawal has passed, the alcohol-dependent individual can best be helped by a combination of chemotherapy and psychotherapy. Chemotherapy should include continued therapy for any remaining metabolic problems, infection, and fluid or electrolyte imbalance. In addition, antianxiety-antidepressant drugs such as imipramine (Tofranil), doxepin hydrochloride (Sinequan) or amitriptyline (Elavil) will help offset anxiety and depression. The practitioner should instruct the patient about the action of any drug given, and the reason for its administration should be explained. Vitamin and mineral supplements are usually indicated to correct long-standing dietary inadequacies. Disulfiram (Antabuse), which is a chemical deterrent to the consumption of alcohol, is effective in the treatment of some alcoholics because it interferes with the metabolism of alcohol and causes nausea, vomiting and hypotension, the symptoms of which are so unpleasant that the patient eschews alcohol in order to avoid them. Aversion treatment is accomplished by administering an emetic and then having the patient drink alcohol. The extreme nausea and vomiting that result will create a strong revulsion for alcohol in some patients.

Psychotherapy on either a group or individual basis may be neither feasible nor available for each alcohol-dependent person. Thus, the psychotherapy given most alcoholics should be that which the practitioner is prepared to give to any anxious, depressed patient. The therapeutic approach consists of 1) reducing the alcoholic's anxiety sufficiently that he can gain insight into his drug dependence and its consequences, 2) motivating the alcoholic and enabling him to put his knowledge into action, and 3) increasing the alcoholic's self confidence.

In helping the alcoholic to remain temperate once he has experienced withdrawal from the drug, it is essential to understand how the drug was used in everyday living, the meaning that alcohol had for the patient, the events that precipitated alcoholic ingestion, and the extent to which the patient underestimated his problem with alcohol or the impact of his drinking on his family, work, or community.

In general, the alcohol-dependent person needs to increase his tolerance for stress, irritation, frustration, anxiety, or sleeplessness. He can be helped to do this by outlining a typical day in detail, asking him, "At what time do you usually awaken?", "What do you think first?", "What do you do first after you get out of bed?", "What do you do next?", "Then what do you do?" This outlining procedure, if tactfully undertaken, will identify key moments when the temptation to drink is apt to be strongest. Once these key conflict moments are identified, new ways of managing or avoiding them should be discussed. The alcoholic needs help in dealing with conflict. The practitioner should determine what allayed his drinking in previous conflict moments and strengthen the technique that has worked for him in the past. It is important that the alcoholic learn how to relax. It is also important that he learn that putting something out of his mouth (talking) can be just as effective in dealing with frustration and anger as is putting something into his mouth (alcohol).

Fortunately, there are many supportive measures available to the alcohol-dependent person when he becomes able to recognize his need for help. The practitioner could suggest individual or group psychotherapy offered by a nurse, social worker, or physician, membership in Alcoholics Anonymous, diagnostic psychological testing, or guidance from a clergyman.

The patient's family can be of great help, if they are taught how to react more supportively to his unspoken needs. Probably the following phrase best sums up the most effective approach to be assumed by the alcoholic's family members: Don't cover up, shut up. This dictum indicates that relatives should be alert to early signs of problem drinking. One of these is a change in behavior, such as wanting to be alone or away from the family more than usual. When it is obvious that he is drinking, the family should not alibi for him. Further, they should not nag him about drinking, thereby making his alcoholism the focus of all interpersonal interaction. It is desirable to separate family life from his drinking. Family members should not threaten the alcoholic unless they intend to carry out the threat. Family members should talk to and interact with the alcohol-dependent family member when he is sober. During these conversations such comments as "It seems to me that your drinking is out of control" and "You know that we'll cooperate with you if you want to get some help with this problem" will assist the patient to acknowledge his alcoholism and take steps to control it.

Since there is no typical alcohol-dependent person, there is no typical therapy.

The practitioner may be the person best able to determine which of several treatment approaches is best suited for the alcoholic patient with whom she has developed a supportive relationship in the process of treating him for another chronic illness. Once treatment for alcoholism has begun, the practitioner may be the person best suited to coordinate the help given the alcoholic and his family by several different individuals and agencies.

BIBLIOGRAPHY: MANAGEMENT OF THE PATIENT WITH ALCOHOLISM

Conn, H. F., Rakel, R. E., and Johnson, T. W.: *Family Practice.* Philadelphia, W. B. Saunders Co. 1973.
Corrigan, E. M.: *Problem Drinkers Seeking Treatment.* New Brunswick, New Jersey, Rutgers Center of Alcoholic Studies, 1974.
Fort, Joel: *Alcohol: Our Biggest Drug Problem.* New York, McGraw-Hill Book Co., 1973.
Leitenberg, H., ed.: *Handbook of Behavioral Modification.* New York. Appleton-Century-Crofts. 1974.
Mueller, J. F.: Treatment for the alcoholic: Cursing and nursing. Amer. J. Nurs., 74 (2) 245–247, 1974.
Rubington, E.: *Alcohol Problems and Social Control.* Columbus, Ohio, Merrill. 1973.
Wintrobe, M. M., Thorn, G., Adams, R., Bennett, I., Braunwald, E., Isselbacher, K., and Petersdorf, R., Eds.: *Harrison's Principles of Internal Medicine.* 6th ed., New York, McGraw-Hill Book Co., 1970.
U.S. National Institute on Alcohol Abuse and Alcoholism. *Alcohol and Alcoholism Problems, Programs, and Progress.* Washington, D. C., U. S. Government Printing Office. (HSM, 72-9127.) 1972.

13
MANAGEMENT OF THE PATIENT WITH CHRONIC OBSTRUCTIVE PULMONARY DISEASE

The older patient who seeks health care for a respiratory ailment frequently suffers more than one pulmonary disorder. Chronic obstructive pulmonary disease (C.O.P.D.) is a syndrome, encompassing several diseases, in which increased resistance to airflow is the most significant abnormality. The term C.O.P.D. is misleading because, traditionally, the degree of airway obstruction has been estimated by the maximum midexpiratory flow rate, which is dependent upon the degree of resistance to airflow through the pulmonary lumen. However, expiratory air-flow rates are also influenced by the recoil pressure exerted by the lung. In emphysema, for instance, there is no obstruction to air flow through the air passages, but the elastic recoil of the lung is sufficiently decreased that the forced vital capacity exhaled in one second is less than normal, even in the presence of normal airway resistance.

Another physiological principle which accounts for the symptoms of C.O.P.D. is the fact that most of the resistance to air flow in normal lungs occurs in the large (>2 mm.) rather than in the terminal airways. There is only minimal resistance to air flow in the small airways. Therefore, considerable obstruction can exist in the terminal airways before a test of total airway resistance yields abnormal values. Patients usually do not seek treatment for C.O.P.D. until they are already short of breath and have developed irreversible pulmonary pathology.

The term "chronic obstructive pulmonary disease" includes chronic bronchitis, emphysema, asthma, bronchiectasis, bronchiolitis, and heart failure. Chronic bronchitis and emphysema are discussed in this section.

Chronic bronchitis is a functional disease characterized by excessive secretion of mucus. Mucus plugging and mucus gland hyperplasia (which thickens the bronchial mucosa) decreases the diameter of the airway lumen. In spite of this obstruction, since the elastic recoil of the lung is normal, the patient may demonstrate normal expiratory flow rates. Coughing typically produces mucoid sputum in the chronic bronchitic. Bronchovesicular breath sounds can be heard, and on hyperventilation rhonchi and wheezing can be elicited.

Emphysema is characterized by destruction of lung parenchyma and loss of elastic recoil of the lung. The destruction to the lung parenchyma is permanent, disrupting acini and arterioles and producing diffusion and perfusion abnormalities. Abnormal clinical findings include prolonged expiratory phase, increased anterior-posterior diameter, decreased chest-wall movement, decreased motion of the diaphragm (flattening of the diaphragm), decreased intensity of vesicular breath sounds, little or no increase in intensity of breath sounds with hyperventilation, increased respiratory rate, use of accessory muscles of respiration, intercostal retractions, hyperresonant thorax, fine rales at lung bases, and an occasional wheeze.

Laboratory and pulmonary function tests for the patient with chronic emphysema show hypoxemia ($PA_{O_2} \leq 80$ mm. Hg), hypercapnia ($PA_{CO_2} \geq 50$ mm. Hg), decreased diffusing capacity, decrease of elastic recoil of the lungs, decreased expiratory flow rate, increased residual volume, increased total lung capacity, and decreased vital capacity. In Figure 57 some similarities and differences between emphysema and chronic bronchitis are outlined.

In chronic bronchitis the closing volume is often increased even if all other pulmonary function tests are normal and the ventilation-perfusion ratio is decreased (ventilation is decreased, perfusion is normal). However, in chronic bronchitis the diffusing capacity (D_{CO}) and elastic recoil of the lungs are usually normal. Because the expiratory flow rate is usually decreased, the residual volume is increased, but the total lung capacity is normal. Since the residual volume is increased, the vital capacity is decreased.

The pulmonary function tests that best differentiate between chronic bronchitis and emphysema are closing volume (CV) and diffusing capacity (D_{CO}). The D_{CO}, which is diminished in emphysema because of capillary bed destruction, is normal in chronic bronchitis. The closing volume may be increased in chronic bronchitics who otherwise have normal pulmonary function tests. In fact, all the standard tests of pulmonary function are normal in the chronic bronchitic who has mild to moderate peripheral airway obstruction but normal elastic recoil of the lungs. Patients with C.O.P.D. are usually mildly dyspneic, with 30 to 40 per cent loss of normal pulmonary functioning before they seek treatment for their problem.

In severe chronic bronchitis the ventilation-perfusion ratio (Va/Qc) is altered (normal is 4L/min/5L/min = 0.8) and hypoxemia and hypercapnia occur. One result of decreased PA_{O_2} and elevated PA_{CO_2} in both bronchitic and emphysematous individuals is increased production of erythrocytes, with consequent elevation of hematocrit and increased viscosity of the blood. Observable signs of hypoxemia are increased respiratory rate, increased pulse rate, telegraphic speech, use of facial muscles in breathing, fatigue, dizziness, restlessness, muscle incoordination, sweating, confusion, and finally cyanosis or cardiac arrest. Observable signs of hypercapnia include headache, restlessness, dizziness, muscular rigidity, shock, arrhythmias, convulsions and coma.

As degeneration of alveoli continues in emphysema, there is an increase in the dead space, with decreased gas exchange between alveolar air and pulmonary blood, causing increased respiratory work. In the chronic bronchitic, pathologic change in the bronchial walls causes uneven distribution of ventilation, leading to intrapulmonary shunting of blood and arterial hypoxemia. Hypoxemia causes the cardiopulmonary system to increase its work in order to meet the metabolic needs of the body for oxygen. Thus, the pathological changes in emphysema and bronchitis cause a disparity between ventilation and pulmonary capillary perfusion, resulting in increased respiratory work, decreased arterial oxygenation, and increased work load on the heart.

MANAGEMENT OF C.O.P.D.

Health education is the key to both prevention and treatment of chronic obstructive pulmonary disease. It is thought that cigarette smoking contributes significantly to the etiology of both bronchitis and emphysema. When the patient stops smoking some pulmonary function tests return to normal.

The C.O.P.D. patient should understand the anatomy of his pulmonary system; the specific parts of the system which are diseased; the probable cause of the disease, and the improvement that can be expected with treatment; the importance of giving up smoking, and the need for graded exercise, postural drainage, coughing, medications, diet, and prevention of complications. The patient should be advised that his disease is irreversible and gradually degenerative but that therapy can provide improvement in his overall breathing comfort and exercise tolerance. The patient should know the symptoms of hypoxemia and hypercapnia (restlessness, tachycardia, headache, dizziness) in order to avoid acute respiratory or heart failure. If the patient concludes that nothing can improve his dyspnea or other symptoms, he will be prone to depression.

The practitioner's task is to provide enough information about the seriousness of his disease to gain the patient's cooperation in the treatment program, while at the same time withholding information that is apt to frighten or depress him.

The patient's participation in the treatment program is essential. The chief objectives of a respiratory therapy program are to relieve the work of breathing, to enhance tissue oxygenation, to provide immediate and long term relief of symptoms, and to improve the patient's general health.

Bronchial Hygiene

The work of breathing can be reduced by relieving airway obstruction and decreasing airway resistance. Bronchial hygiene to facilitate opening of tracheobronchial passages is accomplished by 1) mobilizing secretion, 2) relieving bronchospasm, and 3) decreasing mucosal edema.

Mobilization of secretions is accomplished by a combination of hydration (orally or by aerosol therapy) and chest physical therapy. Hydration of the tracheobronchial airways by oral intake of 6 to 8 glasses of water per day and by humidification of the environment will decrease sputum viscosity enough

TABLE 1. CHRONIC OBSTRUCTIVE PULMONARY DISEASE: SOME DIFFERENCES BETWEEN CHRONIC BRONCHITIS AND EMPHYSEMA

Disease	Bronchitis	Emphysema
Parameter		
Definition	Chronic overproduction of mucus	Destruction of lung parenchyma
Chief abnormalities	Intrinsic airway disease	Loss of elastic recoil in lung
		Decreased expiratory airflow
Lung compliance	Normal	Increased
Diaphragm	Normal movement	Flattened
$P_{A_{O_2}}$	Hypoxemia, severe	Hypoxemia
$P_{A_{CO_2}}$	Hypercapnia	Hypercapnia
Resistance	Inspiratory resistance is increased in severe bronchitis	Expiratory
Best diagnostic clinical tests to differentiate	Decreased ventilation–perfusion ratio (V/Q)	Decreased elastic recoil
	Increased closing volume (CV)	Decreased diffusing capacity (Dco)
		Increased closing volume
Other tests:		
Total lung capacity (TLC)	Normal	Increased
Vital capacity (VC)	Decreased	Decreased
Residual volume (RV)	Increased	Increased
Volume of air forcefully expired in one second (FEV_1)	Normal or decreased	Decreased

that it can be expectorated. Aerosol (a gas in which water particles are suspended) therapy hydrates the airways by depositing fine particles of water directly on the mucosa. During aerosol administration the patient must breathe deeply and slowly and cough vigorously enough to raise and expectorate the loosened secretions. Proper coughing is achieved by 1) inhaling maximally, 2) pausing at the end of inspiration, 3) closing the glottis by Valsalva maneuver, and 4) continuing to contract the abdominal muscles while abruptly opening the glottis and coughing.

Chest physiotherapy combined with aerosol and/or intermittent positive pressure breathing is beneficial in mobilizing the secretions that obstruct the airways. Postural drainage, chest percussion, and chest cupping and vibration are the methods usually used. Drainage of specific lung segments is promoted by systematically positioning the bronchi so as to drain each lung segment perpendicular to the floor. The patient must be well enough to tolerate having his head lower than his body. Family members can be taught chest vibration and percussion techniques. Chest percussion consists of clapping cupped hands on the chest wall to loosen secretions by vibration. Chest vibration is carried out by firmly pressing the palms of the hands on the chest wall while vibrating the hands and arms.

Bronchospasm can be relieved by administration of bronchodilators via inhalation (aerosol) or by mouth. Bronchodilators are beta adrenergic drugs that relax the smooth muscle surrounding the bronchioles. Most bronchodilators also accelerate the heart. The two most effective and popular bronchodilators are isoproterenol (Isuprel) and isoetharine (Bronkosol). Hand nebulizers are thought to be as therapeutic as IPPB machines for administration of bronchodilators. Racemic epinephrine (Vapo-Nephrin) topically administered as an aerosol both decongests bronchial mucosa and systematically acts as a mild bronchodilator. It has a minimal effect on the heart and blood vessels. Steroids administered either via aerosol or orally may decrease airway obstruction.

Individuals with C.O.P.D. are prone to certain complications as a direct result of their disease. They are poor surgical risks and require intensive preoperative care to provide good bronchial hygiene. Also, they are prone to infections, heart failure, and acute respiratory failure. Infections of the tracheobronchial system are treated with tetracycline or ampicillin. In acute respiratory failure the use of mechanical ventilation may be required.

Breathing Exercises

Over a period of years the patient with chronic obstructive pulmonary disease acquires poor habits of posture and ventilation in an effort to inhale sufficient oxygen. The efforts that patients usually select to offset their dyspnea are effective on a short-term basis but detrimental to long-term, good ventilation. Breathing retraining is essential. Patients who hunch over, raise the shoulders, and push the head forward in an effort to improve ventilation need to be taught diaphragmatic breathing. In diaphragmatic breathing chest-wall movement is limited while outward movement of the abdomen is maximized. Pursed lip breathing increases resistance upon expiration, thereby forcing the opening of bronchial passages and the exhalation of carbon dioxide. Good posture is necessary for diaphragmatic breathing.

Breathing exercises can be performed at home and should be engaged in at least twice daily. Breathing exercises and a general exercise program can be easily incorporated into the activities of family living.

Exercise and Diet

Patients with C.O.P.D. generally avoid any exercise that causes dyspnea. The result of such limitation of activity is muscle atrophy. When the patient increases his activity, more oxygen is required (an "out of shape" muscle uses more O_2 to perform work than does an exercised muscle), shortness of breath results, and the patient limits his activity still further. After evaluation of the patient's cardiac status, an exercise program should be begun to gradually increase the patient's tolerance for activity. Sometimes in the initial phases of exercise and muscle training, oxygen is given to the patient while he is exercising. Later, when he is more physically fit, the patient will not need oxygen. The program of exercise is individually outlined for each patient and may include a combination of walking outdoors, bicycling, stair climbing, and treadmill walking. In the initial stages of the exercise program, the patient should be supervised to determine whether he is employing proper breathing during exercise, and to evaluate his response to exercise. General improvement in muscle tone and physical fitness will permit many patients with C.O.P.D. to work and to carry out most activities of daily living without severe dyspnea.

If the patient with C.O.P.D. is markedly above his ideal body weight for his age and body build, weight reduction is indicated. Good nutrition and normal body weight facilitate relief of symptoms, while obesity compounds breathlessness. Exercise one hour after meals will enhance the metabolism of foods, as does eating several (4 to 6) smaller meals daily.

Oxygen Use and Administration

Patients with chronic obstructive pulmonary disease cannot adequately deliver oxygen to the blood and tissues. Oxygen ordinarily does not relieve dyspnea and should not be routinely used by patients with airway obstruction. Overuse of oxygen can, in fact, depress respirations. When oxygen therapy is indicated, consideration should be given to the following in selecting the best mode: ability to regulate the percentage of oxygen administered, humidification, patient comfort, risk of oxygen-induced hypoventilation, and need for a ventilator. The goal of oxygen therapy is to maintain the P_{O_2} at about 60 mm. Hg. Frequent monitoring of the P_{O_2}, P_{CO_2} and pH is necessary when a person with C.O.P.D. is receiving oxygen. The Ventura mask will supply precise concentrations of oxygen (24, 28, 35, 40 per cent) and is the choice mode of oxygen administration for most patients with chronic emphysema. The positive end expiratory pressure (PEEP) ventilator or the volume-limited ventilator is the best choice for patients who require mechanical assistance with respiration.

Psychological Counseling and Social Services

The patient with C.O.P.D. should be educated, motivated, and equipped to treat himself at home with periodic evaluation of his progress by a health professional. Some patients require psychological support in addition to that immediately available in the home environment in order to follow the prescribed exercise, diet, and medication orders. If the patient's depression is pronounced, he should be referred for supportive psychological counseling.

Oxygen, medication, and equipment are expensive, and not all individuals who require them for home use are economically able to purchase needed items. It may be necessary for the community's social service agencies to assist the patient with financial problems.

BIBLIOGRAPHY: MANAGEMENT OF THE PATIENT WITH CHRONIC OBSTRUCTIVE LUNG DISEASE

Bates, D. V., Macklem, P. T., and Christie, R. V.: *Respiratory Function in Disease*. Philadelphia, W. B. Saunders Co. 1971.
Brooks, Stewart M.: *Basic Facts of Body Water and Ions*. 3rd ed., New York, Springer, 1973.
Burrows, B. (Ed.): Symposium on Chronic Respiratory Disease. Med. Clin. N. Amer., 57(3) May, 1973.
Comroe, J. H.: *Physiology of Respiration*. 2nd ed. Chicago, Year Book Medical Publishers, 1974.
Conn, H. F., Ed.: *Current Therapy 1975*. Philadelphia, W. B. Saunders Co. 1975.
Davenport, Horace W.: *The ABCs of Acid-Base Chemistry*. 5th ed., Chicago, University of Chicago Press, 1969.
Guyton, Arthur: *Textbook of Medical Physiology*. 4th ed., Philadelphia, W. B. Saunders Co., 1971.
Sencor, J.: *Patient Care in Respiratory Problems*. Philadelphia, W. B. Saunders Co., 1969.
Webb, W. R.: Symposium on Pulmonary Problems in Surgery. Surg. Clin. N. Amer., 54(5) October, 1974.

NORMAL LABORATORY VALUES OF CLINICAL IMPORTANCE

Prepared by REX B. CONN, M.D., *The Johns Hopkins School of Medicine, Baltimore*

NORMAL HEMATOLOGIC VALUES

Acid hemolysis test (Ham)	No hemolysis
Alkaline phosphatase, leukocyte	Total score 14–100
Bleeding time	
Ivy	Less than 5 min.
Duke	1–5 min.
Carboxyhemoglobin	Up to 5% of total
Cell counts	
Erythrocytes: Males	4.6–6.2 million/cu. mm.
Females	4.2–5.4 million/cu. mm.
Children (varies with age)	4.5–5.1 million/cu. mm.
Leukocytes	
Total	5000–10,000/cu. mm.
Differential	*Absolute* *Percentage*
Myelocytes	0/cu. mm. 0
Juvenile neutrophils	150– 400/cu. mm. 3– 5
Segmented neutrophils	3000–5800/cu. mm. 54–62
Lymphocytes	1500–3000/cu. mm. 25–33
Monocytes	285– 500/cu. mm. 3– 7
Eosinophils	50– 250/cu. mm. 1– ˙3
Basophils	15– 50/cu. mm. 0– 0.75
(Infants and children have greater relative numbers of lymphocytes and monocytes)	
Platelets	150,000–350,000/cu. mm.
Reticulocytes	25,000– 75,000/cu. mm.
	0.5–1.5% of erythrocytes
Clot retraction, qualitative	Begins in 30–60 min.
	Complete in 24 hrs.
Coagulation time (Lee-White)	5–15 min. (glass tubes)
	19–60 min. (siliconized tubes)
Cold hemolysin test (Donath-Landsteiner)	No hemolysis
Corpuscular values of erythrocytes	
(Values are for adults; in children, values vary with age)	
M.C.H. (mean corpuscular hemoglobin)	27–31 picogm.
M.C.V. (mean corpuscular volume)	82–92 cu. micra
M.C.H.C. (mean corpuscular hemoglobin concentration)	32–36%
Fibrinogen	200–400 mg./100 ml.
Fibrinolysins	0
Hematocrit	
Males	40–54 ml./100 ml.
Females	37–47 ml./100 ml.
Newborn	49–54 ml./100 ml.
Children (varies with age)	35–49 ml./100 ml.
Hemoglobin	
Males	14.0–18.0 grams/100 ml.
Females	12.0–16.0 grams/100 ml.
Newborn	16.5–19.5 grams/100 ml.
Children (varies with age)	11.2–16.5 grams/100 ml.
Hemoglobin, fetal	Less than 1% of total
Hemoglobin A₂	1.5–3.0% of total
Hemoglobin, plasma	0–5.0 mg./100 ml.
Methemoglobin	0.03–0.13 grams/100 ml.
Osmotic fragility of erythrocytes	Begins in 0.45–0.39% NaCl
	Complete in 0.33–0.30% NaCl
Partial thromboplastin time	60–70 sec.
Kaolin activated	35–45 sec.
Prothrombin consumption	Over 80% consumed in 1 hr.
Prothrombin content	100% (calculated from prothrombin time)
Prothrombin time (one stage)	12.0–14.0 sec.
Sedimentation rate	
Wintrobe: Males	0–5 mm. in 1 hr.
Females	0–15 mm. in 1 hr.
Westergren: Males	0–15 mm. in 1 hr.
Females	0–20 mm. in 1 hr.
(May be slightly higher in children and during pregnancy)	
Thromboplastin generation test	Compared to normal control
Tourniquet test	Ten or fewer petechiae in a 2.5 cm. circle after 5 min. with cuff at 100 mm. Hg

Bone marrow, differential cell count	*Range*	*Average*
Myeloblasts	0.3– 5.0%	2.0%
Promyelocytes	1.0– 8.0%	5.0%
Myelocytes: Neutrophilic	5.0–19.0%	12.0%
Eosinophilic	0.5– 3.0%	1.5%
Basophilic	0.0– 0.5%	0.3%
Metamyelocytes ("juvenile" forms)	13.0–32.0%	22.0%
Polymorphonuclear neutrophils	7.0–30.0%	20.0%
Polymorphonuclear eosinophils	0.5– 4.0%	2.0%
Polymorphonuclear basophils	0.0– 0.7%	0.2%
Lymphocytes	3.0–17.0%	10.0%
Plasma cells	0.0– 2.0%	0.4%
Monocytes	0.5– 5.0%	2.0%
Reticulum cells	0.1– 2.0%	0.2%
Megakaryocytes	0.03– 3.0%	0.4%
Pronormoblasts	1.0– 8.0%	4.0%
Normoblasts	7.0–32.0%	18.0%

Table continues

NORMAL LABORATORY VALUES OF CLINICAL IMPORTANCE (Continued)

NORMAL BLOOD, PLASMA, AND SERUM VALUES

For some procedures the normal values may vary depending upon the methods used.

Acetone, serum	
Qualitative	Negative
Quantitative	0.3–2.0 mg./100 ml.
Aldolase, serum	0.8–3.0 ml.U./ml. (30°) (Sibley-Lehninger)
Alpha amino nitrogen, serum	4–6 mg./100 ml.
Ammonia nitrogen, blood	75–196 mcg./100 ml.
plasma	56–122 mcg./100 ml.
Amylase, serum	80–160 Somogyi units/100 ml.
Ascorbic acid	See Vitamin C
Base, total, serum	145–160 mEq./liter
Bilirubin, serum	
Direct	0.1–0.4 mg./100 ml.
Indirect	0.2–0.7 mg./100 ml. (Total minus direct)
Total	0.3–1.1 mg./100 ml.
Calcium, serum	4.5–5.5 mEq./liter (9.0–11.0 mg./100 ml.) (Slightly higher in children)
Calcium, serum, ionized	2.1–2.6 mEq./liter (4.25–5.25 mg./100 ml.)
Carbon dioxide content, serum	24–30 mEq./liter Infants: 20–28 mEq./liter
Carbon dioxide tension (Pco_2), blood	35–45 mm. Hg
Carotene, serum	50–300 mcg./100 ml.
Ceruloplasmin, serum	23–44 mg./100 ml.
Chloride, serum	96–106 mEq./liter
Cholesterol, serum	
Total	150–250 mg./100 ml.
Esters	68–76% of total cholesterol
Cholinesterase, serum	0.5–1.3 pH units
RBC	0.5–1.0 pH units
Copper, serum	
Male	70–140 mcg./100 ml.
Female	85–155 mcg./100 ml.
Cortisol, plasma	6–16 mcg./100 ml.
Creatine, serum	0.2–0.8 mg./100 ml.
Magnesium, serum	1.5–2.5 mEq./liter (1.8–3.0 mg./100 ml.)
Nitrogen, nonprotein, serum	15–35 mg./100 ml.
Osmolality, serum	285–295 mOsm./liter
Oxygen, blood	
Capacity	16–24 vol. % (varies with Hb)
Content Arterial	15–23 vol. %
Venous	10–16 vol. %
Creatine phosphokinase, serum	
Male	0–50 mI.U./ml. (30°) (Oliver-Rosalki)
Female	0–30 ml.U./ml. (30°) (Oliver-Rosalki)
Creatinine, serum	0.7–1.5 mg./100 ml.
Cryoglobulins, serum	0
Fatty acids, total, serum	190–420 mg./100 ml.
Fibrinogen, plasma	200–400 mg./100 ml.
Folic acid, serum	7–16 nanogm./ml.
Glucose (fasting)	
blood, true	60–100 mg./100 ml.
plasma or serum, true	80–120 mg./100 ml.
Folin	70–115 mg./100 ml.
Haptoglobin, serum	40–170 mg./100 ml.
Hydroxybutyric dehydrogenase, serum	0–180 ml.U./ml. (30°) (Rosalki-Wilkinson) 114–290 units/ml. (Wroblewski)
17-Hydroxycorticosteroids, plasma	8–18 mcg./100 ml.
Icterus index, serum	4–7
Immunoglobulins, serum	
IgG	800–1500 mg./100 ml.
IgA	50–200 mg./100 ml.
IgM	40–120 mg./100 ml.
Iodine, butanol extractable, serum	3.2–6.4 mcg./100 ml.
Iodine, protein bound, serum	3.5–8.0 mcg./100 ml. (May be slightly higher in infants)
Iron, serum	75–175 mcg./100 ml.
Iron binding capacity, total, serum	250–410 mcg./100 ml.
% saturation	20–55%
17-Ketosteroids, plasma	25–125 mcg./100 ml.
Lactic acid, blood	6–16 mg./100 ml.
Lactic dehydrogenase, serum	0–300 ml.U./ml. (30°) (Wroblewski modified) 150–450 units/ml. (Wroblewski) 80–120 units/ml. (Wacker)
Lipase, serum	0–1.5 units (Cherry-Crandall)
Lipids, total, serum	450–850 mg./100 ml.
Alpha$_2$	0.5–0.9 gram/100 ml. 7–14% of total
Beta	0.6–1.1 grams/100 ml. 9–15% of total
Gamma	0.7–1.7 grams/100 ml. 11–21% of total

Tension, PO_2	Venous	60–85% of capacity	
	Arterial	75–100 mm. Hg	
pH, arterial, blood		7.35–7.45	
Phenylalanine, serum		Less than 3 mg./100 ml.	
Phosphatase, acid, serum		1.0–5.0 units (King-Armstrong)	
		0.5–2.0 units (Bodansky)	
		0.5–2.0 units (Gutman)	
		0.0–1.1 units (Shinowara)	
		0.1–0.63 unit (Bessey-Lowry)	
Phosphatase, alkaline, serum		5.0–13.0 units (King-Armstrong)	
		2.0–4.5 units (Bodansky)	
		3.0–10.0 units (Gutman)	
		2.2–8.6 units (Shinowara)	
		0.8–2.3 units (Bassey-Lowry)	
		30–85 milliunits/ml. (I.U.)	
		(Values are higher in children)	
Phosphate, inorganic, serum		3.0–4.5 mg./100 ml.	
		(Children: 4.0–7.0 mg./100 ml.)	
Phospholipids, serum		6–12 mg./100 ml. as lipid phosphorus	
Potassium, serum		3.5–5.0 mEq./liter	
Proteins, serum			
	Total	6.0–8.0 grams/100 ml.	
	Albumin	3.5–5.5 grams/100 ml.	
	Globulin	2.5–3.5 grams/100 ml.	
	Electrophoresis		
	Albumin	52–68% of total	
	Globulin	3.5–5.5 grams/100 ml.	
	Alpha$_1$	2–5% of total	
		0.2–0.4 gram/100 ml.	
Serotonin, platelet suspension		0.1–0.3 mcg./ml. blood	
	serum	0.10–0.32 mcg./ml.	
Sodium, serum		136–145 mEq./liter	
Sulfates, inorganic, serum		0.8–1.2 mg./100 ml. (as S)	
Thyroxine, free, serum		1.0–2.1 nanogm./100 ml.	
Thyroxine binding globulin (TBG), serum		10–26 mcg./100 ml.	
Thyroxine iodine (T$_4$), serum		2.9–6.4 mcg./100 ml.	
Transaminase, serum: SGOT		0.19 mI.U./ml. (30°)	
		(Karmen modified)	
		15–40 units/ml. (Karmen)	
		18–40 units/ml.	
		(Reitman-Frankel)	
	SGPT	0.17 mI.U./ml. (30°)	
		(Karmen modified)	
		6–35 units/ml. (Karmen)	
		5–35 units/ml.	
		(Reitman-Frankel)	
Triglycerides, serum		0–150 mg./100 ml.	
Urea, blood		21–43 mg./100 ml.	
	plasma or serum	24–49 mg./100 ml.	
Urea nitrogen, blood (BUN)		10–20 mg./100 ml.	
	plasma or serum	11–23 mg./100 ml.	
Uric acid, serum			
	Male	2.5–8.0 mg./100 ml.	
	Female	1.5–6.0 mg./100 ml.	
Vitamin A, serum		20–80 mcg./100 ml.	
Vitamin B$_{12}$, serum		200–800 picogm./ml.	
Vitamin C, blood		0.4–1.5 mg./100 ml.	

NORMAL URINE VALUES

Acetone and acetoacetate	0	
Addis count		
Erythrocytes	0–130,000/24 hrs.	
Leukocytes	0–650,000/24 hrs.	
Casts (hyaline)	0–2000/24 hrs.	
Alcapton bodies	Negative	
Aldosterone	3–20 mcg./24 hrs.	
Alpha amino nitrogen	50–200 mg./24 hrs.	
	(Not over 1.5% of total nitrogen)	
Ammonia nitrogen	20–70 mEq./24 hrs.	
Amylase	35–260 Somogyi units/hr.	
Bence Jones protein	Negative	
Bilirubin (bile)	Negative	
Calcium		
Low Ca diet (Bauer-Aub)	Less than 150 mg./24 hrs.	
Usual diet	Less than 250 mg./24 hrs.	
Catecholamines		
Epinephrine	Less than 10 mcg./24 hrs.	
Norepinephrine	Less than 100 mcg./24 hrs.	
Chloride	110–250 mEq./24 hrs.	
	(Varies with intake)	
Chorionic gonadotrophin	0	
17-Hydroxycorticosteroids		
Male	3–9 mg./24 hrs.	
Female	2–8 mg./24 hrs.	
	(Varies with method used)	
5-Hydroxyindole-acetic acid (5-HIAA)		
Qualitative	Negative	
Quantitative	Less than 16 mg./24 hrs.	
17-Ketosteroids		
Male	6–18 mg./24 hrs.	
Female	4–13 mg./24 hrs.	
Osmolality	38–1400 mOsm./kg. water	
pH	4.6–8.0, average 6.0	
	(Depends on diet)	
Phenylpyruvic acid, qualitative	Negative	
Phosphorus	0.9–1.3 gm./24 hrs.	
	(Varies with intake)	
Porphobilinogen		
Qualitative	Negative	
Quantitative	0–0.2 mg./100 ml.	
	Less than 2.0 mg./24 hrs.	
Porphyrins		
Coproporphyrin	50–250 mcg./24 hrs.	

Table continues

NORMAL LABORATORY VALUES OF CLINICAL IMPORTANCE (Continued)

NORMAL URINE VALUES (Continued)

Copper	0–30 mcg./24 hrs.
Creatine	
Male	0–40 mg./24 hrs.
Female	0–100 mg./24 hrs. (Higher in children and during pregnancy)
Creatinine	15–25 mg./kg. of body weight/24 hrs.
Cystine or cysteine, qualitative	Negative
Delta aminolevulinic acid	1.3–7.0 mg./24 hrs.
Estrogens.	Male Female
Estrone	3–8 4–31
Estradiol	0–6 0–14
Estriol	1–11 0–72
Total	4–25 5–100
	(Units above are mcg./24 hours.) (Markedly increased during pregnancy)
Glucose (reducing substances)	Less than 250 mg./24 hrs.
Gonadotrophins, pituitary	5–10 rat units/24 hrs. 10–50 mouse units/24 hrs. (Increased after menopause)
Hemoglobin and myoglobin	Negative
Homogentisic acid, qualitative	Negative
Uroporphyrin	10–30 mcg./24 hrs.
Potassium	25–100 mEq./24 hrs. (Varies with intake)
Pregnanetriol	Less than 2.5 mg/24 hrs. in adults
Protein	
Qualitative	0
Quantitative	10–150 mg./24 hrs.
Sodium	130–260 mEq./24 hrs. (Varies with intake)
Solids, total	30–70 grams/liter, average 50 grams/liter (To estimate total solids per liter, multiply last two figures of specific gravity by 2.66, Long's coefficient)
Specific gravity	1.003–1.030
Sugar	0
Titratable acidity	20–40 mEq./24 hrs.
Urobilinogen	Up to 1.0 Ehrlich unit/2 hrs. (1–3 P.M.)
	0–4.0 mg./24 hrs.
Vanillylmandelic acid (VMA)	1–8 mg./24 hrs.

NORMAL VALUES FOR GASTRIC ANALYSIS

Basal gastric secretion (one hour)

	Concentration	Output
	Mean ± 1 S.D.	Mean ± 1 S.D.
Male	25.8 ± 1.8 mEq./liter	2.57 ± 0.16 mEq./hr.
Female	20.3 ± 3.0 mEq./liter	1.61 ± 0.18 mEq./hr.

After histamine stimulation
Normal	Mean output = 11.8 mEq./hr.
Duodenal ulcer	Mean output = 15.2 mEq./hr.

After maximal histamine stimulation
Normal	Mean output 22.6 mEq./hr.
Duodenal ulcer	Mean output 44.6 mEq./hr.

Diagnex blue (Squibb):	Anacidity 0–0.3 mg. in 2 hrs.
	Doubtful 0.3–0.6 mg. in 2 hrs.
	Normal Greater than 0.6 mg. in 2 hrs.
Volume, fasting stomach content	50–100 ml.
Emptying time	3–6 hrs.
Color	Opalescent or colorless
Specific gravity	1.006–1.009
pH (adults)	0.9–1.5

NORMAL VALUES FOR CEREBROSPINAL FLUID

Cells	Fewer than 5 cu. mm., all mononuclear
Chloride	120–130 mEq./liter (20 mEq./liter higher than serum)
Colloidal gold test	Not more than 1 in any tube
Glucose	50–75 mg./100 ml. (20 mg./100 ml. less than blood)
Pressure	70–180 mm. water
Protein, total	15–45 mg./100 ml.
Albumin	52%
Alpha, globulin	5%
Alpha, globulin	14%
Beta globulin	10%
Gamma globulin	19%

NORMAL VALUES FOR SEMEN

Volume	2–5 ml., usually 3–4 ml.	Count	60–150 million/ml.
Liquefaction	Complete in 15 min.		Below 60 million/ml. is abnormal
pH	7.2–8.0; average 7.8	Motility	80% or more motile
Leukocytes	Occasional or absent	Morphology	80–90% normal forms

NORMAL VALUES FOR FECES

Bulk	100–200 grams/24 hrs.	Nitrogen, total	Less than 2.0 grams/24 hrs.
Dry matter	23–32 grams/24 hrs.	Urobilinogen	40–280 mg./24 hrs.
Fat, total	Less than 6.0 grams/24 hrs.	Water	Approximately 65%

NORMAL VALUES FOR SEROLOGIC PROCEDURES

Anti-hyaluronidase	Less than 1:200. Significant if rising titer can be demonstrated at weekly intervals.	Proteus OX-19 agglutinins	1:80	Negative
			1:160	Doubtful
			1:320	Positive
Anti-streptolysin O titer	Normal up to 1:128. Single test usually has little significance. Rise in titer or persistently elevated titer is significant.	R. A. test (latex)	1:40	Negative
			1:80 –1:160	Doubtful
			1:320	Positive
Bacterial agglutinins	Significant only if rise in titer is demonstrated or if antibodies are absent.	Rose test	1:10	Negative
			1:20 –1:40	Doubtful
			1:80	Positive
Complement fixation tests	Titers of 1:8 or less are usually not significant. Paired sera showing rise in titer of more than two tubes are usually considered significant.	Tularemia agglutinins	1:80	Negative
			1:160	Doubtful
			1:320	Positive
C reactive protein (CRP)	Negative			

Heterophile titer

	Unabsorbed	Absorbed With G.P.	Absorbed With Beef
Normal	1:160	1:10	1:160
Inf. mono.	1:160	1:320	1:10
Serum sickness	1:160	1:5	1:10

Table continues

225

NORMAL LABORATORY VALUES OF CLINICAL IMPORTANCE (Continued)

TOXICOLOGY

Arsenic, blood	3.5–7.2 mcg./100 ml.	Ethanol, blood	Less than 0.005%
Arsenic, urine	Less than 100 mcg./24 hrs.		0.3–0.4%
Barbiturates, serum	0	Marked intoxication	0.4–0.5%
	Coma level: Phenobarbital approximately 11 mg./100 ml.; most other barbiturates 1.5 mg./100 ml.	Alcoholic stupor	Above 0.5%
		Coma	
		Lead, blood	0–40 mcg./100 ml.
		Lead, urine	Less than 100 mcg./24 hrs.
		Lithium, serum	0
			Therapeutic levels 0.5–1.5 mEq./liter
			Toxic levels above 2 mEq./liter
Bromides, serum	0	Mercury, urine	Less than 10 mcg./24 hrs.
	Toxic levels above 17 mEq./liter	Salicylate, plasma	0
Carbon monoxide, blood	Up to 5% saturation	Therapeutic range	20–25 mg./100 ml.
	Symptoms occur with 20% saturation	Toxic range	Over 30 mg./100 ml.
Dilantin, blood or serum	Therapeutic levels 1–11 mcg./ml.	Death	45–75 mg./100 ml.

LIVER FUNCTION TESTS

Bromsulphalein (B.S.P.)	Less than 5% remaining in serum 45 minutes after injection of 5 mg./kg. of body weight
Cephalin cholesterol flocculation	0–1 in 24 hours.
Galactose tolerance	Excretion of not more than 3.0 grams galactose in the urine 5 hours after ingestion of 40 grams of galactose.
Glycogen storage	Increase of blood glucose 45 mg./100 ml. over fasting level 45 minutes after subcutaneous injection of 0.01 mg./kg. body weight of epinephrine.
Hippuric acid	Excretion of 3.0–3.5 grams hippuric acid in urine within 4 hours after ingestion of 6.0 grams sodium benzoate,
	or
	Excretion of 0.7 gram hippuric acid in urine within 1 hour after intravenous injection of 1.77 grams sodium benzoate.
Thymol turbidity	0–5 units.
Zinc turbidity	2–12 units.

PANCREATIC (ISLET) FUNCTION TESTS

Glucose tolerance tests	Patient should be on a diet containing 300 grams of carbohydrate per day for 3 days prior to test.
Oral	After ingestion of 100 grams of glucose or 1.75 grams glucose/kg. body weight, blood glucose is not more than 160 mg./100 ml. after 60 minutes, 140 mg./100 ml. after 90 minutes, and 120 mg./100 ml. after 120 minutes. Values are for blood; serum measurements are approximately 15% higher. Blood glucose does not exceed 200 mg./100 ml.
Intravenous	After infusion of 0.5 gram of glucose/kg. body weight over 30 minutes. Glucose concentration falls below initial level at 2 hours and returns to preinfusion levels in 3 hours or 1 hour. Values are for blood; serum measurements are approximately 15% higher.
Cortisone-glucose tolerance test	The patient should be on a diet containing 300 grams of carbohydrate per day for 3 days prior to test. At 8½ and again 2 hours prior to glucose load patient is given cortisone acetate by mouth (50 mg. if patient's ideal weight is less than 160 lb., 62.5 mg. if ideal weight is greater than 160 lb.). An oral dose of glucose 1.75 grams/kg. body weight, is given and blood samples are taken at 0, 30, 60, 90, and 120 minutes. Test is considered positive if true blood glucose exceeds 160 mg./100 ml. at 60 minutes, 140 mg./100 ml. at 90 minutes, and 120 mg./100 ml. at 120 minutes. Values are for blood; serum measurements are approximately 15% higher.

RENAL FUNCTION TESTS

Clearance tests (corrected to 1.73 sq. meters body surface area)

Glomerular filtration rate (G.F.R.)		
Inulin clearance,	Males	110–150 ml./min.
Mannitol clearance, or	Females	105–132 ml./min.
Endogenous creatinine clearance		
Renal plasma flow (R.P.F.)	Males	560–830 ml./min.
p-Aminohippurate (P.A.H.), or	Females	490–700 ml./min.
Diodrast		
Filtration fraction (F.F.)	Males	17–21%
$FF = \dfrac{G.F.R.}{R.P.F.}$	Females	17–23%
Urea clearance (C_u)	Standard	40–65 ml./min.
	Maximal	60–100 ml./min.

Concentration and dilution — Specific gravity > 1.025 on dry day; Specific gravity < 1.003 on water day

Maximal Diodrast excretory capacity T_{M_D} — Males 43–59 mg./min.; Females 33–51 mg./min.

Maximal glucose reabsorptive capacity T_{M_G} — Males 300–450 mg./min.; Females 250–350 mg./min.

Maximal PAH excretory capacity $T_{M_{PAH}}$ — 80–90 mg./min.

Phenolsulfonphthalein excretion (P.S.P.) — 25% or more in 15 min.; 40% or more in 30 min.; 55% or more in 2 hrs. After injection of 1 ml. P.S.P. intravenously

THYROID FUNCTION TESTS

Protein bound iodine, serum (P.B.I.)	3.5–8.0 mcg./100 ml.
Butanol extractable iodine, serum (B.E.I.)	3.2–6.4 mcg./100 ml.
Thyroxine iodine, serum (T_4)	2.9–6.4 mcg./100 ml.
Free thyroxine, serum	1.4–2.5 nanogram/100 ml.
T_3 (index of unsaturated T.B.G.)	10.0–14.6%
Thyroxine-binding globulin, serum (T.B.G.)	10–26 mcg. T_4/100 ml.
Thyroid-stimulating hormone, serum (T.S.H.)	0 up to 0.2 milliunits/ml.
Radioactive iodine (I^{131}) uptake (R.A.I.)	20–50% of administered dose in 24 hrs.
Radioactive iodine (I^{131}) excretion	30–70% of administered dose in 24 hrs.
Radioactive iodine (I^{131}), protein bound	Less than 0.3% of administered dose per liter of plasma at 72 hrs.
Basal metabolic rate	Minus 10% to plus 10% of mean standard

GASTROINTESTINAL ABSORPTION TESTS

d-Xylose absorption test — After an 8 hour fast 10 ml./kg. body weight of a 5% solution of d-xylose is given by mouth. Nothing further by mouth is given until the test has been completed. All urine voided during the following 5 hours is pooled, and blood samples are taken at 0, 60, and 120 minutes. Normally 26% (range 16–33%) of ingested xylose is excreted within 5 hours, and the serum xylose reaches a level between 25 and 40 mg./100 ml. after 1 hour and is maintained at this level for another 60 minutes.

Vitamin A absorption test — A fasting blood specimen is obtained and 200,000 units of vitamin A in oil is given by mouth. Serum vitamin A level should rise to twice fasting level in 3 to 5 hours.

INDEX

Note: In this Index, page numbers in *italic* type refer to illustrations.

Abdomen, physical examination of, 86–100
    assisting patient in, 87
    auscultation in, 90–91
    inspection in, 88–90
    palpation in, 91–93, *92*
    percussion in, 91
    pubic hair distribution in, 89
    skin in, 89
    superficial veins in, 89–90
    symmetry in, 88–89
Abdominal aorta, palpation of, 97
Abdominal organs, position of, *88*
Abdominal quadrants, contents of, 87
Abducens nerve, function of, 118
Acetone test, in urinalysis, 135
Achilles reflex, testing of, 125, *126*
Acne rosacea, nose in, 53
Acoustic nerve, function of, 119
Acromegaly, facial structure in, 40
    tongue size in, 57
Addison's disease, discolorations of buccal mucosa in, 57
Agnosia, 117
Albumin test, in urinalysis, 135–136
Alcoholism, management of patient with, 208–213
    history in, 210
    laboratory findings in, 211
    physical examination in, 210
    psychotherapy in, 212
    withdrawal treatment in, 211
    physiological aspects of, 209–210
    psychological aspects of, 209
    social impact of, 208
Allergies, in past medical history, 26
Alveoli, degeneration of, in emphysema, 216
Aphasia, global, 116
    receptive, 117
    sensory, 117
Appendix, palpation of, 97
Apraxia, 117
Arms, palpation of, 109
    physical examination of, 109–111
Arteriosclerosis, hypertension and, 170
    retinal, 49, *49*
Arthritis. See specific types; e.g., *Osteoarthritis, Rheumatoid Arthritis.*

Arthritis deformans. See *Rheumatoid arthritis.*
Atherosclerosis, obliterative, in diabetes, 182
Athlete's foot, 114
Auscultation, in cardiac examination, 81–83, *82*
    in chest examination, 75–76
        adventitious sounds in, 76–77
        breath sounds in, 75, 76
    in examination of abdomen, 90–91
    method of, in physical examination, 37
Axillae, examination of, 109

Back, physical examination of, 107–109
    skin disorders of, 108
Ballottement, in physical examination, 35
Basal metabolic rate, in obesity, 202
Basophils, 132
Biceps reflex, testing of, 123, *124*
Birthmarks, in physical examination, 40
Bladder, urinary, palpation of, 98
Blood, symptoms in, in medical history, 30
    table of normal values for, 222
Blood chemistry studies, blood urea nitrogen, 142
    creatinine, 143
    protein-bound iodine, 144
    serum bilirubin, 143
    serum cholesterol determination, 139
    serum electrolyte, calcium, 140
        chloride, 141
        magnesium, 141
        phosphate, 141
        potassium, 140
        sodium, 139
    serum glucose determination, 137–138
    serum iron, 144
    serum proteins, 141–142
    uric acid determination, 142–143
Blood pressure, high. See *Hypertension.*
    taking of, in hypertension, 171
Blood serum protein, 141–142
Blood urea nitrogen, 142
Body language, in health interviewing, 4
Borborygmi, 90

Bowel sounds, in examination of abdomen, 90
Breast(s), carcinoma of, 67
  inspection of, positions for, 63, *63*, 65
  mass in, 66
  palpation of, 64–66
  physical examination of, 63–67
    positions of nipples in, 63
    skin in, 64
  pigeon, 69
  self-examination of, 67
  symptoms in, in medical history, 30
  tissues of, consistency of, 67
Bronchitis, chronic. See *Chronic bronchitis*.
Bronchospasm, in chronic obstructive pulmonary disease, 217
Buccal mucosa, disorders of, 57
Bulbar conjunctiva, examination of, 44

Candida albicans, tongue disorder with, 57
Carcinoma, of breast, 67
  rectosigmoid, 100
  thyroid, 62
Cardiac. See also *Heart*.
Cardiac arrhythmia, descriptive gestures of patient with, 4
Cardiac cycle, events of, 84–85
Cardiac dullness, 81
Cardiac examination, 78–86
  auscultation in, 81–83, *82*
  heart sounds in, 83–84
  inspection in, 79
  palpation in, 79–80, *80*
  percussion in, 80–81
Cardiac murmurs, 85–86
  diastolic, 86
  systolic, 86
Cardiac work load, reduction of, 197
Cardiovascular system, symptoms in, in medical history, 30
Carotid artery, examination of, 60–61, *60*
Cerebellum, function of, 120–121
Cerebrospinal fluid, table of normal values for, 224
Cervical polyps, 106
Cervix, examination of, 104–106, *106*
Cheilosis, in riboflavin deficiency, 42
Chest. See also *Thorax* and *Lungs*.
Chest percussion, in chronic obstructive pulmonary disease, 217
Chest x-ray, 147
Cheyne-Stokes respirations, in congestive heart failure, 195
Childhood disease, in past medical history, 26
Cholesterol, 139
Chronic arthritis, management of patient with, 184–191
Chronic bronchitis, 214
  differential diagnosis of, emphysema in, 215, 217
  pulmonary function tests in, 215
Chronic obstructive pulmonary disease, management of patient with, 214–219
  breathing exercises in, 218

Chronic obstructive pulmonary disease, management of patient with (*Continued*)
  bronchial hygiene in, 216
  exercise and diet in, 218–219
  oxygen use and administration in, 219
  patient education in, 216
  psychological counseling in, 219
  social services in, 219
  types of, 214
Colon, palpation of, 97–98
Conductive hearing loss, 51
C.O.P.D. See *Chronic obstructive pulmonary disease*.
Cornea, examination of, 44
Coronary artery disease, obesity and, 202
Coronary occlusion, descriptive gestures of patient with, 4
Coughing, in examination of lungs, 77
Creatinine, 143
Crepitus, in osteoarthritis, 185

Data, recording of, Medicare and, 160
  purpose of, 159
Dermatitis, stasis, 112
Dermatophytosis, 114
Diabetes mellitus, complications of, 181–183
  diagnosis of, 178
  diet in, 179–180
  insulin therapy in, 180–181
  obesity and, 202
  oral hypoglycemic agents in, 180
  pathophysiology of, 176–177, *177*, *178*
  patient assessment in, 179
  serum glucose determination in, 138
  symptoms and signs of, 177–178
Diastasis recti, 98
Diet, in diabetes mellitus, 179–180
  in obesity, 205
Diuresis, in diabetes mellitus, 177
  in chronic congestive heart failure, 198
Dorsalis pedis pulse, palpation of, 112, *113*
Drug therapy, in chronic congestive heart failure, 197–198
  in diabetes mellitus, 180–181
  in hypertension, 173–174
  in obesity, 206
  in osteoarthritis, 187
  in rheumatoid arthritis, 190
Dullness, cardiac, 81
  in chest percussion, 75
Dyspnea, in heart failure, 194
  obesity and, 202

Ear(s), examination of, 51–53
  otoscope in, 51
  symptoms in, in medical history, 30
Eardrum, examination of, 51
Electrocardiogram, 147–149, *148*
  in hypertension, 172
Emotional stress, and hypertension, 169
  differential diagnosis of, chronic bronchitis in, 215, 217
  pulmonary function tests in, 215

Endocrine system, symptoms in, in medical history, 30
Eosinophils, 132
Epididymitis, 102
Epispadias, 102
Erythrocyte sedimentation rate, 132
　in osteoarthritis, 186
Erythrocytes, counting of, errors in, 131
　life span of, 131
　normal range of, 130
　tests of, 130–132
Examination. See also *Physical examination.*
　roentgenographic, 146–147
Exercise therapy, in obesity, 206
Exophthalmos, eyes in, 42
　facial expression in, 39
Extremities, physical examination of, 109–114
　lower, 111–114
　upper, 109–111
Eye(s), examination of, 42–51
　funduscopic, 46–51, *46–50*
　ophthalmoscopic, 46–51, *46–50*
　Snellen chart in, *43*
　test of ocular motion in, 43
　examination of bulbar conjunctiva of, 44
　fundus of, normal, *47*
　in exophthalmos, 42
　nystagmus of, 43
　strabismus of, 43
　symptoms in, in medical history, 30
Eye movements, and anxiety, 150
Eyelids, edema of, in nephritis and nephrosis, 44

Face, symptoms in, in medical history, 30
Facial expression, assessment of, 150
　in various diseases, 39–40
Facial hair, in physical examination, 41
Facial nerve, function of, 119
Facial skin, in physical examination, 40
Facial tissue, hydration of, 40
　lipomas in, 41
　swelling of, 41
Family health history, in health interview, 21–22
Feces, table of normal values for, 224
Femoral hernia, palpation of, 99–100
Flatness, in chest percussion, 75
Folliculitis, 42
Fremitus, pleural friction, 73
　rhonchal, 73
　tussive, 73
　vocal, 72

Gag reflex, 58
Gallbladder, palpation of, 94
Gastric analysis, table of normal values for, 224
Gastrointestinal absorption, tests of, 227
Gastrointestinal system, symptoms in, in medical history, 30

Genitalia, examination of, female, 103–107, *104, 105*
　male, 101–102
Geographic tongue, 57
Glans penis, inflammation of, 101
Glaucoma, cupping of optic disc in, 48, *48*
Global aphasia, 116
Glossopharyngeal nerve, function of, 120
Gluconeogenesis, 176
Glucose test, in urinalysis, 135
Glycosuria, in diabetes mellitus, 178
Goiter, thyroid gland in, 62
Granulocytes, 132
Gums, disorders of, in vitamin C deficiency, 56

Hands, examination of, 110
Head, physical examination of, 38–58
　symptoms in, in medical history, 30
Health interview, active listening in, 5
　appearance of nurse in, 2
　assessing health needs and strengths in, 152–153
　attitude of support in, 11
　careful selection of terms in, 7–8
　chief complaint of patient in, 3
　　clarification of, 16–17
　direct questioning in, 18
　emphasis on current patient concerns in, 5–6
　environment for, 2
　establishing communication in, 3–4
　guidelines for, 3
　health history of patient's family in, 21–22
　health of patient's children in, 22
　history of present illness in, 17–21
　interpersonal distance in, 10–11
　investigating symptoms in, description of, 19
　　development of, 18
　　duration of, 18
　　other symptoms involved, 20
　　periodicity of, 20
　　precipitating causes for, 18
　nonverbal communication in, 4
　nurse-patient relationship in, 10
　of repressed patient, 4
　past history in, 24–29
　patient comfort in, 2
　patient reluctance in, 3
　personal history in, 22–24
　preliminary patient assessment in, 150–152
　purpose of, 1
　review of body systems in, 29–31
　review of identifying data before, 15
　supportive phraseology in, 7–8
　sympathy of nurse in, 4
　symptoms in, location of, 19
　　severity of, 19
　techniques of, 1–12
　validating information received, 8
　verifying information received, 8–9
　withholding of advice and opinion in, 9–10

Hearing, tests of, 51, *52*, *53*, 54
    Weber, 53, 54
Hearing loss, types of, 51
Heart. See also *Cardiac*.
    boot-shaped, in hypertension, 171
    in diabetes mellitus, 182
Heart failure, backward, 193
    causes of, 193
    chronic congestive, Cheyne-Stokes respirations in, 195
        complications of, 199
        management of patient with, 192–199
        mechanism of, 193
        treatment of, 196–199
    definition of, 192
    dyspnea in, 194
    forward, 193
    heart dilation in, 196
    heart sounds in, 195
    high output, 192
    left, 193
    rales in, 195
    symptoms of, 194
Heart sounds, 83–84
Hematocrit, 131
Hematologic values, normal, table of, 221
Hemoglobin, measuring of, 131
Hemolytic jaundice, serum bilirubin in, 143
Hemorrhage, gastrointestinal, stool in, 146
Hernia, palpation of, 98–100, *99*
Herpes simplex, 42
Hypercapnia, in emphysema, 215
Hypercholesterolemia, in diabetes mellitus, 177
Hyperglycemia, in diabetes mellitus, 176
Hyperresonance, in chest percussion, 75
Hypertension, definitions of, 170
    diagnosis of, 170–172
    effects of, 170
    emotional stress and, 169
    management of patient with, 168–175
    mortality in, 168
    obesity and, 202
    pathophysiology of, 168–169, *169*
    renal, 168
    retinal changes in, 49, *49*, *50*
    treatment of, general, 172–173
        drug, 173–174
Hyperventilation, causes of, 70
Hypoglossal nerve, function of, 120
Hypoglycemia, in alcoholism, 209
Hypospadias, 102
Hypoxemia, in emphysema, 215

Illness prevention, early signs of psychological disequilibrium in, 155
    levels of need in, primary, 154–155
        secondary, 155–156
        tertiary, 156
    psychological crisis in, 154
Illnesses, in past medical history, 27
    mental and emotional, 28
Immunization, in illness prevention, 154
Incisional hernia, palpation of, 98
Inguinal hernia, palpation of, 99, *99*
Injuries, in past medical history, 28

Inoculations, in past medical history, 26
Inspection, in cardiac examination, 79
    in examination of abdomen, 88–90
Insulin reaction, 181
Insulin shock, 181
Insulin therapy, in diabetes mellitus, complications of, 181
Intention tremor, in cerebellar disease, 121
Iodine, protein-bound, 144
Iris, examination of, 44

Jaundice, obstructive, stool in, 145
Joints, in rheumatoid arthritis, 187
    osteoarthritic changes in, 185
Jugular vein, external, distention of, 60
Juvenile onset obesity, 203

Kahn flocculation test, 137
Ketoacidosis, in diabetes, 181
Ketone bodies, 176
Ketonuria, in diabetes mellitus, 178
Kidneys, palpation of, 94–95, *94*
    tests of function of, 227
Kolmer complement fixation test, 137
Koplik's spots, in measles, 57

Laboratory tests and special examinations, 129–149
Large intestine, palpation of, 97–98
Larynx, examination of, 61
    symptoms in, in medical history, 30
Legs, deformities of, 114
    examination of, 111–114
    palpation of, 112, *113*
    swelling of, 111–112
Leukemia, leukocytes in, 133
Leukocyte count, in osteoarthritis, 186
Leukocytes, normal range of, 132
    types of, 132
Liver, palpation of, 93, *94*
    tests of function of, 226
Levels of illness prevention, 153–154
Liver disease, obesity and, 202
Lungs, physical examination of, 67–78
    auscultation in, 75–76
    breathing pattern in, 70
    chest wall expansion in, 71, *72*
    coughing in, 77
    inspection in, 69–70
    percussion in, 73–75, *74*
Lung parenchyma, destruction of, in emphysema, 215
Lymph nodes, palpation of, axillary, 67, 109
    cervical, 59
    inguinal, 112
    popliteal, 112
Lymphocytes, 132

Malnutrition, in alcoholism, 209
Maslow's hierarchy of needs, 152–153, *153*

Mazzini flocculation test, 137
Measles, Koplik's spots in, 57
Medical history, accuracy of, informant and, 16
  content of, 13-32
  day to day activities in, 24
  education in, 22
  family health history in, 21-22
  financial status in, 24
  history of alcohol, drugs, and tobacco in, 23
  history of present illness in, 17-21
    history of treatment given in, 21
    patient's thoughts concerning, 21
  length of, 13
  military history in, 23
  occupation in, 23
  outline of content, 14
  past, allergies in, 26
    childhood diseases in, 26
    history of inoculations in, 26
    information included, 25
    injuries in, 28
    mental and emotional illness in, 28
    method of exploring, 25-26
    obstetrical, 28
    previous illnesses in, 27
    purpose of, 24
    surgical operations in, 27
  purposes of, 13
  recording of, present vs. past history in, 21
  recording of chief complaint in, 17
  recording of negative findings in, 20
  review of body systems in, 29-31
    outline for, 30-31
  social and recreational, 23
  summarization of, 31-32
Medical record, problem-oriented, in planning patient care, 164-167
  Medicare and, 160
  problem list for, 161, *162*
  progress notes in, 163
  steps in, 161
Medicare, and recording of health data, 160
Mental illness, in past medical history, 28
Mixed hearing loss, 51
Moles, 42
Mongolism, tongue size in, 57
Monocytes, 132
Mouth, physical examination of, 56-58
  mouth odor in, 58
  symptoms in, in medical history, 30
Muscles, wasting of, in rheumatoid arthritis, 188
Muscle coordination, testing of, 121
Muscle strength, tests of, 122
Muscle tone, neurological evaluation of, 122
Musculoskeletal system, symptoms in, in medical history, 31
Myopia, size of pupils in, 45

Nasal passages, examination of, 54
Nasal septum, examination of, 55
Neck, physical examination of, 58-63
  symptoms in, in medical history, 30
Nephritis, edema of eyelids in, 44

Nephrosis, edema of eyelids in, 44
Nervous system, symptoms in, in medical history, 31
Neurological examination, 114-128
  cerebellar function in, 120-121
  cranial nerve function in, 117-120
  level of consciousness in, 115
  memory in, 116
  mood in, 115
  motor function in, 121-122
  muscle function in, 121-122
  reflexes in, 123
  sensory perception in, 126-128
  test of complex functions in, 116-117
Neutrophils, 132
Nose, in acne rosacea, 53
  in rhinitis, 53
  physical examination of, 53-56
  saddle, in syphilis, 53
  symptoms in, in medical history, 30
Nystagmus, 43

Obesity, and coronary artery disease, 202
  determination of degree of, 201-202
  dyspnea in, 202
  etiology of, 200-201
  family eating patterns in, 204
  hazards of, 202
  juvenile onset, 203
  laboratory tests in, 204
  management of patient with, 200-207
  metabolic changes in, 202-203
  treatment plan for, 205
Observation, method of, in physical examination, 34-35
Obstetrical history, in past medical history, 28
Oculomotor nerve, function of, 118
Olfactory nerve, function of, 117
Ophthalmoscope, in eye examination, 46-51, *46-50*
Optic disc, choking of, in papilledema, 48, *48*
  cupping of, in glaucoma, 48, *48*
Optic nerve, function of, 117-118
Oropharynx, examination of, 58
Osteoarthritis, blood findings in, 186
  crepitus in, 185
  joint changes in, 185
  pathophysiology of, 184-185
  treatment of, 186-187
Otoscope, in ear examination, 51

Palate, examination of, 58
Palpation, in cardiac examination, 79-80, *80*
  in examination of abdomen, 91-93, *92*
  in examination of head and neck, 39
  in examination of thorax, 71-73
  method of in physical examination, 34-35
  of abdominal aorta, 97
  of appendix, 97
  of arms, 109
  of axillary lymph nodes, 67
  of breasts, 64-66

Palpation (*Continued*)
  of carotid artery, 61-62
  of cervical lymph nodes, 59
  of colon, 97-98
  of dorsalis pedis pulse, 112, *113*
  of gallbladder, 94
  of hernia, 98-100, *99*
  of kidneys, 94-95, *94*
  of liver, 93, *94*
  of pancreas, 96
  of posterior tibial pulse, 112, *113*
  of small intestine, 97
  of spine, 109
  of spleen, 95-96, *95*
  of stomach, 96
  of thyroid gland, 61-62, *62*
  of trachea, 72
  of urinary bladder, 98
  of uterine tube, 107
  of uterus, 107
Pancreas, in diabetes mellitus, 176
  palpation of, 96
Pancreatic islets, tests of function of, 226
Pancreatitis, stool in, 146
Papanicolaou smear test, 104, 144-145
Papilledema, choking of optic disc in, 48
Paralysis agitans, masklike facies in, 39
Parathyroid glands, 63
Parkinson's disease, pill-rolling tremor in, 122
Parotid gland, swelling of, in parotitis, 59
Patellar reflex, testing of, 125, *125*
  planning of, problem-oriented medical record in, 164-167
  self-determination in, 9
Pelvis, physical examination of, 100-107
Penis, examination of, 101
Peptic ulcer, descriptive gestures of patient with, 4
Perceptive hearing loss, 51
Percussion, in cardiac examination, 80-81
  in chest examination, 73-75, *74*
    sounds in, 75
  in chronic obstructive pulmonary disease, 217
  in examination of abdomen, 91
  in physical examination, method of, 35-37, *36*
  of spine, 108, 109
  of stomach, 96
Peristalsis, 90
Peritoneal friction rub, 90
Pharynx, symptoms in, in medical history, 30
Pheochromocytoma, and hypertension, 169
Phlebothrombosis, 112
pH test, in urinalysis, 134
Physical examination, ballottement in, 35
  cardiac, 78-86
  electrocardiogram in, 147-149, *148*
  general procedure for, 33-38
  in hypertension, 171
  method of auscultation in, 37
  method of observation in, 34
  method of palpation in, 34-35
  method of percussion in, 35-37, *36*
  neurological, 114-128
  of abdomen, 86-100

Physical examination (*Continued*)
  of arms, 109-111
  of back, 107-109
  of breasts, 63-67
  of ear, 51-53
  of extremities, 109-114
  of eyes, 42-51
  of face, 39-42
    facial expression in, 39-40
  of feet, 112, *113*
  of female genitalia, 103-107, *104*, *105*
  of hands, 110
  of head and neck, 38-63
  of legs, 111-114
  of lungs, 67-78
  of male genitalia, 101-102
  of mouth, 56-58
  of neck, 58-63
  of nose, 53-56
  of pelvis, 100-107
  of prostate, 100, *101*
  of shoulders, 111
  of spine, 108-109
  of thorax, 63-86
  overall survey in, 38
  overview of, 33-38
  rectal, 100, *101*
  roentgenographic, 146-147
  taking of measurements in, 37-38
  teeth in, 56
  vital signs in, 37-38
Pigeon breast, 69
Pityriasis rosea, of back, 108
Polydipsia, in diabetes mellitus, 177
Polyphagia, in diabetes mellitus, 177
Polyps, cervical, 106
Pleural effusion, in congestive heart failure, 195
Pleural friction rub, 77
Prostate, examination of, 100, *101*
Protein-bound iodine, 144
Psoriasis, of back, 108
Psychosocial assessment, and intervention, 150-158
  health balance in, 156-158, *157*
  levels of illness prevention in, 153-154
  of health needs and strengths, 152-153
  preliminary, 150-152
Pubic hair, distribution of, in examination of abdomen, 89
Pulse, in congestive heart failure, 195
  posterior tibial, palpation of, 112, *113*
Pupils, Argyll Robertson, 45
  examination of, 45
  testing light reflex of, 45, *45*

Qualitative tests, 129
Quantitative tests, 130

Radial reflex, testing of, 124
Rales, 77
  and hypertension, 171
  in congestive heart failure, 195
Receptive aphasia, 117
Rectal examination, 100, *101*

INDEX

Reflexes, testing of, in neurological examination, 123
Renal function tests, 227
Reproductive system, symptoms in, in medical history, 31
Resonance, in chest percussion, 75
Respiratory system, symptoms in, in medical history, 30
Retinal arteriosclerosis, 49, 49
Rheumatoid arthritis, diagnosis of, 188–189
    joint changes in, 187
    muscle wasting in, 188
    pathophysiology of, 187
    treatment of, 189–180
Rheumatoid spondylitis, 188
Rhinitis, nasal passages in, 54–55
    nose in, 53
Rhonchi, 76
Riboflavin deficiency, cheilosis in, 42
Rinne's test of hearing, 51–53, 52, 53
Risus sardonicus, in tetanus, 39

Saddle nose, in syphilis, 53
Salivary ducts, examination of, 57
Screening tests, 129
Scrotum, examination of, 102
Semen, table of normal values for, 225
Sensory aphasia, 117
Sensory perception, testing of, deep pain, 126
    loss of sensation, 127
    position, 127
    temperature, 126
    two-point touch, 127
    vibratory, 127
Serologic procedures, table of normal values for, 225
Serum bilirubin, 143
Serum cholesterol determination, 139
Serum glucose determination, 137–138
Serum iron, 144
Shock, insulin, 181
Shoulder, examination of, 111
Sinuses, paranasal, examination of, 55, 55
    symptoms in, in medical history, 30
Skin, in examination of abdomen, 89
    in examination of face, 40
    in medical history, 29
    in physical examination, 40
    of back, disorders of, 108
Small intestine, palpation of, 97
Smoking, and hypertension, 173
Snellen eye chart, 43
Specific gravity test, in urinalysis, 134
Speech, assessment of, 151
Spinal accessory nerve, function of, 120
Spine, examination of, 108–109
    palpation of, 109
    percussion of, 108, 109
Spleen, palpation of, 95–96, 95
Spondylitis, rheumatoid, 188
Stasis dermatitis, 112
Stensen's duct, examination of, 57
Stethoscope, in physical examination, 37
Stomach, palpation of, 96
    percussion of, 96

Stool, in gastrointestinal hemorrhage, 146
    in obstructive jaundice, 145
    in pancreatitis, 146
Stool examination, test for occult blood in, 146
Strabismus, 43
Stretch reflex, testing of, 123
Stridor, 77
Surgical operations, in past medical history, 27
Syphilis, peg-shaped teeth in, 56
    saddle nose in, 53
    serologic tests for, 137

Tearing, excessive, 44
Teeth, examination of, 56
    infections of, 56–57
    malposition of, 56
    peg-shaped, in syphilis, 56
Testes, examination of, 102
Tests, biochemical, in hypertension, 172
    blood chemistry, 137–144
    for chronic obstructive pulmonary disease, 215
    hemogram, red cell studies, 130–132
        white cell studies, 132–133
    in obesity, 204
    Papanicolaou smear, 144–145
    pulmonary function, in bronchitis and emphysema, 215
    qualitative, 129
    quantitative, 130
    screening, 129
    serologic, for syphilis, 137
    stool examination, 145–147
    tuberculin skin sensitivity, 136
    urinalysis, 133–137
        in hypertension, 171
Tetanus, risus sardonicus in, 39
Thorax, anterior, common reference points, 68, 68
    physical examination of, 63–86
        auscultation in, 75–77
        chest wall expansion in, 71, 72
        coughing in, 77
        inspection in, 69–70
        palpation in, 71–73
        percussion in, 73–75, 74
Thyroid carcinoma, 62
Thyroid function tests, 227
Thyroid gland, in goiter, 62
    palpation of, 61, 62, 62
Thyrotoxicosis, auscultation in, 62
Tongue, examination of, 57
    pathologic lesions of, 57
    tremor of, 57
Tonsils, examination of, 58
Toxicology, table of normal values for, 226
Trachea, examination of, 61, 61
    palpation of, 72
Triceps reflex, testing of, 123, 124
Trigeminal nerve, function of, 118
Trochlear nerve, function of, 118
Tuberculin skin sensitivity test, 136
Tussive fremitus, 73

Umbilical hernia, palpation of, 98
Uric acid, 142–143
Urinalysis, acetone test in, 135
  albumin test in, 135–136
  glucose test in, 135
  in hypertension, 171
  methods of specimen collection in, 133–134
  microscopic examination in, 136
  pH test in, 134
  specific gravity in, 134
Urinary bladder, palpation of, 98
Urinary casts, 136
Urinary system, symptoms in, in medical history, 30
Urine, table of normal values for, 223–224
Uterine tube, palpation of, 107
Uterus, examination of, 104–106, *105*
  palpation of, 107

Vaginal examination, 104, *104, 105*
Vagus nerve, function of, 120
Varicocele, 102

Varicose veins, 112
VDRL flocculation test, 137
Viscerotonia, 90
Vital signs, in physical examination, 37–38
Vitamin C deficiency, gum disorders in, 56
Vocal fremitus, testing for, 72

Warts, 42
Wasserman test, for syphilis, 137
Weber test of hearing, 53, 54
Wharton's duct, examination of, 57
Wheezing, 77

X-ray, in diabetes mellitus, 183
  in hypertension, 171
  in osteoarthritis, 186
  in physical examination, 146–147
  in rheumatoid arthritis, 188
  of chest, 147
    in congestive heart failure, 196